Review Questions & Answers For Veterinary Technicians

Edited by

Paul W. Pratt, VMD

Production Manager:
Elisabeth S. Stein

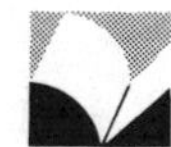

American Veterinary Publications, Inc.
5782 Thornwood Drive
Goleta, CA 93117

This book is for review purposes only. The publisher and authors make no warrant as to results for readers using this book in preparing for scholastic, licensure or certification examinations. While every effort has been made to ensure the accuracy of the information contained herein, the publisher and authors are not legally responsible for errors or omissions. Drug selection, drug dosages, diagnostic methods and treatment methods mentioned in this book are in accord with those in use at the time of publication. However, readers should consult drug package inserts and current veterinary texts and journals for current diagnostic and therapeutic recommendations.

Library of Congress Card Number: 93-70152

ISBN 0-939674-44-0

Printed in the United States of America

Authors

Introduction

Joann Colville, DVM
Associate Professor, Department of Veterinary and Microbiological Sciences, North Dakota State University, Fargo, ND 58105

Anatomy

Donald R. Adams, PhD
Professor, Department of Veterinary Anatomy, College of Veterinary Medicine, Iowa State University, Ames, IA 50011

Fredric L. Frye, DVM, MS
Fellow, Royal Society of Medicine, Former Clinical Professor of Medicine, Department of Medicine, School of Veterinary Medicine, University of California, Davis, CA 95616

Nani G. Ghoshal, GVSc, PG, DTVM, Dr Med Vet, PhD, FRZS
Professor, Department of Veterinary Anatomy, College of Veterinary Medicine, Iowa State University, Ames, IA 50011

Alexander de Lahunta, DVM, PhD, Dipl ACVIM
James Law Professor, Department of Anatomy, College of Veterinary Medicine, Cornell University, Ithaca, NY 14853

Sheryl J. Morgan, DVM, PhD, Dipl ACVP
Veterinary Pathologist, Division of Drug Safety Evaluation, Abbott Laboratories, D-469, AP-13A, One Abbott Park Road, Abbott Park, IL 60064

Animal Welfare and Ethics

Paul W. Pratt, VMD
Editor and Publisher, American Veterinary Publications, 5782 Thornwood Drive, Goleta, CA 93117

Anesthetic Nursing

Colin I. Dunlop, BVSc, Dipl ACVA
Associate Professor, Department of Clinical Sciences, College of Veterinary Medicine, Colorado State University, Fort Collins, CO 80526

Hui-Chu Lin, DVM, MS
Assistant Professor, Large Animal Surgery and Medicine, College of Veterinary Medicine, Auburn University, Auburn, AL 36849

John C. Thurmon, DVM, MS, Dipl ACVA
Professor, Chief of Anesthesiology, Department of Veterinary Clinical Medicine, College of Veterinary Medicine, University of Illinois, Urbana, IL 61801

Behavior

Katherine Albro Houpt, VMD, PhD
Professor, Animal Behavior Clinic, College of Veterinary Medicine, Cornell University, Ithaca, NY 14853

Care of Aquarium Fish

Terry W. Campbell, DVM, MS, PhD
1752 Big Oak Lane, Kissimmee, FL 32741

Care of Cage/Aviary Birds

Richard C. Blomquist, DVM
414 Franklin Avenue, Franklin Square, NY 11010

Continued

Branson W. Ritchie, DVM, PhD
Assistant Professor, College of Veterinary Medicine, University of Georgia, Athens, GA 30602

Care of Food Animals

Trevor R. Ames, DVM, MS, Dipl ACVIM
Professor, Department of Clinical and Population Sciences, College of Veterinary Medicine, University of Minnesota, St. Paul, MN 55108

Katherine N. Bretzlaff, DVM, PhD, Dipl ACT
Associate Professor, Department of Large Animal Medicine and Surgery, College of Veterinary Medicine, Texas A&M University, College Station, TX 77843

Ronnie G. Elmore, DVM, MS, Dipl ACT
Associate Dean, Dean's Office, College of Veterinary Medicine, Kansas State University, Manhattan, KS 66506

Norman L. Gates, DVM, MPH
Extension Sheep Specialist, College of Veterinary Medicine, Washington State University, Pullman, WA 99164

Steven C. Henry, DVM
Abilene Animal Hospital, 320 NE 14th Street, Abilene, KS 67410

Thomas H. Herdt, DVM, MS, Dipl ACVIM, Dipl ACVN
Associate Professor, Department of Large Animal Clinical Sciences, College of Veterinary Medicine, Michigan State University, East Lansing, MI 48824

Linda R. Krcatovich, LVT
Food Animal Technician, Large Animal Clinic, College of Veterinary Medicine, Michigan State University, East Lansing, MI 48824

Dan G. Morrical, MS, PhD
Extension Veterinarian and Sheep Specialist, Department of Animal Science, Iowa State University, 109 Kildee, Ames, IA 50011

Dale R. Nelson, DVM, MS
Professor, Department of Food Animal Medicine and Surgery, College of Veterinary Medicine, University of Illinois, Urbana, IL 61801

G. Michael H. Shires, BVSc, MS, MRCVS, Dipl ACVS
Dean and Professor, College of Veterinary Medicine, University of Tennessee, POB 1071, Knoxville, TN 37901

Barbara E. Straw, DVM, PhD
Professor, Department of Veterinary Science, University of Nebraska, Lincoln, NE 68583

Eric P. Tulleners, DVM, Dipl ACVS
Associate Professor, Chief of Surgery, School of Veterinary Medicine, New Bolton Center, University of Pennsylvania, Kennett Square, PA 19348

David C. Van Metre, DVM
Resident, Department of Large Animal Medicine, School of Veterinary Medicine, University of California, Davis, CA 95616

Continued

Charles E. Wallace, DVM, MS, Dipl ACVS
Associate Professor, Department of Large Animal Medicine, College of Veterinary Medicine, University of Georgia, Athens, GA 30602

Care of Horses

A.N. Baird, DVM, MS
Assistant Professor, Department of Large Animal Medicine and Surgery, College of Veterinary Medicine, Auburn University, Auburn, AL 36849

John P. Caron, DVM, MVS, Dipl ACVS
Associate Professor, Department of Large Animal Clinical Sciences, College of Veterinary Medicine, Michigan State University, East Lansing, MI 48824

Benjamin J. Darien, DVM, MS, Dipl ACVIM
Assistant Professor, Department of Medical Sciences, School of Veterinary Medicine, University of Wisconsin, Madison, WI 53706

Susan Clark Eades, DVM, PhD, Dipl ACVIM
Assistant Professor, Department of Large Animal Medicine, College of Veterinary Medicine, University of Georgia, Athens, GA 30602

Ann M. Lamar, LVT
Technician II, Large Animal Teaching Hospital, College of Veterinary Medicine, Michigan State University, East Lansing, MI 48824

James N. Moore, DVM, PhD, Dipl ACVS
Professor, Department of Large Animal Medicine, College of Veterinary Medicine, University of Georgia, Athens, GA 30602

Karen A. Moriello, DVM, Dipl ACVD
Associate Professor, Department of Medical Sciences, College of Veterinary Medicine, University of Wisconsin, Madison, WI 53706

Mary Rose Paradis, DVM, MS, Dipl ACVIM
Chief of Staff, Hospital for Large Animals, School of Veterinary Medicine, Tufts University, North Grafton, MA 01536

Care of Laboratory Animals

W. Sheldon Bivin, DVM, PhD, Dipl ACLAM
Director, Division of Laboratory Animal Medicine, School of Veterinary Medicine, Louisiana State University, Baton Rouge, LA 70803

Care of Marine Mammals

Roberto Aguilar, DVM
Senior Veterinary Resident, The Raptor Center, University of Minnesota, 1920 Fitch Avenue, St. Paul, MN 55105

Terry W. Campbell, DVM, MS, PhD
1752 Big Oak Lane, Kissimmee, FL 32741

Leslie A. Dierauf, VMD
United States House of Representatives, Committee on Merchant Marine and Fisheries, Washington, DC 20515

Tina Gemeinhardt, DVM
Huff Animal Hospital, 1512 56th Street, Delta, BC, Canada V4L 2A8

Continued

David Huff, DVM
Huff Animal Hospital, 1512 56th Street, Delta, BC, Canada V4L 2A8

James D. Letcher, DVM
Associate Veterinarian, Lincoln Park Zoological Gardens, 2200 North Cannon Drive, Chicago, IL 60614

Care of Poultry and Wild Fowl

Edwin M. Odor, DVM, MAM, Dipl ACPV
Senior Scientist, Research and Education Center, University of Delaware, Route 2, Box 47, Georgetown, DE 19947

Care of Small Animals

Kenneth C. Bovée, DVM, MS
Bower Professor, Department of Medicine, School of Veterinary Medicine, University of Pennsylvania, Philadelphia, PA 19104

Ronald M. Bright, DVM, MS, Dipl ACVS
Professor, Director of Surgical Services, Department of Urban Practice, College of Veterinary Medicine, POB 1071, University of Tennessee, Knoxville, TN 37901

Dennis E. Brooks, DVM, PhD, Dipl ACVO
Associate Professor, Ophthalmology Service Chief, Department of Small Animal Clinical Sciences, College of Veterinary Medicine, University of Florida, Gainesville, FL 32610

Philip A. Bushby, DVM, MS, Dipl ACVS
Professor, Academic Program Director, College of Veterinary Medicine, Mississippi State University, Mississippi State, MS 39762

Susan M. Cotter, DVM, Dipl ACVIM
Professor, Department of Medicine, School of Veterinary Medicine, Tufts University, North Grafton, MA 01536

Sharon K. Fooshee, DVM, MS
Animal Health Center of Franklin, 400 Eddy Lane, Franklin, TN 37064

Joseph Harari, DVM, MS, Dipl ACVS
Assistant Professor, Department of Veterinary Clinical Medicine and Surgery, College of Veterinary Medicine, Washington State University, Pullman, WA 99164

Evan T. Keller, DVM, MPVM
Resident, Department of Medical Sciences, School of Veterinary Medicine, University of Wisconsin, Madison, WI 53706

Joe N. Kornegay, DVM, PhD, Dipl ACVIM
Professor, Department of Companion Animal and Special Species Medicine, College of Veterinary Medicine, North Carolina State University, Raleigh, NC 27606

Dennis W. Macy, DVM, MS, Dipl ACVIM
Professor, Department of Biomedical Sciences, College of Veterinary Medicine, Colorado State University, Fort Collins, CO 80523

N. Sydney Moise, DVM, MS, Dipl ACVIM
9748 Arden Road, Trumansburg, NY 14886

Continued

Karen A. Moriello, DVM, Dipl ACVD
Associate Professor, Department of Medical Sciences, College of Veterinary Medicine, University of Wisconsin, Madison, WI 53706

James K. Roush, DVM, MS, Dipl ACVS
Assistant Professor, Department of Clinical Sciences, College of Veterinary Medicine, Kansas State University, Manhattan, KS 66506

Fred W. Scott, DVM, PhD, Dipl ACVM
Professor, Director of Cornell Feline Health Center, Department of Microbiology, Immunology and Parasitology, College of Veterinary Medicine, Cornell University, Ithaca, NY 14853

Robert G. Sherding, DVM, Dipl ACVIM
Professor, Head of Small Animal Medicine, Department of Veterinary Clinical Sciences, College of Veterinary Medicine, Ohio State University, Columbus, OH 43210

Carrie B. Waters, DVM
Resident, Department of Veterinary Clinical Sciences, School of Veterinary Medicine, Purdue University, West Lafayette, IN 47907

Michael D. Willard, DVM, MS, Dipl ACVIM
Professor, Department of Small Animal Medicine and Surgery, College of Veterinary Medicine, Texas A&M University, College Station, TX 77845

Care of Zoo and Exotic Animals

Roberto Aguilar, DVM
Senior Veterinary Resident, The Raptor Center, University of Minnesota, 1920 Fitch Avenue, St. Paul, MN 55105

Katherine Hudelson, DVM
Tucson Wildlife Rehabilitation Center, 316 East Waverly, Tucson, AZ 85705

James D. Letcher, DVM
Associate Veterinarian, Lincoln Park Zoological Gardens, 2200 North Cannon Drive, Chicago, IL 60614

Daniel H. Nielsen, DVM
Box V, New Berlin, NY 13411

Georganna Ranglack, DVM, PhD
Coordinator of Research, Audubon Park Zoo, 6500 Magazine Street, New Orleans, LA 70118

Dorcas O. Schaeffer, DVM, MS, Dipl ACLAM
Assistant Professor, Division of Laboratory Animal Medicine, School of Veterinary Medicine, Louisiana State University, Baton Rouge, LA 70803

Susan K. Wells-Mikota, DVM
Director of Veterinary Services and Research, Freeport McMoran Species Survival and Research Center, Audubon Park Zoo, 6500 Magazine Street, New Orleans, LA 70118

Peregrine L. Wolff, DVM
Director of Animal Health, Minnesota Zoological Garden, 1300 Zoo Boulevard, Apple Valley, MN 55124

Continued

Clinic Administration and Client Relations	*Alan H. Bush, DVM* Modular Management Systems, Route 5, Box 43, Big Pine Key, FL 33043
	John B. McCarthy, DVM, MBA Suite 710, 1101 Vermont Avenue, NW, Washington, DC 20005
	Paul M. Newman, DVM 6770 Colorno Court, Rancho Cucamonga, CA 91701
	Priscilla K. Stockner, DVM, MS, MBA President, Stockner & Associates, 340 State Place, Escondido, CA 92029
Dentistry	*Gordon J. Baker, BVSc, PhD, MRCVS, Dipl ACVS* Professor, Head of Equine Medicine & Surgery, Department of Veterinary Clinical Medicine, College of Veterinary Medicine, University of Illinois, Urbana, IL 61801
	Robert B. Wiggs, DVM, Dipl AVDC Director, Dallas Dental Service Animal Clinic, 12600 Coit Road, Dallas, TX 75251
Diagnostic Imaging and Recordings	*John M. Bowen, DVM, PhD* Associate Dean, Dean's Office, College of Veterinary Medicine, University of Georgia, Athens, GA 30602
	Connie M. Han, RVT Imaging Technologist, Veterinary Teaching Hospital, School of Veterinary Medicine, Purdue University, West Lafayette, IN 47907
	William R. Klemm, DVM, PhD Professor, Department of Veterinary Anatomy and Public Health, College of Veterinary Medicine, Texas A&M University, College Station, TX 77843
	Paul W. Pratt, VMD Editor and Publisher, American Veterinary Publications, 5782 Thornwood Drive, Goleta, CA 93117
	Donald E. Thrall, DVM, PhD, Dipl ACVR Professor, Department of Anatomy, Physiological Sciences and Radiology, College of Veterinary Medicine, North Carolina State University, Raleigh, NC 27606
	Larry Patrick Tilley, DVM, Dipl ACVIM 220-50 Hartland, Hollis Hills, NY 11427
Epidemiology and Public Health	*John S. Reif, DVM, MS* Professor, Department of Epidemiology and Public Health, College of Veterinary Medicine, Colorado State University, Fort Collins, CO 80521
	George T. Woods, DVM, MPH, MS Professor Emeritus, Department of Veterinary Microbiology, Public Health and Research, College of Veterinary Medicine, University of Illinois, Urbana, IL 61801
Ethics and Law	*Rodrick W. Lewis, DVM, JD* Associate Attorney, Warner, Norcross and Judd, 900 Old Kent Building, 111 Lyon Street NW, Grand Rapids, MI 49503

Continued

Mark D. Steele, Esquire
95360 Overseas Hwy, Suite 1, Key Largo, FL 33037

Hematology and Cytology

Rick L. Cowell, DVM, MS, Dipl ACVP
Associate Professor, Department of Veterinary Pathology, College of Veterinary Medicine, Oklahoma State University, Stillwater, OK 74078

W. Jean Dodds, DVM
President, HEMOPET, 938 Stanford Street, Santa Monica, CA 90403

Brad L. Hines, DVM
Intern, Department of Small Animal Surgery and Medicine, College of Veterinary Medicine, Auburn University, Auburn, AL 36830

Immunology

Ian Tizard, BVMS, PhD
Professor, Department of Veterinary Pathobiology, College of Veterinary Medicine, Texas A&M University, College Station, TX 77843

Laboratory Procedures

Barry T. Mitzner, DVM
President, Southeast Vetlab, 3865 Shipping Avenue, Miami, FL 33146

Rose E. Raskin, DVM, PhD, Dipl ACVP
Assistant Professor, Department of Physiological Sciences, College of Veterinary Medicine, University of Florida, Gainesville, FL 32610

Microbiology

Gordon R. Carter, DVM, MS, DVSc, Dipl ACVM
Professor Emeritus, Department of Pathobiology, Virginia-Maryland Regional College of Veterinary Medicine, Virginia Polytechnic Institute, Blacksburg, VA 24061

Muhammed Ikram, DVM, MS, PhD
Animal Health Technology Program, Fairview College, Box 3000, Fairview, Alberta, Canada T0H 1L0

Necropsy

Paul W. Pratt, VMD
Editor and Publisher, American Veterinary Publications, 5782 Thornwood Drive, Goleta, CA 93117

Nutrition

Linda D. Baker, VMD, Dipl ACVN
Lecturer, Department of Clinical Studies, School of Veterinary Medicine, New Bolton Center, University of Pennsylvania, Kennett Square, PA 19348

Edward A. Moser, VMD, MS, Dipl ACVN
Veterinary Nutrition Specialists, 83 Schuckler Drive, North East, MD 21901

Rebecca L. Remillard, DVM, PhD, Dipl ACVN
Clinical Nutritionist, Angell Memorial Animal Hospital, 350 S. Huntington Avenue, Boston, MA 02130

Parasitology

Dwight D. Bowman, PhD, MS
Assistant Professor, Department of Microbiology, Immunology and Parasitology, College of Veterinary Medicine, Cornell University, Ithaca, NY 14853

Continued

Pharmacology and Pharmacy Procedures	*Lloyd E. Davis, DVM, PhD, Dipl ACVCP* Professor, Department of Veterinary Clinical Medicine, College of Veterinary Medicine, University of Illinois, Urbana, IL 61801
	Sue Hudson Duran, RPh, MS Assistant Professor, Director of Pharmacy, Department of Large Animal Surgery and Medicine, Auburn University, Auburn, AL 36849
Physical Restraint	*Teresa F. Sonsthagen, RVT* Instructor, Veterinary Technology, Department of Veterinary Science, North Dakota State University, Fargo, ND 58105
Physiology	*James E. Breazile, DVM, PhD* Professor, Director of Laboratory Animal Resources, College of Veterinary Medicine, Oklahoma State University, Stillwater, OK 74078
	Thomas P. Colville, DVM, MS Director, Veterinary Technology Program, Department of Veterinary and Microbiological Sciences, North Dakota State University, Fargo, ND 58105
Preventive Medicine	*Paul C. Bartlett, DVM, PhD, MPH, Dipl ACVPM* Associate Professor, Department of Large Animal Clinical Sciences, College of Veterinary Medicine, Michigan State University, East Lansing, MI 48823
	Craig Nash Carter, DVM, MS, PhD, Dipl ACVPM Adjunct Professor, Head of Epidemiology and Informatics, Department of Veterinary Public Health, College of Veterinary Medicine, Texas A&M University, POD 3040, College Station, TX 77841
	Johnny D. Hoskins, DVM, PhD, Dipl ACVIM Professor, Department of Veterinary Clinical Sciences, School of Veterinary Medicine, Louisiana State University, Baton Rouge, LA 70803
Principles of Disease	*Ronald D. Hunt, DVM* Professor, New England Regional Primate Research Center, Harvard Medical School, POB 9102, Southborough, MA 01772
Reproduction	*Thomas J. Burke, DVM, MS* Professor, Department of Veterinary Clinical Medicine, College of Veterinary Medicine, University of Illinois, Urbana, IL 61801
	Stanley M. Dennis, BVSc, PhD, FRCVS, FRCPath, Dipl ACT Professor Emeritus, School of Veterinary Medicine, Ross University, POB 334, St. Kitts, West Indies
	Maarten Drost, DVM Professor, College of Veterinary Medicine, University of Florida, Gainesville, FL 32610
	Bruce E. Eilts, DVM, MS, Dipl ACT Associate Professor, Department of Veterinary Clinical Sciences, School of Veterinary Medicine, Louisiana State University, Baton Rouge, LA 70803

Continued

Fredric L. Frye, DVM, MS
Fellow, Royal Society of Medicine, Former Clinical Professor of Medicine, Department of Medicine, School of Veterinary Medicine, University of California, Davis, CA 95616

Michael B. Paster, DVM
Avalon Animal Hospital and Bird Clinic, 22404 S. Avalon Boulevard, Carson, CA 90745

Roderick C. Tubbs, DVM, MS, Dipl ACT
Swine Veterinarian, Commercial Program, Assistant Professor, Department of Surgery, College of Veterinary Medicine, University of Missouri, Columbia, MO 65211

Steven D. Van Camp, DVM, Dipl ACT
Associate Professor, Department of Food Animal and Equine Medicine, College of Veterinary Medicine, North Carolina State University, Raleigh, NC 27606

Christine S.F. Williams, BVSc, MRCVS, Dipl ACLAM
Director, Laboratory Animal Resources, College of Veterinary Medicine, Clinical Center C, Michigan State University, East Lansing, MI 48824

Surgical Nursing

Thomas P. Colville, DVM, MS
Director, Veterinary Technology Program, Department of Veterinary and Microbiological Sciences, North Dakota State University, Fargo, ND 58105

Robert L. Leighton, VMD, Dipl ACVS
Professor Emeritus, Department of Surgery, School of Veterinary Medicine, University of California, Davis, CA 95616

Terminology

Paul W. Pratt, VMD
Editor and Publisher, American Veterinary Publications, 5782 Thornwood Drive, Goleta, CA 93117

Toxicology

Gary D. Osweiler, DVM, MS, PhD, Dipl ABVT
Professor, Veterinary Diagnostic Laboratory, College of Veterinary Medicine, Iowa State University, Ames, IA 50011

Preface

This review book was developed to help candidates prepare for scholastic and certification examinations. While the book is not a definitive text, it can help candidates organize their preparations, and detect areas in which more study is required.

I am indebted to our group of 112 contributors, who have taken the time from their busy professional and personal lives to carefully craft questions on their respective subject areas. Their enthusiasm and ingenuity in developing challenging questions are evident throughout the book. While I had considered myself fairly well read in our field, I was humbled by the depth and breadth of knowledge illustrated in their questions.

This book contains over 2,100 questions, with accompanying answers. We have gone to great effort to root out all errors and ambiguous statements. Despite these precautions, however, a number of flaws undoubtedly have escaped notice.

We would be grateful if readers would notify us of any errors, ambiguities or questionable statements in this book. We also encourage readers to send their comments/criticism on any aspect of this book. In this way we can improve the quality of future editions. For your convenience, a postage-paid Comments form is included at the back of the book.

Paul W. Pratt, VMD
Editor and Publisher

Contents

Continued

Continued

Continued

Introduction

J. Colville

Veterinary technicians in any phase of their education or professional career can benefit from *Review Questions & Answers For Veterinary Technicians.*

This is not a textbook, nor is it meant to supplant textbooks. Rather, it is a guide designed to help readers review, in convenient form, current information on the various subject areas within the scope of a veterinary technician's duties.

Who Should Use This Book?

Technician Students: Technician students can use this book as a review in preparing for final examinations, as each course is concluded.

New Graduates: Graduates can use this book at the conclusion of their technician education program in preparing for the Veterinary Technician National Examination, and in preparing for certification examinations required by many states and provinces (see the following section on Certification of Veterinary Technicians).

Practicing Technicians: Graduates now working in veterinary practice will find this book useful in continuing education. Graduates re-entering the profession will find the book helpful in updating their knowledge on various topics. Finally, technicians moving to a new locale can use this book to prepare for the certification examination in their new state or province.

What Is Covered In This Book?

Review Questions & Answers For Veterinary Technicians covers nearly every aspect of veterinary medicine. Over 2,100 questions have been divided into the following subject areas:

Anatomy: These questions relate to gross anatomy of all body tissues, and include some questions on microscopic anatomy. Species covered include small animals (dogs, cats), monogastric ungulates (horses, pigs), ruminants (cattle, sheep, goats), and avian/exotics (birds, reptiles).

Anesthetic Nursing: Emphasis is placed on knowledge of equipment, techniques and agents used to anesthetize animals. Included are questions on sedation, tranquilization, and general, local and spinal anesthesia.

Behavior: Questions on normal and abnormal behavior of domestic species are included in this section.

Care of Cage/Aviary Birds: These questions relate to diseases and husbandry of cage/aviary birds.

Care of Food Animals, Care of Horses, Care of Small Animals: These 3 sections contain questions on nursing care of animals with infectious, noninfectious or surgical diseases. Questions cover history taking, physical examination, diagnostic techniques, medical care, preoperative preparation, postoperative care and emergency care.

Care of Laboratory Animals: These questions relate to diseases and husbandry of common laboratory species.

Care of Poultry: These questions relate to diseases and husbandry of domestic fowl and wild waterfowl.

Care of Zoo Animals, Exotic Animals, Marine Mammals and Aquarium Fish: These questions relate to diseases and care of zoo species, companion exotic species, marine mammals and aquarium fish.

Clinic Administration and Client Relations: These questions relate to clinic management and personal interaction with clients.

Cytology: This section includes questions on cytologic evaluation of various types of specimens.

Dentistry: This section includes questions on dental anatomy, terminology, periodontal disease, prophylaxis, floating, extraction, endodontics, orthodontics and other dental procedures.

Diagnostic Imaging and Recordings: Questions in this section relate to equipment and techniques used in radiography, ultrasonography, endoscopy, electrocardiography, electroencephalography and electromyography.

Epidemiology and Public Health: These questions relate to the dynamics of disease in animal populations, zoonoses, and meat and milk hygiene.

Ethics, Law and Animal Welfare: Ethical, legal and animal welfare issues in veterinary medicine are explored in this section.

Hematology: This section includes questions on hematopoiesis, blood and bone marrow cell morphology and coagulation.

Laboratory Procedures: These questions concern laboratory analyses, including fecal examination, urinalysis, blood chemistry assays, heartworm tests, immune-based diagnostic tests, skin scrapings, blood smears, enzymology and antimicrobial sensitivity tests.

Microbiology: These questions relate to morphology, physiology, culture and identification of bacteria, fungi and viruses of veterinary importance.

Necropsy: Included are questions on techniques used in necropsy of domestic animals.

Nutrition: Nutritional requirements and feeding domestic animals are the focus of this section.

Parasitology: These questions relate to the life cycle, pathologic effects and identification of arthropods, protozoans and helminths of veterinary importance.

Pharmacology and Pharmacy Practices: These questions concern the actions of various classes of drugs, calculation of dosages and dilutions, and procedures used in the pharmacy.

Physical Restraint: These questions relate to equipment and methods used to physically restrain domestic animals.

Physiology: This section covers the function of the various body systems.

Preventive Medicine: This section focuses on procedures used to prevent disease in domestic species, including use of biologics, anthelmintics, disinfectants and quarantine.

Principles of Disease: These questions relate to pathologic processes in various body systems.

Reproduction: This section includes questions on reproductive physiology, function and disease in male and female animals.

Surgical Nursing: These questions concern wound healing and infection, antimicrobial use, hemostasis, asepsis, sterilization, instruments, suture materials, drains and dressings.

Terminology: This section reviews surgical, medical, anatomic and directional terms, terms used in microbiology and pharmacology, and universally accepted abbreviations.

What Types of Questions Are Included In This Book?

The questions in this book were prepared by highly qualified authors, including technician educators, content-area specialists and experienced clinicians. The questions have been carefully constructed to test factual knowledge, reasoning skills and clinical judgment. They will also help pinpoint deficiencies in a candidate's studies. These questions are original, and none have been knowingly "recycled" from previous national or state certification examinations.

All of the questions in this book are multiple choice. This format was chosen because it is most commonly used in certification examinations. Also, it is similar to the format used in the Veterinary Technician National Examination (VTNE). Questions in the VTNE present 4 answer choices; questions in this book present 5 answer choices. Each question has only 1 correct answer.

Multiple-choice questions offer several advantages. Many questions covering a broad range of subjects can be presented in a limited testing period. Also, multiple-choice examinations can be quickly and accurately graded (often by automated optical scanner). Finally, a candidate's answers to multiple-choice questions are not subject to differences of interpretation by the grading examiner, as in essays.

Questions are presented in several styles:

Completion: Together with the question stem, the appended answer forms a complete sentence. For example,

1. The last nucleated stage of maturing mammalian erythrocytes is the:

a. rubricyte
b. metarubricyte
c. reticulocyte
d. mature erythrocyte
e. prorubricyte

(The correct answer is b.)

Selection: The question is presented as a complete sentence, and the reader selects the best answer. For example,

2. Which stage of maturing mammalian erythrocytes is the last nucleated stage?

a. rubricyte
b. metarubricyte
c. reticulocyte
d. mature erythrocyte
e. prorubricyte

(The correct answer is b.)

Association: Several answer choices are listed, followed by a series of questions relating to these choices. For example,

a. prorubricyte
b. metarubricyte
c. reticulocyte
d. erythrocyte
e. rubricyte

3. The final stage of erythrocyte maturation.

4. The last nucleated stage of maturing erythrocytes.

5. The first non-nucleated stage of maturing erythrocytes.

6. The earliest functional stage of maturing erythrocytes.

7. The stage of maturing erythrocytes ***least*** *commonly seen in peripheral blood.*

(Correct answers: 3. d, 4. b, 5. c, 6. e, 7. a)

Case History: A clinical case is described, and questions pertain to case management. For example,

Questions 8 through 11

A 3-month-old mixed-breed puppy is presented because of diarrhea and coughing. The puppy was recently obtained from an animal shelter, and has been vaccinated (DHLP) but never dewormed. The puppy has a dull haircoat and slight fever, but is well hydrated, alert and playful.

8. The most appropriate initial procedure is to:

a. make thoracic and abdominal radiographs
b. perform a physical examination
c. obtain blood samples for serum chemistry assays
d. perform an electrocardiographic examination
e. euthanize the puppy because of probable distemper

9. You examine a fecal sample and find roundworm eggs. The drug most likely to be prescribed by the veterinarian for deworming this puppy is:

a. niclosamide
b. piperazine
c. sulfadimethoxine
d. praziquantel
e. fenbendazole

10. Considering this dog's history and origin, the most likely cause of the coughing is:

a. infectious tracheobronchitis
b. lungworm infection

c. heartworm disease
d. congenital heart defect
e. tracheal collapse

11. The most reasonable course of action by the veterinarian is to:

a. hospitalize the puppy for elimination of adult heartworms
b. hospitalize the puppy for angiocardiographic studies
c. deworm the puppy and dispense antibacterials
d. hospitalize the puppy for intravenous antibacterial and fluid therapy
e. administer dexamethasone and dispense prednisolone

Answers

8. **b** This first step can help guide subsequent diagnostic procedures and treatments.

9. **b** None of the other drugs listed is appropriate for treating roundworm infection.

10. **a** "Kennel cough" is a common problem in commingled dogs obtained from pounds and shelters.

11. **c** This treatment should resolve these relatively minor problems.

How To Use This Book

This book is meant to be used in reviewing for final examinations or certification examinations. Before you begin a section, review your texts and course notes pertaining to that subject area. Then, approach each section as you would an actual examination:

- *Carefully read each question.* Look for such key words as "most," "best," "least," "always," "never" and "except." Consider only the facts presented in the question, and don't make assumptions and inferences that may not be true.
- *Carefully evaluate each answer choice.* Each question has only 1 correct answer, with 4 incorrect answers or "distractors." If more than 1 answer choice appears to be correct, closely examine them for clues that would eliminate any as incorrect.

  Most of the questions ask you to find a single correct answer among 4 incorrect answers. However, some questions ask you to find an *exception*. For these questions, the answer you are seeking is the single *incorrect* answer among 4 *correct* answers.
- *Select an answer* by circling the letter preceding your answer choice. If you do not wish to mark the book, use the blank answer sheets in the back of the book for practice tests.
- *Compare your answers with the correct answers.* The correct answers are listed separately at the end of each section. Many answers are accompanied by an explanation as to why a specific answer is correct or incorrect.
- *Identify your "weak" areas.* If you cannot correctly answer most of the questions in a particular subject area, it may be wise to spend extra time reviewing that subject before your actual examination. If you do not understand the rationale of why certain answers are correct or incorrect, consult the references in the Recommended Reading list at the beginning of each section.

Preparing for final examinations and certification examinations can be an intimidating task. Faced with stacks of textbooks and lecture notes, you may find it difficult to know where to begin and how to study in an organized, productive fashion. Also, anxiety about state and national certifying examinations can interfere with your preparations.

We hope *Review Questions & Answers For Veterinary Technicians* will assist you in preparing for examinations and in updating your knowledge on the many subject areas of veterinary medicine. Good luck in your preparations.

According to Earl Nightingale, "Luck is what happens when preparedness meets opportunity." You have always had the opportunity to succeed. With this book, you can better prepare for success.

Joann Colville, DVM
Department of Veterinary and Microbiological Sciences
North Dakota State University
Fargo, North Dakota

Certification of Veterinary Technicians

J. Colville

The American Veterinary Medical Association (AVMA) sponsors the Veterinary Technician National Examination (VTNE). The AVMA's Veterinary Technician Testing Committee is responsible for developing new examinations. Each year the Committee develops 2 new forms of the VTNE.

The VTNE consists of 200 multiple-choice questions in 3 knowledge areas: Basic Sciences (30%), Animal Care and Management (20%), and Clinical Sciences (50%).The examination is designed to assess essential job-related knowledge at the entry level.

The VTNE is prepared by the Professional Examination Service under contract to the AVMA. It is available for purchase by state and provincial licensing boards.

The VTNE is currently used by a number of states and provinces to certify veterinary technicians. Candidates should contact the licensing board of the state or province in which they desire certification to obtain information on the requirements for certification.

Candidates moving from one state to another can have their VTNE test score reported to their new state by contacting the Interstate Reporting Service, Professional Examination Service, 475 Riverside Drive, New York, NY 10015; telephone (212) 870-3169.

United States

For the convenience of technicians seeking information on certification, the addresses of state licensing boards follow:

Alabama

Executive Officer
Board of Veterinary Medicine
PO Box 1767
Decatur AL 35602

Alaska

Division of Occupational Licensing
Department of Commerce & Economic Development
PO Box D-LIC
Juneau AK 99881

Arizona

Executive Director
Veterinary Medical Examining Board
Room 410
1645 W. Jefferson
Phoenix AZ 85007

Arkansas

Executive Secretary
Arkansas Veterinary Medical Examining Board
1 Natural Resources Drive
Little Rock AR 72215

California

Executive Officer
Board of Examiners in Veterinary Medicine
Suite 6
1420 Howe Ave.
Sacramento CA 95825

Colorado

Colorado Veterinary Medical Association
Suite 701
1780 S. Bellaire
Denver CO 80222

Connecticut
Connecticut Association of Animal Health Technicians
2500 Black Road Turnpike
Fairfield CT 06430

Delaware
Board of Veterinary Medicine
PO Box 1401
Dover DE 19903

District of Columbia
Board of Veterinary Examiners
Room 923
614 H St. NW
Washington DC 20001

Florida
Veterinary Technician Committee
Florida Veterinary Medical Association
PO Box 2092
Sebring FL 33871

Georgia
Executive Director
166 Pryor St. SW
Atlanta GA 30303

Hawaii
Executive Secretary
Board of Veterinary Examiners
Box 3469
1010 Richards St.
Honolulu HI 96801

Idaho
Board of Veterinary Medicine
PO Box 7249
Boise ID 83707

Illinois
Veterinary Licensing and Disciplinary Board
Department of Professional Regulation
320 W. Washington
Springfield IL 62786

Indiana
Board Director
Health Professions Bureau
Suite 1020
1 American Square
Indianapolis IN 46282

Iowa
Secretary
Board of Veterinary Medicine
2nd Floor
Wallace Building
Des Moines IA 50319

Kansas
Registration Board
Box 121
Colby KS 67701

Kentucky
Board of Veterinary Examiners
PO Box 456
Frankfort KY 40602

Louisiana
Animal Health Technician Certification Committee
Department of Agriculture/Animal Science
Northwestern State University of Louisiana
Natchitoches LA 71497

Maine
Division of Licensing and Enforcement
Department of Professional and Financial Regulation
State House Station 35
Augusta ME 04333

Maryland
Secretary
State Board of Veterinary Medical Examiners
50 Truman Hwy.
Annapolis MD 21401

Massachusetts
Technician Committee
Massachusetts Veterinary Medical Association
200 Westboro Rd.
North Grafton MA 01536

Michigan
Licensing Administrator
Board of Veterinary Medicine
Department of Licenses & Registration
PO Box 30018
Lansing MI 48909

Minnesota
Veterinary Technician Committee
Minnesota Veterinary Medical Association
2469 University Ave.
St. Paul MN 55114

Mississippi
Executive Secretary
Board of Veterinary Medicine
209 S. Lafayette St.
Starkville MS 39759

Missouri
Executive Director
Veterinary Medical Board
PO Box 633
Jefferson City MO 65102

Montana
Board of Veterinary Medicine
Department of Commerce
Lower Level, Arcade Building
111 N. Last Chance Gulch
Helena MT 59620

Nebraska
Director
Bureau of Examining Boards
Department of Health
PO Box 95007
Lincoln NE 68509

Nevada
Board of Veterinary Medical Examiners
Suite 246
1005 Terminal Way
Reno NV 89502

New Hampshire
Secretary-Treasurer
Board of Veterinary Medicine
Caller Box 2042
Concord NH 03302

New Jersey
Board of Veterinary Medical Examiners
PO Box 45020
Newark NJ 07101

New Mexico
Executive Director
Board of Veterinary Examiners
Suite 400-C
1650 University Blvd. NE
Albuquerque NM 87102

New York
Executive Secretary
Board of Veterinary Medical Examiners
Room 3043
Cultural Education Center
Albany NY 12230

North Carolina
Executive Director
Veterinary Medical Board
PO Box 12587
Raleigh NC 27605

North Dakota
Veterinary Medical Examining Board
c/o Livestock Sanitary Board
State Capitol
Bismarck ND 58505

Ohio
Executive Secretary
Veterinary Medical Board
16th Floor
77 S. High St.
Columbus OH 43266

Oklahoma
Board of Veterinary Medical Examiners
Suite C
5104 N. Francis
Oklahoma City OK 73118

Oregon
Executive Secretary
Veterinary Medical Examining Board
PO Box 231
Portland OR 97207

Pennsylvania
Chairman
Board of Veterinary Medicine
PO Box 2649
Harrisburg PA 17104

Rhode Island
Administrator
Division of Professional Regulation
Department of Health
Room 104
3 Capitol Hill
Providence RI 02908

South Carolina
Secretary-Treasurer
Board of Veterinary Medical Examiners
PO Box 11293
Columbia SC 29211

South Dakota
Executive Secretary
Board of Veterinary Medical Examiners
411 S. Fort St.
Pierre SD 57501

Tennessee
Registration Boards Administrator
Board of Veterinary Medical Examiners
283 Plus Park Blvd.
Nashville TN 37217

Texas
Texas Veterinary Medical Association
Suite 201
6633 Hwy. 290 East
Austin TX 78723

Utah
Division of Occupational and Professional Licensing
PO Box 45802
Salt Lake City UT 84145

Vermont
State Veterinary Board
Office of Professional Regulations
109 State St.
Montpelier VT 05609

Virginia
Board of Veterinary Medicine
1601 Rolling Hills Dr.
Richmond VA 23229

Washington
Program Manager
Veterinary Board of Governors
PO Box 1099
Olympia WA 98504

West Virgina
Executive Secretary
Board of Veterinary Medicine
712 McCorkle Ave.
South Charleston WV 25303

Wisconsin
Bureau Director
Veterinary Examining Board
PO Box 8935
Madison WI 53708

Wyoming
Animal Technician Committee
Wyoming Veterinary Medical Association
Box 84
Castleford ID 83321

Canada

Technicians interested in practicing in Canadian provinces should contact those licensing boards at the following addresses:

Alberta
Secretary-Treasurer
Board of Veterinary Medical Examiners
#100
8615 149th St.
Edmonton, Alberta T5R 1B3

British Columbia
Board of Veterinary Medical Examiners
Suite 155
1200 W. 73rd Ave.
Vancouver, British Columbia V6P 6G5

Manitoba
Registrar
Veterinary Medical Board
Agricultural Services Complex
545 University Crescent
Winnipeg, Manitoba R3T 5S6

New Brunswick
Secretary-Treasurer
Board of Veterinary Medical Examiners
PO Box 1065
Moncton, New Brunswick E1C 8P2

Nova Scotia
Board of Veterinary Medical Examiners
Agricultural Centre
Kentville, Nova Scotia B4N 1J5

Ontario
Registrar
College of Veterinarians
Suite 24-25
340 Woodlawn Rd. West
Guelph, Ontario N1H 2X1

Quebec
General Director and Secretary
Board of Veterinary Medical Examiners
Suite 200
795 Avenue du Palais
St. Hyacinthe, Quebec J2S 5C6

Saskatchewan
Secretary-Treasurer
Board of Veterinary Medical Examiners
Suite 11
1025 Boychuk Dr.
Saskatoon, Saskatchewan S7H 5B2

Section 1

Anatomy

D.R. Adams, A. de Lahunta, F.L. Frye, N.G. Ghoshal, S.J. Morgan

Recommended Reading

Adams DR: *Canine Anatomy.* Iowa State University Press, Ames, 1986.
Baumel JJ *et al: Nomina Anatomica Avium.* Academic Press, New York, 1979.
Constantinescu GM: *Clinical Dissection Guide for Large Animals.* Mosby Year Book, St. Louis, 1991.
Cooper JE and Jackson OF: *Diseases of the Reptilia.* Academic Press, New York, 1981.
de Lahunta A and Habel RE: *Applied Veterinary Anatomy.* Saunders, Philadelphia, 1986.
Dyce KM *et al: Textbook of Veterinary Anatomy.* Saunders, Philadelphia, 1987.
Dyce KM and Wensing CJG: *Essentials of Bovine Anatomy.* Lea & Febiger, Philadelphia, 1971.
Evans HE and Christensen GC: *Miller's Anatomy of the Dog.* 2nd ed. Saunders, Philadelphia, 1979.
Frye FL: *Biomedical and Surgical Aspects of Captive Reptile Husbandry.* 2nd ed. Krieger Publishing, Melbourne, FL, 1991.
Getty R: *Sisson and Grossman's Anatomy of the Domestic Animals.* Saunders, Philadelphia, 1975.
Harrison GJ and Harrison LR: *Clinical Avian Medicine and Surgery.* Saunders, Philadelphia, 1986.
Jennings PB: *The Practice of Large Animal Surgery.* Saunders, Philadelphia, 1984.
King AS and McLelland J: *Form and Function in Birds.* Academic Press, New York, 1979.
King AS and McLelland J: *Outlines of Avian Anatomy.* Bailliere Tindall, London, 1975.
Marcus LC: *Veterinary Biology and Medicine of Captive Amphibians and Reptiles.* Lea & Febiger, Philadelphia, 1981.
Nickel R *et al: Anatomy of Domestic Birds.* Verlag Paul Parey, Berlin, 1977.
Nickel R *et al: The Viscera of the Domestic Mammals.* 2nd ed. Verlag Paul Parey, Berlin, 1979.
Nickel R *et al: The Anatomy of the Domestic Animals.* Vol 1. Verlag Paul Parey, Berlin, 1986.
Petrak ML: *Diseases of Cage and Aviary Birds.* 2nd ed. Lea & Febiger, Philadelphia, 1982.
Sack WO: *Essentials of Pig Anatomy.* Veterinary Textbooks, Ithaca, NY, 1982.
Sack WO: *Rooney's Guide to the Dissection of the Horse.* 6th ed. Veterinary Textbooks, Ithaca, NY, 1991.
Smallwood JE: *A Guided Tour of Veterinary Anatomy.* Saunders, Philadelphia, 1992.
Stashak TS: *Adams' Lameness in Horses.* 4th ed. Lea & Febiger, Philadelphia, 1987.

Practice answer sheet is on page 345.

Correct answers are on pages 11-14.

Questions

1. *The primary action of the triceps brachii is to:*

   a. flex the shoulder
   b. extend the shoulder
   c. flex the elbow
   d. extend the elbow
   e. abduct the thoracic limb

2. *The paired muscle that opens the jaw is the:*

   a. buccinator
   b. masseter
   c. digastricus
   d. temporalis
   e. medial pterygoid

3. *Most growth in height of a young dog occurs in the distal portion of the humerus and femur. This growth occurs in the:*

   a. physes
   b. metaphyses
   c. diaphyses
   d. articular cartilages
   e. primary ossification centers

4. *Accommodation for near and far vision is accomplished by contraction or relaxation of muscles in the:*

   a. ciliary body
   b. conjunctiva
   c. iris
   d. limbus
   e. retina

5. *The cervical vertebra with large ventrolaterally projecting transverse processes, each subdivided into 2 projections, is the:*

   a. first cervical vertebra
   b. second cervical vertebra
   c. third cervical vertebra
   d. sixth cervical vertebra
   e. seventh cervical vertebra

6. *The ligamentum nuchae:*

   a. assists in extension of the cervical vertebrae
   b. is present in cats
   c. attaches to the nuchal crest of the skull in dogs
   d. arises, in dogs and cats, from the last 5 cervical and first thoracic vertebrae
   e. is in contact, in dogs and cats, with all cervical vertebrae

7. *An intervertebral disk is* **least** *likely to rupture:*

   a. dorsally
   b. between vertebrae in the 11th thoracic to 4th lumbar area
   c. where it contacts an intercapital ligament
   d. into the vertebral canal
   e. at vertebral levels with adjacent longus colli muscles

8. *Which joint has the* **least** *developed collateral ligaments?*

   a. shoulder
   b. elbow
   c. antebrachiocarpal joint
   d. stifle
   e. proximal interphalangeal joint

9. *Which structure is normally located in the right half of a dog's body?*

   a. descending duodenum
   b. descending colon
   c. spleen
   d. gastric fundus
   e. mid-cervical portion of the esophagus

10. *In a normal dog or cat, an incision through the ventral abdominal wall into the peritoneal cavity, between the umbilicus and urinary bladder, would first reveal the:*

    a. jejunum
    b. descending colon

c. ureter
d. greater omentum
e. transverse colon

11. *In dogs, which tooth has the greatest number of roots?*

a. 4th upper premolar
b. 2nd upper premolar
c. canine
d. 2nd lower premolar
e. 1st lower premolar

12. *A segment of bowel with blood vessels coursing along both its mesenteric and antimesenteric borders is the:*

a. ascending duodenum
b. terminal portion of the ileum
c. transverse colon
d. descending colon
e. rectum

13. *Anal sacs:*

a. do not occur in cats
b. occupy the space between coccygeus and levator ani muscles
c. empty their secretions into the rectum
d. are situated between the external and internal anal sphincters
e. are encased in fat and fascia of the ischiorectal fossae

14. *A dog swallows a sharp bone. If the bone subsequently penetrates the parietal portion of the stomach, it would also most likely:*

a. enter the omental bursa
b. puncture the gallbladder
c. pierce the left ventricle of the heart
d. pierce the liver
e. tear through the greater omentum

15. *The fourth upper premolar (shearing tooth or carnassial tooth) in dogs has how many roots?*

a. the number varies with the individual dog
b. 2 lateral and 2 medial
c. 2 lateral and 1 medial
d. 1 medial and 2 lateral
e. 1 medial and 1 lateral

16. *The middle ear cavity normally drains into the:*

a. frontal sinus
b. external auditory meatus
c. nasopharynx
d. laryngopharynx
e. nasal cavity

17. *When the lungs are fully inflated, their caudolateral margins extend caudally to about the transverse level of the:*

a. 6th thoracic vertebra
b. 8th thoracic vertebra
c. 10th thoracic vertebra
d. 12th thoracic vertebra
e. 2nd lumbar vertebra

18. *The accessory lobe of the right lung is curled around the:*

a. esophagus
b. aorta
c. caudal vena cava
d. trachea
e. right azygos vein

19. *A tear or rip in a dog's thoracic diaphragm, between the diaphragmatic openings of the esophagus and caudal vena cava, would most likely permit:*

a. lung tissue to collapse
b. lung tissue to enter the abdominal cavity
c. abdominal viscera to enter the pericardial cavity
d. liver lobes to enter the right pleural cavity
e. liver lobes to enter the left pleural cavity

Correct answers are on pages 11-14.

20. *Passing a nasogastric tube through the nasal cavity is difficult in carnivores because the:*

a. epiglottis occludes the nasopharyngeal lumen
b. vomer divides the nasopharyngeal meatus into 2 channels
c. ethmoid conchae project into the ventral nasal meatus
d. dorsal conchae end caudally in a cul de sac
e. ventral conchae are highly branched

21. *In a resting dog that is not panting or swallowing, the apex or tip of the epiglottis is normally positioned in the:*

a. laryngopharynx
b. oropharynx
c. intrapharyngeal ostium
d. piriform recess
e. laryngeal vestibule

22. *The ureters open into the urinary bladder through its:*

a. apex
b. dorsocranial surface
c. dorsocaudal surgace
d. ventrocranial surface
e. ventrocaudal surface

23. *In male dogs, the erectile tissue at the proximal end of the glans penis that is an integral part of the "tie" during copulation is the:*

a. bulbus glandis
b. penile frenulum
c. corpus spongiosum penis
d. corpus cavernosum penis
e. ischiocavernosus

24. *The portion of the penis that is in direct contact with and surrounds the urethra is the:*

a. os penis
b. bulbus glandis
c. corpus cavernosum penis
d. corpus spongiosum penis
e. pars longa glandis

25. *The round ligament of the uterus:*

a. is a remnant of the umbilical artery
b. is a remnant of the umbilical vein
c. spans the distance from the uterine horn to the inguinal canal
d. attaches the ovary to the uterus
e. contains the uterine branch of the ovarian artery

26. *The vagina is positioned:*

a. directly dorsal to the rectum
b. directly ventral to the urethra
c. within the pubovesicular excavation
d. within the rectogenital excavation
e. ventral to the perineal body

27. *From dorsal to ventral, pelvic structures are arranged in the order of:*

a. vagina, rectum, urethra
b. vagina, urethra, rectum
c. rectum, urethra, vagina
d. rectum, vagina, urethra
e. urethra, rectum, vagina

28. *The ovarian bursa:*

a. is a membranous sac totally separating the ovary from the peritoneal cavity
b. is composed of membranes within which most of the uterine tube is located
c. contains the round ligament of the uterus
d. contains the suspensory ligament of the ovary
e. is not present in cats

29. *Which vessel carries the* ***least*** *amount of blood to an organ, such as the heart, lungs, gut, liver, pancreas, urinary bladder or uterus?*

a. internal thoracic artery
b. celiac artery
c. cranial mesenteric artery

d. caudal mesenteric artery
e. portal vein

30. In adult animals, remnants of the arterial blood supply to the fetal placenta supply blood to the:

a. liver
b. duodenum
c. jejunoileum
d. linea alba
e. urinary bladder

31. Incomplete occlusion of the cephalic vein during venipucture allows venous blood to continue flowing from the cranial surface of the antebrachium toward the heart, through the:

a. axillobrachial vein
b. omobrachial vein
c. median vein
d. median cubital vein
e. accessory cephalic vein

*32. Which vein does **not** normally drain directly into the right atrium?*

a. right pulmonary vein
b. cranial vena cava
c. caudal vena cava
d. great cardiac vein
e. right azygos vein

33. The coronary arteries are branches of the:

a. pulmonary trunk
b. aorta
c. right atrium
d. left atrium
e. brachiocephalic trunk

34. Pulsating blood spurting from a laceration across the ventral cervical region would most likely be from the:

a. external jugular vein
b. internal jugular vein
c. subclavian artery
d. common carotid artery
e. vertebral artery

35. In a normal animal, a substance injected into the left external jugular vein would pass sequentially through the:

a. left atrium, left ventricle, lung, right atrium and right ventricle
b. left atrium, left ventricle, aorta, left coronary artery, heart muscle and great cardiac vein
c. right atrium, right ventricle, aorta, liver, caudal vena cava and left atrium
d. right atrium, right ventricle, pulmonary trunk, lung, pulmonary veins and left atrium
e. linguofacial vein, facial vein and deep facial vein

36. Which portion of the heart is most closely adjacent to the dome of the thoracic diaphragm?

a. left ventricle
b. right ventricle
c. apex of the ventricles
d. right atrium
e. left atrium

*37. Venous blood from which structure does **not** first drain into the liver before passing into the heart?*

a. pancreas
b. spleen
c. adrenal gland
d. descending colon
e. stomach

38. Fats that are digested and absorbed into lacteals are then carried most directly into the:

a. hepatic vein
b. portal vein
c. right azygos vein
d. cisterna chyli
e. lumbar trunk

Correct answers are on pages 11-14.

39. The thoracic duct:

a. drains into the cisterna chyli
b. drains lymph from the pelvic limbs, tail and intestines
c. drains the pulmonary and tracheobronchial lymph nodes
d. crosses the lateral surface of the pericardium
e. enters the right azygos vein

*40. Which structure is **not** contained within the mediastinum?*

a. thymus
b. thoracic portion of the esophagus
c. thoracic portion of the trachea
d. heart
e. thoracic portion of the caudal vena cava

*41. Concerning positional relationships, which statement is **least** accurate?*

a. The esophagus is dorsal to the tracheal carina.
b. In the midcervical region, the esophagus is dorsolateral to the trachea and on the left.
c. The trachealis muscle is located within the dorsal portion of the trachea.
d. The pylorus of the stomach and cranial portion of the duodenum are located toward the left side of the abdominal cavity.
e. The prostate gland is ventral to the rectum.

42. The lacrimal gland:

a. is ventral to the eyeball
b. is lateral to the eyeball
c. secretes fluid that enters the conjuntival sac through the caudal surface of the third eyelid
d. secretes fluid that enters the anterior chamber of the eye
e. secretes fluid that drains from the orbital region into the nasal vestibule

*43. Cats do **not** have a:*

a. clavicle
b. lateral laryngeal ventricle
c. gastrocnemius muscle
d. supracondylar foramen in the distal portion of the humerus
e. gallbladder

*44. Which structure evidences the **least** difference in fetal and adult positions?*

a. testis
b. thoracic diaphragm
c. thyroid gland
d. trapezius
e. cranial preputial muscle

45. A fracture through the distomedial portion of a cat's humerus would most likely involve direct injury to the:

a. cephalic vein
b. radial nerve
c. median nerve
d. ulnar nerve
e. head of the radius

46. Distal to the fetlock joint, which of the following represents the normal dorsal-palmar or dorsal-plantar relationship of the digital vessels and nerve on the medial and lateral aspects of the proximal phalanx?

a. digital vein, artery and nerve
b. digital artery, vein and nerve
c. digital nerve, artery and vein
d. digital artery, nerve and vein
e. digital vein, nerve and artery

47. Among the following joints of the vertebral column, which has the most movement?

a. intercentral joint or intervertebral symphysis
b. lumbar intertransverse joint
c. lumbosacral intertransverse joint
d. lumbosacral joint
e. sacroiliac joint

48. Which of the following sites is used for cerebrospinal fluid collection in the horse?

a. lumbosacral joint
b. first intercaudal joint
c. sacrocaudal joint
d. sacroiliac joint
e. intersacral joint

49. *The hoof receives its nutrient blood supply via the:*

a. corium
b. horny laminae
c. collateral cartilages of the distal phalanx
d. digital cushion
e. white line or zone

50. *Occlusion or stenosis of which of the following is most likely to cause an immediate backflow of blood into the liver of a horse?*

a. aortic valve
b. mitral or bicuspid (left atrioventricular) valve
c. pulmonic valve
d. tricuspid (right atrioventricular) valve
e. common bile duct

51. *A horse has a "full mouth," that is, all of its incisors are in wear. The upper corner incisors have a "hook." There is an indication of a faint dental star on the central incisor. What is the approximate age of this horse?*

a. 5 years
b. 6 years
c. 8 years
d. 7 years
e. 18 years

52. *In closed castration of stallions, the incision does* ***not*** *involve the:*

a. skin
b. cremaster fascia
c. internal spermatic fascia
d. parietal layer of the vaginal tunic
e. external spermatic fascia

53. *Concerning the ovaries of mares, which statement is* ***least*** *accurate?*

a. They are located in the sublumbar region.
b. They are large and bean shaped.
c. Ovulation usually occurs at the ovarian fossa.
d. They are suspended by the mesovarium.
e. Ruptured follicles can ovulate from any surface of the ovary.

54. *An obstruction of the left atrioventricular (mitral) valve would first be manifested as retrograde accumulation of blood in the:*

a. liver
b. right ventricle
c. left ventricle
d. lungs
e. cervical and cephalic regions

55. *The first permanent tooth to erupt in horses is the:*

a. first (central) incisor tooth
b. first cheek tooth
c. first molar tooth
d. canine tooth
e. first upper premolar tooth

56. *To focus on near objects,:*

a. lens curvature increases and the ciliary muscles relax
b. tension on the suspensory ligaments of the lens decreases and the ciliary muscles relax
c. tension on the suspensory ligaments of the lens increases and the ciliary muscles contract
d. lens curvature increases and tension on the suspensory ligaments of the lens increases
e. the ciliary muscles contract and lens curvature increases

57. *Concerning the cheek teeth, which statement is most accurate?*

a. They number 6 on the upper arcade on each side (3 premolars and 3 molars).
b. All of them have roots that are vertical in respect to the alveolar border of the maxilla.
c. The molars are present in deciduous dentition.
d. They have roots that project into the maxillary paranasal sinus, with the exception of the first and second cheek teeth.
e. They should not be floated in young animals.

Correct answers are on pages 11-14.

58. The tympanic cavity, which houses the auditory ossicles and communicates with the nasopharynx by means of the auditory (eustachian) tube, is a part of the:

a. external ear
b. middle ear
c. internal ear
d. auditory vesicles
e. guttural pouch

59. The oval window of the inner ear is covered by the:

a. base of the stapes
b. head of the incus
c. long crus of the incus
d. tensor tympani muscle
e. tympanic membrane

60. Jugular venipuncture is more safely performed in the cranial half of the neck because the external jugular vein is separated from the common carotid artery by the:

a. sternocephalicus muscle
b. omohyoideus muscle
c. sternothyroideus muscle
d. omotransversarius muscle
e. longus capitis muscle

61. Light passes from outside of the eye through the structures and media of the eye in which sequence?

a. cornea, aqueous humor, lens, vitreous humor and retina
b. cornea, aqueous humor, anterior chamber, lens, posterior chamber and retina
c. cornea, anterior chamber, iris, aqueous humor, lens and retina
d. cornea, pupil, iris, lens, vitreous humor and retina
e. cornea, anterior chamber, aqueous humor, lens, posterior chamber and retina

62. A nasogastric tube can be conveniently passed through the:

a. dorsal nasal meatus
b. middle nasal meatus
c. ventral nasal meatus
d. common nasal meatus
e. frontal nasal meatus

*63. In suckling newborn pigs, occasionally the "needle teeth" are clipped to prevent injury to the sow's nipples. In this process, which tooth is **not** clipped?*

a. deciduous "corner" incisor of the upper dental arcade
b. deciduous canine of the upper dental arcade
c. deciduous "corner" incisor of the lower dental arcade
d. deciduous canine of the lower dental arcade
e. deciduous first incisor of the upper dental arcade

64. In boars, which teeth are used as defensive weapons?

a. incisors
b. canines
c. premolars
d. molars
e. wolf teeth

65. During collection of blood from the cranial vena cava of pigs, the right side is preferred so as to avoid injury to the:

a. thyroid gland, left brachiocephalic artery and thymus
b. left phrenic nerve, thymus and heart
c. thoracic duct, thyroid gland and left phrenic nerve
d. heart, left phrenic nerve and thymus
e. left brachiocephalic artery, thymus and thoracic duct

*66. Concerning the kidneys of pigs, which statement is **least** accurate?*

a. They are smooth externally but lobated internally.
b. A hilus is present.
c. A renal pelvis is absent.
d. Renal calices are present.

e. They are bean shaped, flattened and covered by a capsule.

67. *In estimating the age of an animal, various characteristics of teeth are considered, such as form, number, type, structure and periods of eruption. Which surface of the teeth is frequently used in determining age in ruminants?*

a. labial surface
b. lingual surface
c. buccal surface
d. contact surface
e. occlusal surface

68. *To avoid invading the frontal paranasal sinus, calves should be dehorned:*

a. before 4 months of age
b. at about 6 months of age
c. at about 8 months of age
d. before 1 year of age
e. after 18 months of age

69. *The scent glands of goats are modified sebaceous glands that, unless resected or cauterized, produce a repulsive musky odor in milk and meat. Which site contains an abundance of these scent glands?*

a. chin region
b. dorsum of the trunk
c. interdigital space
d. inguinal region
e. caudomedial to the base of the horn

70. *In domestic ruminants, the relative size of the omasum varies. Concerning the size of the omasum and reticulum, which statement is most accurate?*

a. The omasum is larger than the reticulum in cattle but smaller than the reticulum in sheep and goats.
b. The omasum is slightly smaller than the reticulum in cattle.
c. The omasum is much larger than the reticulum sheep and goats.
d. The omasum is approximately half as large as the reticulum in cattle.
e. The omasum and reticulum are of relatively equal size in all ruminants.

71. *Which of the following is the "true" or "glandular" stomach in ruminants and does **not** form a part of the forestomach?*

a. rumen
b. reticulum
c. omasum
d. abomasum
e. ruminoreticular complex

72. *Blood from which organ does **not** drain into the caudal vena cava?*

a. liver
b. stomach
c. testis
d. kidney
e. adrenal (suprarenal) gland

73. *In a 3-year-old cow, which dental findings are most likely to be observed?*

a. a visible "neck" at the gum line on the permanent inferior (lower) central incisors (I_1)
b. inferior (lower) deciduous canine (DC/I_4) teeth still present, with recent eruption of the third permanent inferior incisors (I_3)
c. only the permanent inferior (lower) central incisors (I_3) present and in wear, with all other incisors deciduous
d. all incisor teeth still firmly anchored into their alveoli, allowing no movement of the teeth on digital manipulation
e. recent eruption of the superior (upper) corner incisors

74. *In which species would unilateral pleuritis be **least** likely to spread to the opposite pleural hemicavity to cause generalized pleuritis?*

a. both small and large ruminants
b. ox and goat
c. sheep and goat
d. ox and sheep
e. sheep only

Correct answers are on pages 11-14.

75. Concerning uterine caruncles, which statement is ***least*** *accurate?*

a. They are endometrial sites for the attachment of fetal membranes.
b. They are present in ruminants.
c. They form placentomes for fetal-maternal interface, in conjunction with fetal cotyledons.
d. They remain constant in position but enlarge greatly during pregnancy.
e. They tend to change position but remain the same size during pregnancy.

76. Concerning the median caudal (coccygeal) artery of the ox, which statement is ***least*** *accurate?*

a. The median caudal artery is commonly used for evaluating the pulse.
b. The median caudal artery is the caudal extension of the median sacral artery, which, in turn, is the continuation of the abdominal aorta.
c. The median caudal artery courses within the hemal arch of the ventral crest of the caudal vertebrae, which are sometimes fused, enclosing the artery.
d. The median caudal artery is too deep for pulse evaluation but can be used for collection of arterial blood for blood gas analysis.
e. Blood samples are frequently taken from the median caudal vessels.

77. Stenosis (occlusion) of which heart valve is most likely to cause an immediate backflow of blood into the lungs in ruminants?

a. aortic valve
b. pulmonary valve
c. left atrioventricular valve
d. right atrioventricular valve
e. pulmonoaortic valve

78. Though there are many types of feathers and their intermediate forms, which type covers predominantly the entire body?

a. contour feather
b. down feather
c. filoplume feather
d. bristle feather
e. powder feather

79. Concerning the crop or ingluvies, which statement is most accurate?

a. It is a diverticulum of the air sac at the thoracic inlet.
b. It lies on the left side of the neck in chickens, on the right side in parakeets, and on both sides in pigeons.
c. In hoatzin, it consists of a thoracic and an abdominal part.
d. In pigeons and doves, it produces "crop milk" during incubation, under the influence of prolactin.
e. It is extremely muscular and not very distensible.

80. Which structure is ***absent*** *from the large intestine of birds?*

a. cecum
b. colon
c. rectum
d. colorectum
e. coprodeum

81. Which air sac is single (unpaired)?

a. abdominal air sac
b. cervical air sac
c. caudal thoracic air sac
d. clavicular air sac
e. cranial thoracic air sac

82. Concerning the reproductive system in birds, which statement is ***least*** *accurate?*

a. Males are heterogametic and determine the sex of offspring.
b. The left reproductive organs in adult females are only functional in most birds.
c. The rudiments of the right ovary and oviduct persist and remain nonfunctional.
d. Usually the right ovary remains in an ambisexual or bisexual state.
e. If disease renders the left ovary nonfunctional, the right ovary may compensate for this loss of function.

83. Which segment of the oviduct produces the albumen of birds' eggs?

a. vagina
b. isthmus
c. folliculorum
d. magnum
e. stapus

84. Cosmetic "pinioning" is occasionally performed in adult birds to prevent flight. Which type of feather is clipped in this procedure?

a. down feather
b. primary contour feather
c. secondary contour feather
d. semiplume feather
e. filoplume feather

85. Male lizards and snakes have paired copulatory organs called:

a. claspers
b. paracloacal spurs
c. hemipenes
d. cloacal vents
e. vasa deferentia

86. In reptiles, the feces pass from the colon and rectum into the:

a. antrum
b. vestibule
c. coprodeum
d. urodeum
e. cecum

87. Some pythons and boas, and all pit vipers have labial or facial pit organs as part of their sensory apparatus. These structures are sensitive to:

a. light
b. touch
c. atmospheric pressure
d. sound
e. heat

88. Which of the following is most likely to occur with sciatic nerve injury?

a. walking on the dorsal surface of the hind paw
b. inability to support weight on the pelvic limb
c. inability to flex the hip to advance the pelvic limb
d. analgesia on the medial side of the crus
e. analgesia on the proximocaudal aspect of the thigh

89. Which tissue is normally vascular?

a. cornea
b. lens
c. hyaline cartilage
d. elastic cartilage
e. bone

*90. Concerning the intestinal tract, which statement is **least** accurate?*

a. Villi serve to increase the surface area for absorption.
b. In the normal maturation process, epithelial cells migrate distally along the contour of the villi.
c. Peyer's patches are found only in the ileum.
d. On sections stained with hemotoxylin and eosin, mucus within the epithelial-cell cytoplasm appears as large, round, clear vacuoles.
e. Brunner's glands are present in the duodenum.

Answers

1. **d** One head of the triceps brachii arises from the caudal surface of the scapula and would have flexor action on the shoulder. All 4 heads of the triceps brachii insert by means of a common tendon on the olecranon and have a primary role in extension of the elbow joint.

2. **c** The digastricus is composed of a caudal and a rostral portion, each having separate cranial innervation. The digastricus, which extends from the base of skull to the caudoventral surface of the mandible, acts to open the lower jaw. The masseter, temporalis and pterygoid muscles all elevate (close) the lower jaw, while the buccinator tightens the cheek pouch.

3. **a** Primary ossification centers are established in the diaphyses of long bones before birth. Secondary centers of ossification are initiated in the epiphyses and in some osseous prominences during the first several months of postnatal life. The epiphyseal plate, or physis, is the zone of tissue between the epiphysis and diaphysis. It consists of several regions: nonproliferating cartilage zone, pro- liferating cartilage zone, zone of hypertrophy and maturation, and a zone of calcification. When the physis ceases to proliferate, the epiphyseal plate becomes calcified and bone lengthening ceases.

4. **a** Muscles of the ciliary body cause stretching or relaxation of the lens of the eye.

5. **d** The 1st cervical vertebra, or atlas, has very large, undivided transverse processes. The 6th cervical vertebra, with dorsal and ventral subdivisions of each transverse process, is easy to identify on radiographs. Novices may mistake the ventral subdivision in radiographs for a foreign body.

6. **a** Epaxial muscles in the cervical region are responsible for extending or dorsally bending the cervical vertebrae. The ligamentum nuchae provides an elastic force that permits the lowered head to be raised relatively easily.

7. **c** The heads of each pair of ribs 1 to 10 articulate against the intervertebral spaces between the 7th cervical and 10th thoracic vertebrae. An intercapital ligament passes from the head of the rib on one side, over the intervertebral disk, to the head of the rib on the opposite side. Caudal to the 10th thoracic vertebra, the heads of the ribs articulate progressively further caudally, coming to be positioned against the body of one vertebra rather than on an intervertebral disk and adjacent bodies. The heads of these caudal several ribs are not connected to those on the other side by intercapital ligaments.

8. **a** Collateral ligaments, right and left, develop in the fibrous capsule of hinge joints. The more flexible a joint is for rotation, circumduction and swiveling functions, the less well developed are the collateral ligaments.

9. **a**

10. **d** The superficial leaf of the greater omentum normally extends caudally, from the greater curvature of the stomach all the way to the urinary bladder before reflecting cranially as the deep leaf of the greater omentum. Before one can examine the jejunoileum or transverse colon, the caudal end of the omentum must be lifted and retracted cranially.

11. **a**

12. **b** From an embryologic viewpoint, the stomach, terminal ileum and cecum are unusual in having vascularity on both the dorsal and ventral surfaces.

13. **d**

14. **d** The parietal area of the stomach is that portion lying adjacent to the liver. Though an ingested bone might penetrate the gallbladder, the greatest area of contact is with the liver.

15. **c**

16. **c**

17. **d** The caudal peripheral margin, or basal margin, of the caudal lobes of the right and left lungs extends into the acutely angled costo-diaphragmatic recess. This recess is immediately cranial and parallel to the costal arch.

18. **c** The plica vena cava extends to the right and dorsally from the mediastinum, forming the mediastinal recess as a subdivision of the right pleural cavity. The dorsal margin of the plica, containing the caudal vena cava and right phrenic nerve, indents the right accessory lobe of the lung.

19. **d** Intraabdominal pressure is normally much higher than intrathoracic pressure. As a result of this pressure differential, abdominal organs move into the thoracic compartment with herniation of the thoracic diaphragm. Because the right pleural space is much larger than the left, and the caudal mediastinum deflects to the left to line the diaphragm as diaphragmatic pleura, abdominal organs move into the right pleural space if they penetrate the central or right portion of the thoracic diaphragm.

20. **e**

21. **c** Except for brachycephalic dogs, in which the soft palate projects caudally beyond the epiglottis, the normal position of the tip of the epiglottis during quiet respiration is dorsal to the caudal free edge of the soft palate.
22. **c**
23. **a**
24. **d**
25. **c**
26. **e** The perineal body is the fibromuscular tissue, caudal to the pelvic cavity, that interconnects the ventral wall of the rectum/anal canal and the dorsal wall of the vagina.
27. **d**
28. **b**
29. **a**
30. **e** The umbilical arteries that supply blood to the apex of the urinary bladder are the remnants of the fetal arterial blood supply from the placenta.
31. **d** The median cubital vein interconnects the cephalic and median veins. Because it contains no valves, the median cubital vein carries blood from the cephalic vein to the median vein unless the median cubital is occluded by applying traction caudally on the skin at the cranial surface of the elbow.
32. **a** The pulmonary veins drain into the left atrium. The right azygos vein sometimes drains into the right atrium, though it usually enters the cranial vena cava.
33. **b** The right and left coronary arteries arise from the initial portion of the ascending aorta.
34. **d**
35. **d**
36. **a**
37. **c**
38. **d**
39. **b** Lymph from the pelvic limbs, tail and intestines is collected into the cisterna chyli and passed on through the thoracic duct to the venous system.
40. **e**
41. **d**
42. **e**
43. **b**
44. **c**
45. **c** In cats, the median nerve and brachial artery pass through the supracondylar foramen on the medial side of the humerus. Any damage to this bone in this region could also damage the median nerve.
46. **a**
47. **d**
48. **a**
49. **a**
50. **d**
51. **d**
52. **d**
53. **e**
54. **d**
55. **e**
56. **e**
57. **d**
58. **b**
59. **a**
60. **b**
61. **a**
62. **c**
63. **e**
64. **b**
65. **c**
66. **c**
67. **e**
68. **a**
69. **e**
70. **a**
71. **d**
72. **b**
73. **b**
74. **b**
75. **e**
76. **d**
77. **c**
78. **a**
79. **d**
80. **b**
81. **d**
82. **a**
83. **d**

84. **c**

85. **c** Hemipenes are the paired copulatory organs of male snakes and lizards.

86. **c** In reptiles, feces pass from the colon/rectum into the coprodeum.

87. **e** The facial or labial pit organs of some snakes are highly sensitive to temperature differences and are used to help locate food or predators.

88. **a** Walking on the dorsal surface of the hind paw results from damage to the peroneal branch of the sciatic nerve to the extensors of the digits.

89. **e** Bone is normally vascular. The other tissues listed are vascular only under pathologic conditions.

90. **c** Peyer's patches, though most prominent in the ileum, are found in other portions of the small intestine, particularly the jejunum.

Notes

Section 2

Anesthetic Nursing

C.I. Dunlop, H-C. Lin, J.C. Thurmon

Recommended Reading

Hall LW and Clarke KW: *Veterinary Anaesthesia.* 9th ed. Bailliere Tindall, London, 1992.

Haskins SC and Klide AM: Opinions in small animal anesthesia. *Vet Clin No Am* (Small Anim Pract) 22:245-502, 1992.

Lumb WV and Jones EW: *Veterinary Anesthesia.* 2nd ed. Lea & Febiger, Philadelphia, 1984.

Muir WW and Hubbell JA: *Handbook of Veterinary Anesthesia.* Mosby Year Book, St. Louis, 1989.

Muir WW and Hubbell JA: *Equine Anesthesia.* Mosby Year Book, St. Louis, 1991.

Riebold TW. Principles and techniques of equine anesthesia. *Vet Clin No Am* (Equine Pract) 6:485-741, 1990.

Thurman JC: Anesthesia. *Vet Clin Co Am* (Food Animal Pract) 2:485-741, 1990.

Short CE: *Principles and Practice of Veterinary Anesthesia.* Williams & Willkins, Baltimore, 1987.

Short CE and Poznak AV: *Animal Pain.* Churchill Livingstone, New York, 1992.

Practice answer sheet is on page 347.

Questions

1. *When using a non-rebreathing system with halothane or isoflurane, the O_2 flow rate should be:*

   a. 2.5-3 times the minute ventilation
   b. 4 times the minute ventilation
   c. 5 times the minute ventilation
   d. 6 times the minute ventilation
   e. equal to the minute ventilation

2. *Concerning the rebreathing bag on an anesthetic machine (circle system), which statement is **least** accurate?:*

   a. It acts as a reservoir bag from which the animal may breath O_2 and anesthetic gas.
   b. It can be used to manually support respiration.
   c. It allows visual assessment of the respiratory rate.
   d. It acts to trap carbon dioxide expired by the animal.
   e. It allows visual assessment of the tidal volume.

Correct answers are on pages 25-27.

3. *Concerning the endotracheal tube, which statement is* ***least*** *accurate?*

   a. It serves as a source of infection if not properly disinfected.
   b. If permitted to protrude excessively out of the mouth, it can extend the dead space.
   c. When inserted too deeply, it can cause bronchial cannulation, collapsing the opposite lung if anesthesia is prolonged.
   d. Inflating the cuff too tightly can restrict blood flow to the mucous membrane where the cuff contacts the trachea, resulting in ulceration.
   e. An endotracheal tube should be placed in all animals receiving injectable anesthetics.

4. *Soda lime absorbs 100 ml of CO_2/g. In a 30-lb dog producing 3 ml of CO_2/lb/min, 600 g of soda lime will last about:*

   a. 6 hours
   b. 11 hours
   c. 15 hours
   d. 22 hours
   e. 30 hours

5. *Concerning use of oxygen in pressurized tanks, which statement is* ***least*** *accurate?*

   a. The tank must be equipped with a pressure regulator to reduce the pressure so that it can be used safely in an anesthetic machine.
   b. To work effectively, most anesthetic machines must receive a gas supply at a pressure of 100 lb/square inch.
   c. A single-stage regulator permits regulation of the line pressure as gas flows to the anesthetic machine flow meters.
   d. Single-stage regulators are set to work automatically at slightly less than 50 lb/square inch.
   e. The regulator provides the safe operating pressure for the flow meter of the anesthetic machine.

6. *Anesthetic vaporizers located within the breathing circuit:*

   a. are designed for precision administration of anesthetics
   b. are designed for anesthetics that vaporize poorly or have low potency
   c. can be used safely with halothane
   d. cannot be used safely with methoxyflurane
   e. show the anesthetic concentration by the number located on the top of the Ohio #8 vaporizer (*eg*, 1=1%, 2=2%, etc)

7. *Vaporizers located outside the rebreathing circuit:*

   a. are designed to administer anesthetics of either low or high potency
   b. cannot be used safely with methoxyflurane
   c. permit the patient to breath through them
   d. are referred to as nonprecision vaporizers
   e. are more economical to purchase and use than those located within the circuit

8. *Mistaken placement of the incorrect gas cylinder on an anesthetic machine is prevented by:*

   a. color-coded identification
   b. pin-coded cylinder valve bodies
   c. the diameter-coded cylinder valve outlet
   d. the cylinder lable
   e. the cylinder tag

9. *What size of O_2 cylinder is attached directly to the anesthetic machine?*

   a. E
   b. F
   c. G
   d. H
   e. I

10. *An "H" O_2 cylinder with a pressure reading of 2200 lb/square inch is considered full at standard room temperature and pressure, and contains about:*

    a. 500 L
    b. 700 L
    c. 5000 L
    d. 7000 L
    e. 70,000 L

11. Which anesthetic machine part is used to calculate flow of gases to the anesthetic machine and patient?

a. flow meter
b. regulator
c. pressure gauge
d. gas cylinder
e. vaporizer

12. An example of a precision bubble-through vaporizer located out of the breathing system in which any of the available liquid anesthetics can be used is the:

a. Fluotec Mark III
b. Ohio #8
c. Vapor
d. Copper Kettle
e. Stevens

13. When using an O_2 flow meter, gas flow should be read at the:

a. bottom of the ball or the center of other types of indicators
b. center of the ball or the top of other indicators
c. bottom of the ball or the top of other indicators
d. top of any indicator
e. center of any indicator

14. The numbers associated with the control lever on the top of an Ohio #8 vaporizer show:

a. the concentration of anesthetic in the vaporizing chamber
b. the concentration of anesthetic exiting the vaporizer
c. the relative percentage of anesthetic (oxygen and anesthetic gas) flowing through the vaporizing chamber
d. the relative percentage of carbon dioxide gas flowing through the vaporizing chamber
e. a close estimate of the anesthetic concentration being inspired by the patient

15. Used or depleted soda lime is:

a. hard and bluish
b. soft and white
c. hard and white
d. soft and bluish
e. hard and pink

16. In comparing the effects of acepromazine and xylazine,:

a. acepromazine causes vasoconstriction
b. xylazine causes alpha-1 blockade
c. acepromazine initially causes hypertension
d. acepromazine produces profound analgesia
e. xylazine produces profound analgesia and deep sedation

17. In which species are opiates most likely to causes an excitatory response?

a. pigs and dogs
b. horses and pigs
c. dogs and cattle
d. cats and horses
e. cats and dogs

18. Atropine:

a. should be given as a preanesthetic to all patients
b. is totally effective in controlling bradycardia
c. is totally effective in controlling salivation in ruminants
d. can be safely given to horses that have not been fasted
e. is an anticholinergic acting centrally and peripherally, generally preventing bradycardia caused by vagovagal reflexes

19. An agent that can be given intravenously for humane euthanasia of dogs is:

a. succinylcholine
b. strychnine
c. magnesium sulfate
d. guaifenesin
e. sodium pentobarbital

Correct answers are on pages 25-27.

20. A 10% solution of thiopental contains the drug at a concentration of:

a. 0.1 mg/ml
b. 1 mg/ml
c. 10 mg/ml
d. 100 mg/ml
e. 1000 mg/ml

21. In horses, xylazine typically causes:

a. second-degree atrioventricular blockade
b. sinus tachycardia
c. atrial fibrillation
d. ventricular bigeminy
e. ventricular tachycardia

22. The initial sign of local anesthetic toxicity in goats is:

a. opisthotonos with seizure
b. widespread erythema
c. sudden cardiovascular collapse
d. vomiting
e. nystagmus

23. Injection of xylazine into the carotid artery of horses causes:

a. sweating
b. vomiting
c. diarrhea
d. sudden collapse
e. excitement

24. Concerning differences between isoflurane and halothane, which statement is most accurate?

a. The anesthetic level can be changed more quickly with isoflurane than with halothane.
b. Isoflurane causes greater sensitization of the heart to catecholamines than does halothane.
c. Isoflurane is much less volatile than halothane.
d. Biodegradation occurs to a far lesser degree with halothane than with isoflurane.
e. Halothane causes greater vasodilation and less myocardial depression than isoflurane.

25. Acepromazine, a phenothiazine tranquilizer, causes hypotension by:

a. blockade of beta-1 receptors
b. blockade of beta-2 receptors
c. blockade of alpha-1 receptors
d. decreasing cardiac output
e. agonism of beta-2 receptors

26. The agent most commonly associated with severe hypotension in horses is:

a. diazepam
b. droperidol
c. xylazine
d. detomidine
e. acepromazine

27. Which of the following is the characteristic breathing pattern induced by ketamine administration?

a. slow, deep breathing
b. Cheyne-Stokes breathing
c. tachypnea
d. apneustic breathing
e. hyperventilation

*28. In what situation is use of ketamine anesthesia **unsuitable**?*

a. muscle trauma
b. bradycardia
c. hypotension
d. castration of a cat
e. intraocular surgery

29. The agent most likely to produce adequate chemical restraint of vicious dogs is:

a. xylazine
b. morphine with acepromazine

c. morphine
d. acepromazine
e. diazepam with tripellenamine

30. Which of the following is the most likely reason for prolonged ketamine anesthesia (delayed recovery) in cats?

a. hyperthermia
b. low total plasma protein level
c. metabolic alkalosis
d. inadequate urinary clearance
e. hepatic dysfunction

31. Innovar-Vet is a combination of:

a. tiletamine and zolazepam
b. droperidol and fentanyl
c. meperidine and fentanyl
d. detomidine and fentanyl
e. diazepam and ketamine

32. The drug that is a complete narcotic antagonist is:

a. tolazoline
b. doxapram
c. naloxone
d. yohimbine
e. nalbuphine

33. Which drug is the most potent analgesic?

a. fentanyl
b. meperidine
c. xylazine
d. butorphanol
e. morphine

34. Which drug combination is used to produce neuroleptanalgesia?

a. tranquilizers and barbiturates
b. tranquilizers and narcotics
c. sedatives and hypnotics
d. tranquilizers and muscle relaxants
e. narcotics and muscle relaxants

35. About how long does it take for halothane to reach equilibrium between the pulmonary alveoli and vessel-rich organs in an animal that is breathing normally?

a. 15 minutes
b. 30 minutes
c. 45 minutes
d. 1 hour
e. 2 hours

36. Using an inhalant anesthetic with a minimum alveolar concentration (MAC) of 1.0, the percentage of patients that do **not** *move when subjected to a painful stimulus is:*

a. 10%
b. 25%
c. 50%
d. 75%
e. 100%

37. Accidental massive overdose of xylazine can be effectively treated with intravenous fluids and:

a. naloxone
b. detomidine
c. tolazoline
d. doxapram
e. epinephrine

38. Concerning use of atropine and glycopyrrolate as anticholinergic preanesthetics, which statement is most accurate?

a. Atropine does not cross the blood-brain barrier.
b. Atropine crosses the blood-brain barrier more slowly than glycopyrrolate and has only peripheral effects.
c. Atropine is longer acting than glycopyrrolate.
d. Glycopyrrolate crosses the blood-brain barrier in larger amounts than atropine and has primarily central effects.
e. Glycopyrrolate crosses the blood-brain barrier more slowly than atropine and has primarily peripheral effects.

Correct answers are on pages 25-27.

39. The inhalant anesthetic that induces the ***least*** *cardiovascular depression during general anesthesia is:*

a. halothane
b. methoxyflurane
c. enflurane
d. isoflurane
e. desflurane

40. The inhalant anesthetic that ***does not*** *require a vaporizer for administration is:*

a. halothane
b. methoxyflurane
c. nitrous oxide
d. enflurane
e. isoflurane

41. In cats, the sedative effect of xylazine can be effectively reversed with the alpha antagonist:

a. doxapram
b. naloxone
c. butorphanol
d. buprenorphine
e. tolazoline

42. Postanesthetic myositis is most likely to occur in:

a. horses
b. pigs
c. dogs
d. rabbits
e. cattle

43. Malignant hyperthermia associated with inhalant anesthesia is most likely to be encountered in:

a. pigs
b. cats
c. dogs
d. rabbits
e. sheep

44. Postoperative pain may result in any of the following ***except:***

a. hypoventilation
b. hypoxia
c. alkalosis
d. acidosis
e. hyperventilation

45. A high $PaCO_2$ in a patient during anesthesia suggests:

a. hyperventilation
b. metabolic alkalosis
c. hypoventilation
d. metabolic acidosis
e. respiratory alkalosis

46. High caudal epidural anesthesia is ***contraindicated*** *in:*

a. dogs
b. cats
c. pigs
d. horses
e. cattle

47. Which of the following is most suitable for use in castration of horses?

a. guaifenesin
b. phenobarbital
c. xylazine with ketamine
d. acepromazine with diazepam
e. droperidol with fentanyl

48. The species with 7 lumbar vertebrae is the:

a. horse
b. sheep
c. ox
d. dog
e. pig

49. The species in which you are ***least*** *likely to insert the needle into the subarachnoid space when giving a lumbosacral injection is the:*

a. horse
b. dog
c. pig
d. goat
e. ox

50. The normal resting heart rate for a healthy Thoroughbred horse is:

a. 42-60 beats/minute
b. 64-78 beats/minute
c. 28-40 beats/minute
d. 80-100 beats/minute
e. 112-120 beats/minute

51. When attempting endotracheal intubation under light anesthesia, laryngospasm is most likely to occur in:

a. horses
b. cattle
c. sheep
d. cats
e. dogs

52. Continuous positive-pressure ventilation is ***contraindicated*** *in patients with:*

a. acute pulmonary edema
b. diffuse emphysema
c. neonatal respiratory distress syndrome
d. peripheral circulatory failure
e. asthma

53. When using a guaifenesin-ketamine-xylazine combination, the smallest amount of xylazine is required in:

a. dogs
b. pigs
c. horses
d. cats
e. ruminants

54. Balanced anesthesia is characterized by:

a. sedation, analgesia and muscle relaxation
b. narcosis, analgesia and muscle relaxation
c. neuroleptanalgesia
d. hypnosis and muscle relaxation
e. tranquilization, analgesia and muscle relaxation

55. In rabbits, injectable anesthetics are best injected into the:

a. femoral vein
b. jugular vein
c. auricular vein
d. cephalic vein
e. right ventricle

56. In rabbits,:

a. atropine effectively controls salivation
b. the safety margin between the anesthetic and lethal dose of pentobarbital is very narrow
c. pentobarbital is a potent analgesic
d. the trachea is easily intubated under light pentobarbital anesthesia
e. intravenous fluid infusion is not recommended during anesthesia

57. Concerning ketamine anesthesia in birds, which statement is ***least*** *accurate?*

a. A dosage of 30-40 mg/kg IM is required for such diagnostic procedures as radiography and laparoscopy.
b. Ketamine may be given IV to large birds.
c. Induction is smooth and muscle relaxation is enhanced when ketamine is combined with diazepam.
d. There are considerable species variations in the response to ketamine, and owls appear to be especially sensitive.
e. Injectable anesthesia is the method of choice for lengthy or involved surgical procedures in birds.

58. Concerning anesthesia in birds, which statement is ***least*** *accurate?*

a. Inhalant anesthetics are best delivered with a non-rebreathing system, such as a Bain apparatus.
b. The trachea of birds is easily intubated.
c. Birds do not have a larynx.
d. As compared with mammals, birds have a higher lung surface-to-volume ratio and a thinner blood-air barrier, making it more efficient for gas exchange.
e. Birds require more time to recover from inhalation anesthesia than do mammals.

Correct answers are on pages 25-27.

59. *The most common change in acid-base status in an anesthetized patient is:*

a. metabolic acidosis
b. metabolic alkalosis
c. respiratory alkalosis
d. respiratory acidosis
e. mixed acid-base disturbance

60. *The most reliable indication of the depth of anesthesia and well-being of birds is:*

a. respiratory rate and character and ventilatory response to stimulation
b. electrocardiographic pattern
c. blood gas and acid-base status
d. palpebral reflex present in deep anesthesia
e. pedal reflex present in deep anesthesia

61. *Which inhalant anesthetic is considered most desirable for birds?*

a. ether
b. nitrous oxide
c. isoflurane
d. methoxyflurane
e. halothane

62. *When using injectable agents for restraint and analgesia in small animals, xylazine combined with an opioid is useful because this combination:*

a. produces no detrimental cardiovascular effect
b. does not depress respiration
c. is completely compatible with ketamine
d. does not alter the dosage requirement of other drugs that might be used
e. has specific antagonists that can nearly completely reverse the depressant effects, if necessary

63. *Primates are most easily intubated if positioned in:*

a. dorsal recumbency
b. left lateral recumbency
c. right lateral recumbency
d. sternal recumbency
e. the prone position

64. *The larynx of primates is considered:*

a. very sensitive to stimulation, making it difficult to intubate
b. about as sensitive to stimulation as that of a dog
c. weakly sensitive to stimulation, making intubation rather simple
d. the primary cause of difficult intubation because of its proximity to the uvula
e. easy to intubate because of its shape and location

65. *The agent of choice for anesthesia of reptiles is:*

a. xylazine
b. thiopental
c. pentobarbital
d. ketamine
e. acepromazine

66. *In horses anesthetized with xylazine and ketamine,:*

a. xylazine should be given before ketamine
b. ketamine should be given before xylazine
c. the drugs should be mixed and given simultaneously
d. xylazine should be given before ketamine, and both drugs should be preceded by acepromazine
e. the order of drug administration is of no consequence

67. *In general anesthesia of ruminants, the animal should:*

a. be fasted for 3 days previously
b. be intubated with an appropriately sized endotracheal tube
c. have a stomach tube placed in the rumen to prevent gas accumulation
d. receive atropine as a preanesthetic
e. be maintained in dorsal recumbency

68. In horses, the trachea is generally intubated:

a. using a guide tube
b. blindly during inspiration
c. by the tactile method
d. using a laryngoscope
e. only after the larynx has been sprayed with lidocaine

69. Abolition of the awareness of pain is referred to as:

a. hypnosis
b. sedation
c. narcosis
d. analgesia
e. tranquilization

70. Deep anesthesia with isoflurane generally depresses ventilation and causes CO_2 retention. Clinical management of this problem should include:

a. IV infusion of sodium bicarbonate
b. assisted or controlled ventilation
c. IV fluid administration
d. acepromazine as a preanesthetic drug
e. a lighter plane of anesthesia and assisted or controlled ventilation

71. If a patient inhales 50% N_2O at the standard temperature and pressure, the partial pressure of N_2O in the alveolus should be approximately:

a. 180 mm of Hg
b. 355 mm of Hg
c. 450 mm of Hg
d. 460 mm of Hg
e. 760 mm of Hg

72. Shock is initially treated with:

a. rapid infusion of fluids
b. epinephrine
c. dobutamine
d. alpha-2 antagonists
e. corticosteroids

73. All anesthetic machines should be equipped with:

a. a static electricity arrestor
b. an electrocardiograph
c. a waste gas scavenging system
d. a blood pressure monitor
e. a nitrous oxide flow meter and flush valve

74. The normal resting heart rate and respiratory rate of cats are:

a. 40-60 beats/minute, 10-15 breaths/minute
b. 60-90 beats/minute, 40-60 breaths/minute
c. 60-80 beats/minute, 10-20 breaths/minute
d. 110-150 beats/minute, 20-40 breaths/minute
e. 150-200 beats/minute, 40-60 breaths/minute

75. When inducing anesthesia in a Greyhound dog, the barbiturate of choice is:

a. thiamylal
b. thiopental
c. pentobarbital
d. methohexital
e. phenobarbital

*76. Which of the following is **not** an objective of preanesthetic medication?*

a. alleviate or minimize pain
b. facilitate handling
c. minimize undesirable postanesthetic recovery complications
d. increase reflex autonomic activity
e. decrease the dose of parenteral anesthetic induction drugs

77. One milliliter of 10% solution of a drug contains how many milligrams of that drug?

a. 10 mg/ml
b. 20 mg/ml
c. 1.0 mg/ml
d. 0.1 mg/ml
e. 100 mg/ml

Correct answers are on pages 25-27.

78. *If you administer 350 ml of a 5% solution of guaifenesin to a 250-kg pony, how many mg/kg would be administered?*

a. 35
b. 250
c. 70
d. 10
e. 100

79. *Following anesthetic induction with thiopental in a dog, you intubate the animal and administer halothane and oxygen via a circle system. The dog immediately becomes apneic. The most appropriate course of action is to:*

a. institute intermittent positive-pressure ventilation at 12 breaths/min, at a volume of 100 ml/kg
b. turn off the halothane because the dog is deeply anesthetized
c. stimulate upper airway reflexes by gently moving the endotracheal tube backward and forward
d. institute intermittent positive-pressure ventilation at 2-3 breaths/min, at a volume of 10 ml/kg
e. administer another one-quarter dose of thiopental because the dog's apnea is due to light anesthesia

80. *Concerning use of thiopental in cats, which statement is most accurate?*

a. Thiopental should not be used in cats because they are more sensitive to the drug and more prone to toxicity than dogs.
b. It can be given intramuscularly or subcutaneously to cats.
c. It is an appropriate choice for uremic, dehydrated cats.
d. It is associated with excessive muscle tone, so diazepam should also be administered.
e. It can cause increased laryngeal reflexes and coughing, especially at light anesthetic levels.

81. *Ketamine is a good choice for anesthetic induction in a:*

a. cat with an elevated blood urea nitrogen level and a history of chronic renal failure
b. dog that has been hit by a car and has evidence of head trauma
c. cat with hyperthyroidism and a resting heart rate of 200 beats/min
d. brachycephalic dog with upper airway obstruction
e. male cat with a history of urethral obstruction

82. *The intravenous anesthetic with the shortest anesthetic recovery time is:*

a. thiopental
b. ketamine with diazepam
c. pentobarbital
d. tiletamine with zolazepam
e. propofol

83. *To produce epidural anesthesia in a dog, a local anesthetic drug should be injected at the:*

a. sacrococcygeal junction to avoid recumbency
b. junction of the 5th and 6th lumbar vertebrae to ensure mixing with cerebrospinal fluid
c. lumbosacral space, between the periosteum and dura mater
d. lumbosacral space, between the pia mater and arachnoid
e. lumbosacral junction, between the pia mater and arachnoid

84. *Which inhalation agent is most potent?*

a. halothane
b. nitrous oxide
c. isoflurane
d. methoxyflurane
e. propofol

85. *Mask induction of anesthesia using inhalation agents is:*

a. the best way to induce anesthesia in a patient with an upper airway obstruction
b. best accomplished using a volatile anesthetic that is highly soluble in blood, such as methoxyflurane

c. best accomplished using a volatile anesthetic that is relatively insoluble in blood, such as halothane
d. not influenced by the adequacy of ventilation
e. less expensive than routine parenteral anesthetic inductions

86. *Nitrous oxide:*

a. has no analgesic activity
b. should not be used in concentrations less than 80%
c. is not sufficiently potent to produce anesthesia in dogs
d. should only be used with halothane
e. should be used in closed-circuit anesthesia

87. *Inhalation anesthesia can be induced more rapidly in neonatal animals than adults because neonates:*

a. are relatively smaller but have a proportionately larger surface area to body weight
b. contain less body water
c. become hypothermic, so less anesthetic is required
d. have relatively greater alveolar ventilation and cardiac output
e. have a relatively larger larynx

88. *The reading on the pressure gauge gives no indication of quantity of gas remaining in the cylinder for which agent?*

a. nitrogen
b. oxygen
c. helium
d. halothane
e. nitrous oxide

89. *What is the color of cylinders used for nitrous oxide, and what is the pressure in a full cylinder?*

a. green; 2,200 psi
b. blue; 750 psi
c. orange; 2,000 psi
d. green; 750 psi
e. blue; 2,200 psi

90. *The pressure in a nitrous oxide cylinder decreases when:*

a. the cylinder is half full
b. the cylinder is one-fourth full
c. all of the liquid nitrous oxide has vaporized, which occurs when the tank is nearly empty
d. the cylinder is heated
e. the cylinder is initially opened, then the pressure gradually decreases until the tank is empty of pressure

---

Answers

1. **a**
2. **d**
3. **e**
4. **b**
5. **b**
6. **b**
7. **a**
8. **b**
9. **a**
10. **d**
11. **a**
12. **d**
13. **b**
14. **c**
15. **a**
16. **e**
17. **d**
18. **e**
19. **e**
20. **d**

21. **a**
22. **a**
23. **d**
24. **a**
25. **c**
26. **e**
27. **d**
28. **e**
29. **b**
30. **d**
31. **b**
32. **c**
33. **a**
34. **b**
35. **a**
36. **c**
37. **c**
38. **e**
39. **e**
40. **c**
41. **e**
42. **a**
43. **a**
44. **c**
45. **c**
46. **d**
47. **c**
48. **d**
49. **b**
50. **c**
51. **d**
52. **d**
53. **e**
54. **b**
55. **c**
56. **b**
57. **e**
58. **e**
59. **d**
60. **a**
61. **c**
62. **e**
63. **a**
64. **a**
65. **d**
66. **a**
67. **b**
68. **b**
69. **d**
70. **e**
71. **b**
72. **a**
73. **c**
74. **d**
75. **d**
76. **d** Premedication agents, such as atropine, are used to minimize undesirable reflex autonomic activity.
77. **e** A 10% solution = 10 g/100 ml = 10,000 mg/100 ml = 100 mg/ml.
78. **c** 350 ml x 50 mg/ml = 17,500 mg/250 kg = 70 mg/kg.
79. **d** Apnea is commonly seen following thiopental induction of anesthesia, especially with a high inspired oxygen level. Giving 2-3 normal breaths per minute ensures that the patient remains oxygenated, receives some halothane and allows the arterial carbon dioxide to rise to a level sufficient to stimulate spontaneous ventilation. If no halothane were administered, this dog would be awake in 10-15 minutes. Propofol also causes postinduction apnea.
80. **e** Thiobarbiturates cause perivascular irritation and tissue sloughing, and are associated with prolonged recovery in dehydrated, emaciated, hypoproteinemic animals. They produce relatively good muscle relaxation at anesthetic doses.
81. **d** Rapid induction of anesthesia and maintenance of laryngeal function are desirable in brachycephalic dogs. In addition, a rapid recovery is desirable. Though not producing the fastest induction and smoothest recovery (thiopental or propofol would be better), ketamine would be acceptable.
82. **e**

83. **c** The epidural space is located immediately outside of the dura mater.

84. **d** MAC values for these anesthetics in dogs: 0.9 volume % for halothane, 215 volume % for nitrous oxide and 1.4 volume % for isoflurane, versus 0.23 volume % for methoxyflurane. Propofol is not an inhalational anesthetic agent.

85. **c** Mask inductions are slow (undesirable if rapid airway control is desirable), with speed of induction dependent on drug solubility (insoluble agents produce faster induction) and ventilation (hyperventilation produces faster induction). Mask induction can be expensive, especially with isoflurane (about $5 for induction in a dog).

86. **c** The minimum alveolar concentration (MAC) of nitrous oxide in dogs is approximately 215 volume %, so under normal conditions (1 atmosphere of pressure), it cannot alone produce anesthesia.

87. **d** Uptake of anesthetic is improved with increased ventilation. The "centralized" circulation of neonates ensures rapid delivery of anesthetic to the brain.

88. **e** Nitrous oxide is a liquid when stored under pressure at room temperature. Halothane is a vapor, not a gas, and therefore is not stored under pressure. Gases that can be liquefied at room temperature are purchased by weight. Pressure is an accurate index of quantity for nonliquefiable compressed gases.

89. **b**

90. **c** The pressure in the cylinder begins to drop when all of the liquid nitrous oxide has been vaporized and the gas loses pressure. Cylinders must be watched thereafter for rapid emptying. Another cause of decreased pressure is chilling of the cylinder.

Notes

Notes

Section 3

Behavior

K.A. Houpt

Recommended Reading

Beaver BV: *Feline Behavior: A Guide for Veterinarians.* Saunders, Philadelphia, 1992.
Campbell WE: *Behavior Problems in Dogs.* 2nd ed. American Veterinary Publications, Goleta, CA, 1992.
Hart BL: *The Behavior of Domestic Animals.* Freeman, New York, 1985.
Hart BL and Hart LA: *Canine and Feline Behavioral Therapy.* Lea & Febiger, Philadelphia, 1985.
Houpt KA: *Domestic Animal Behavior for Veterinarians and Animal Scientists.* Iowa State University Press, Ames, 1991.
Marder AR and Voith VL: Advances in companion animal behavior. *Vet Clin No Am* (Small Anim Pract) 21:203-420, 1991.

Practice answer sheet is on page 349.

Questions

1. *You are presented with a cat that is eliminating throughout the house and near but not in the litterbox. To determine the underlying cause of this behavior, the client should be asked:*

   a. whether there have been any changes in the household
   b. the reason the cat was chosen as a pet
   c. whether the cat is urinating, defecating or both
   d. whether the cat has been declawed
   e. how the cat was housebroken

2. *Spraying can be differentiated from nonspraying urination in that, with spraying, the urine is typically deposited:*

   a. on electronic equipment
   b. on a noncarpeted floor
   c. on a carpeted floor
   d. on a vertical surface
   e. near the litterbox

3. *Spraying is most common in:*

   a. single-cat households
   b. multi-cat households containing all males
   c. multi-cat households containing all females
   d. multi-cat households containing 2 males and 1 or more females
   e. multi-cat households containing 2 females and 1 or more males

Correct answers are on pages 34-35.

4. *A probable cause of a healthy cat's failure to urinate in the litterbox is:*

   a. jealousy
   b. vindictiveness
   c. boredom
   d. substrate preference
   e. loss (of memory) of housebreaking

5. *The first step in treating a cat that eliminates outside the litterbox is to:*

   a. improve litterbox hygiene
   b. confine the cat in a cage
   c. prescribe diazepam
   d. punish the cat
   e. substitute a covered litterbox

6. *An efficient means of determining which litter substrate a cat will use is to:*

   a. offer several choices of litter simultaneously
   b. offer several choices of litter sequentially
   c. mix new litter with the old and gradually add a greater percentage of new litter
   d. confine the cat with the new litter
   e. mix the old litter with the new litter and gradually add a greater percentage of the old litter

7. *An indication that the litter substrate is the source of an elimination problem is suggested by the cat's:*

   a. perching on the side or corner of the litterbox to eliminate
   b. eliminating in the shower or bathtub
   c. eliminating on beds or clothing
   d. attempts to go outdoors
   e. spraying urine on furniture and curtains

8. *Experiments have shown that the litter substrate preferred by most cats is:*

   a. plain clay
   b. deodorized clay
   c. clumping litter
   d. sawdust
   e. newspaper

9. *A single cat that defecates outside the litterbox may be less likely to do so if:*

   a. the type of litter is changed
   b. the type of litterbox is changed
   c. another litterbox is added
   d. another cat is added
   e. the carpet is removed

10. *Cats that prefer to eliminate on rugs may use a litterbox with:*

    a. a hood
    b. a wide wooden frame surrounding it
    c. an aluminum foil lining
    d. a carpeted frame surrounding it
    e. a plastic mat under it

11. *An effective means of treating urination outside the litterbox in multiple-cat households is:*

    a. increasing the number and location of litterboxes
    b. replacing the carpeting
    c. making the place where the cat urinates aversive to the animal
    d. punishing the offending cat
    e. providing a companion dog

12. *A urinary tract problem is most likely to be the underlying cause of inappropriate elimination if the problem involves:*

    a. spraying urine
    b. urinating in a squatting posture outside the litterbox
    c. defecatinig outside the litterbox
    d. urinating and defecating outside the litterbox
    e. defecating and spraying urine outside the litterbox

13. *The medical problem most often associated with urination outside the litterbox is:*

a. diabetes insipidus
b. diabetes mellitus
c. impacted anal sacs
d. urinary tract disease
e. cardiovascular disease

14. In a multiple-cat household, a cat suddenly displays aggression toward another long-term resident that has recently returned from hospitalization at a veterinary clinic. The underlying cause of this aggression is most likely:

a. a new infant in the household
b. a new adult (person) in the household
c. a new type of litter substrate that the aggressive cat dislikes
d. the aggressive cat's inability to chase a squirrel it sees through a window
e. a change in the odor or appearance of the victimized cat

15. A dog demonstrating territorial aggression is most likely to bite:

a. a family member entering the house
b. a stranger entering the house
c. a stranger punishing the dog
d. a family member pushing the dog off the couch
e. another dog during a walk in the park

16. A male dog demonstrating sexual aggression is most likely to bite:

a. a male family member entering the house
b. a female stranger entering the house
c. a male stranger punishing the dog
d. a female family member punishing the dog
e. another male dog during a walk in the park

17. To determine the type of aggression shown by a dog, the owner should be asked:

a. when the aggression occurred
b. who was the victim
c. his or her reaction to the aggression
d. why the dog was aggressive
e. where the dog was purchased

18. A dog is most likely to be aggressive toward the owner when the owner:

a. lets the dog out of the house
b. enters the house, yard or car
c. gives the dog a food reward
d. pets the dog on the head
e. throws a toy for the dog to fetch

19. Aggressive behavior in a dog can be initiated or exacerbated by all of the following ***except:***

a. household with few visitors
b. fear, hostility or aggression commonly shown by family members toward outsiders
c. including the dog in social interaction with guests
d. teasing or aggression by outsiders
e. encouragement of hostility toward outsiders

20. A dog is most likely to be aggressive toward a stranger when the stranger:

a. is walking his or her own dog nearby
b. enters the house, yard or car
c. gives the dog a food reward
d. is standing near the owner
e. throws a toy for the dog to fetch

21. Castration reduces urine marking in approximately:

a. 98% of male dogs
b. 80% of male dogs
c. 50% of male dogs
d. 20% of male dogs
e. 2% of male dogs

22. In dogs, fear of thunder is most likely to be manifested in:

a. puppies
b. juvenile dogs
c. young adults
d. middle-aged adults
e. old adults

Correct answers are on pages 34-35.

23. *The behavioral problem for which young dogs (less than 2 years old) are most likely to be presented for treatment is:*

a. aggression
b. phobia
c. destructiveness
d. urine marking
e. barking

24. *The owners of a dog return home to find that the animal has chewed up a valuable Oriental carpet. They punish the dog severely. Such delayed punishment for destructive behavior usually:*

a. resolves destructive behavior
b. leads to inappropriate elimination
c. exacerbates destructive behavior
d. teaches the dog to be aggressive
e. leads to problem barking

25. *The breed of dog most likely to exhibit destructive behavior is the:*

a. Malamute
b. Cocker Spaniel
c. Doberman Pinscher
d. Golden Retriever
e. Pomeranian

26. *In order of increasing severity of therapy, treatment for problem barking may include:*

a. behavior modification, ultrasonic collar, shock collar, physical punishment
b. ultrasonic collar, behavior modification, shock collar, physical punishment
c. vocal cordectomy, physical punishment, shock collar, behavior modification
d. vocal cordectomy, shock collar, ultrasonic collar, behavior modification
e. behavior modification, ultrasonic collar, shock collar, vocal cordectomy

27. *The breed of dog most frequently presented for treatment of problem barking is the:*

a. Afghan
b. Basenji
c. Collie
d. Sheltie
e. Malamute

28. *The first method one should suggest to the owner of a dog that disturbs the neighbors by continually barking in the yard is to:*

a. keep the dog in the house and take it outside only on a leash
b. use a collar that shocks the dog when it barks
c. use a collar that emits ultrasound when the dog barks
d. have the dog treated by vocal cordectomy
e. have the dog euthanized if it does not respond to heavy sedation

29. *A commercially available collar (Promise Collar, Haltie) for dogs is constructed so that a pull on the leash tightens a loop around the animal's muzzle. Such collars have been effective in curtailing aggression in some dogs in that:*

a. the owner can rapidly produce hypoxemia in the dog
b. the pressure produces pain, which decreases aggression
c. the dog immediately assumes a submissive position
d. the dog is rewarded by pressure on its muzzle
e. the dog is given a subordinating signal, with the owner at a safe distance

30. *To be most effective in suppressing undesirable behavior, punishment must be administered to the animal within:*

a. a millisecond of the offending behavior
b. seconds of the offending behavior
c. 1-2 minutes of the offending behavior
d. 1 hour of the offending behavior
e. 1-2 days of the offending behavior

31. *"Snapping" (champing or tooth clapping) is an equine behavior shown by:*

a. stallions after investigating urine
b. mares in anestrus
c. geldings investigating foals

d. foals approaching a stallion
e. socially dominant adult horses

32. The flehmen response is an equine behavior shown by:

a. stallions after investigating urine
b. mares in anestrus
c. geldings investigating foals
d. foals approaching a stallion
e. socially dominant adult horses

33. When food, water or shelter is limited, the horses most likely to gain access are:

a. stallions with a harem of mares
b. mares under 3 years of age
c. geldings of any age
d. foals over 3 months of age
e. socially dominant adult horses

34. Self-mutilation or flank biting in horses is most likely to occur in:

a. stallions in a herd situation
b. stallions housed in individual stalls
c. geldings housed in individual stalls
d. mares housed in individual stalls
e. mares in a herd situation

35. One can sometimes predict the gender of a foal based upon the mare's behavior during pregnancy. Concerning such predictions, which statement is most accurate?

a. Mares showing aggressive behavior during pregnancy are usually carrying colts.
b. Mares showing aggressive behavior during pregnancy are usually carrying fillies.
c. Mares showing estrus during pregnancy are usually carrying fillies.
d. Mares showing estrus during pregnancy are usually carrying colts.
e. Primiparous mares are more likely to be carrying fillies.

36. In pigs, tail biting is most likely to occur when:

a. pigs in dirt lots are stimulated by estrual sows
b. pigs on concrete floors are stimulated by fresh corn
c. pigs in dirt lots are stimulated by fresh corn
d. pigs on concrete floors are stimulated by fresh blood
e. sows are in farrowing crates

37. Just before farrowing, sows may demonstrate:

a. nest building
b. self-mutilation
c. tail biting
d. stereotypic biting or champing
e. piglet stealing

38. Just before lambing, ewes may demonstrate:

a. nest building
b. self-mutilation
c. wool biting
d. stereotypic biting or champing
e. lamb stealing

39. The breed of cat most likely to chew or suck woolen cloth is the:

a. Abyssinian
b. Maine Coon Cat
c. Siamese
d. Persian
e. Manx

40. A dairy farmer tells you that he saw one of his cows mounting another cow. You should appropriately advise the farmer that he should:

a. arrange for insemination of the mounting cow immediately
b. arrange for insemination of the mounted cow and the mounting cow immediately
c. arrange for insemination of the mounted cow immediately
d. arrange for insemination of the mounted cow immediately and of the mounting cow in a few days
e. arrange for insemination of the mounting cow immediately and of the mounted cow in a few days

Correct answers are on pages 34-35.

41. A client says she is having a problem transporting one of her horses. In a partitioned 2-horse trailer, the horse scrambles or struggles. What is an appropriate recommendation that may resolve this problem?

a. feed the horse in the trailer for 2 weeks before transport
b. activate a remote-controlled shock collar when the horse begins to struggle in the trailer
c. sedate the horse with xylazine before shipping
d. transport the horse in an unpartitioned stock trailer, or remove the partition from the original trailer
e. hobble the horse during transport

42. Pushing ventrally on a sow's back may reflexly evoke a rigid stance. This usually indicates that the sow is:

a. pregnant
b. socially dominant
c. socially subordinate
d. in estrus
e. in diestrus

43. In horses, coprophagia is most likely to occur in:

a. stallions housed in individual stalls
b. anestrual mares and pregnant mares
c. geldings in a herd situation
d. well-fed foals and adult horses fed a deficient diet
e. socially dominant adult horses

44. A mare is most likely to reject attempted suckling by a newborn foal:

a. at the first foaling
b. at the fifth or a later foaling
c. if the foal has been born in a stall
d. if the foal has been born at pasture
e. if the foal is a female born twin to a male

45. Foal rejection by a mare is best managed by:

a. separating the mare and foal and reuniting them every 4 hours for nursing
b. restraining the mare so she cannot injure the foal and leaving them together
c. treating the mare with acepromazine and treating the foal with dopamine
d. leaving the mare and foal together, under natural conditions
e. restraining foal so that nursing only occurs when the mare approaches the foal

---

Answers

1. **c** Treatment of the various types of elimination problems depends upon the underlying cause.
2. **d** Urine on a vertical object indicates that the cat is spraying.
3. **d** The more cats in a household, the greater the likelihood of spraying. The presence of both genders aggravates the situation.
4. **d** A change of litter substrate usually helps. The owner is likely to punish the cat inappropriately if a, b and c are believed to be true.
5. **a** When given a choice, cats use a different (clean) place to eliminate each time.
6. **a** Cats can quickly indicate their preference.
7. **a** A cat that perches may prefer a more stable surface or may perch to avoid touching litter.
8. **c** Most cats tested preferred clumping litter.
9. **c** Some cats prefer to use one box for urination and another for defecation.
10. **d**
11. **a** This is especially helpful in multiple-cat households.

12. **b** Pain associated with urination causes the cat to avoid the site in which pain was experienced (litterbox).
13. **d** Pain associated with urination may cause a cat to avoid the site in which pain was experienced (litterbox). The cat may also urinate outside the litterbox because of urgency.
14. **e** A common cause of aggression is a change in odor or appearance of the other cat.
15. **b** An invader of the territory will be bitten by a dog displaying territorial aggression.
16. **e** Intermale aggression usually occurs between dogs.
17. **b** To determine whether the dog is displaying dominance aggression or territorial aggression, the nature of the victim must be known.
18. **d** Owners may believe they are comforting the dog, but the dog may perceive the action as a challenge of dominance.
19. **c** Including the dog in normal social interaction is unlikely to evoke aggression, whereas keeping the dog away from guests can exacerbate underlying aggression.
20. **b** A strange person's entry into a dog's home territory is most likely to provoke an attack.
21. **c** Approximately half of male dogs stop urinating in the house after castration.
22. **d** The average age at presentation is 5 years.
23. **c** The average age at presentation is 12-18 months.
24. **c** The dog is unable to associate the punishment with its past action, and may become more anxious concerning interaction with the owner.
25. **a** Though any breed of dog may be destructive, northern breeds are believed to be more susceptible.
26. **e** There are several ways to treat problem barking. In general, one should begin with the least invasive technique.
27. **d**
28. **a** It the stimulus is removed, the dog may stop barking.
29. **e** The Promise collar or Haltie presumably acts as a dominant dog would by restricting the dog's muzzle.
30. **b** Punishment must be administered within seconds after the undesirable behavior.
31. **d** Foals click their teeth together when frightened or in an approach-avoidance situation.
32. **a** Stallions sniff urine and then exhibit the flehmen response.
33. **e** Dominance allows preferred access to scarce resources; adults are dominant.
34. **b** Stallions are involved more often than geldings or mares.
35. **c** Mares pregnant with fillies may show signs of estrus.
36. **d** Blood stimulates aggression in pigs. Play leads to true biting.
37. **a** Sows often try to build a nest before parturition.
38. **e** Ewes may steal the lambs of other ewes before parturition.
39. **c** Oriental breeds often demonstrate wool sucking.
40. **d** Cows in proestrus mount estrous cows.
41. **d** If the horse is allowed to stand in a comfortable position in the trailer, the animal may not scramble.
42. **d** This reaction is a sign of estrus in sows.
43. **d**
44. **a** Primiparous mares are most likely to reject foals.
45. **b** Over a period of weeks, the mare may gradually accept the foal.

Notes

Section

4

Care of Aquarium Fish

T.W. Campbell

Recommended Reading

Lewbart GA: Medical management of disorders of freshwater tropical fish. *Compend Cont Ed Pract Vet* 13:968-977, 1991.

Stoskopf MK: *Fish Medicine.* Saunders, Philadelphia, 1993.

Stoskopf MK: Tropical fish medicine. *Vet Clin No Am* (Small Animal Pract) 18:283-474, 1988.

Wallach JD and Boever WJ: *Diseases of Exotic Animals.* Saunders, Philadelphia, 1983.

Whitaker BR: Common disorders of marine fish. *Compend Cont Ed Pract Vet* 13:960-967, 1991.

Practice answer sheet is on page 351.

Questions

1. *Which chemical is used to neutralize chlorine in water to make it safe for use in a fish aquarium?*

   a. sodium hypochlorite
   b. hydrochloric acid
   c. potassium permanganate
   d. sodium thiosulfate
   e. nitrofurazone

2. *Ammonia is present in water in 2 forms: the highly toxic un-ionized form (NH_3) and the relatively nontoxic ionized form (NH_4^+). Which of the following water values is the single most important factor in determining formation of un-ionized ammonia in aquarium water?*

   a. salinity
   b. pH
   c. temperature
   d. pressure
   e. hardness

3. *The disease commonly referred to as "ich," which can affect all species of freshwater fish, is caused by which parasite?*

   a. *Ichthyophthirius multifiliis*
   b. *Ichthyobodo necatrix*
   c. *Ichthyophonus hoferi*
   d. *Aeromonas hydrophilia*
   e. *Tetrahymena pyriformis*

Correct answers are on pages 38-39.

4. *Most tropical marine fish are best maintained in aquarium water with a salinity of:*

a. 20 parts per million
b. 35 parts per million
c. 50 parts per million
d. 20 parts per thousand
e. 35 parts per thousand

5. *Most tropical fish thrive in water at an optimal temperature zone between:*

a. 20 and 23 C (68 and 74 F)
b. 24 and 27 C (76 and 80 F)
c. 28 and 32 C (82 and 89 F)
d. 33 and 37 C (91 and 98 F)
e. 38 and 40 C (100 and 105 F)

6. *Aquarium overcrowding is a common mistake made by new aquarists. The usual guideline given for the maximum number of fish for a correctly functioning aquarium system, in inches of fish body length per gallon of water, is:*

a. 4 inches of fish per gallon of water
b. 2 inches of fish per gallon of water
c. 1 inch of fish per gallon of water
d. 1/2 inch of fish per gallon of water
e. 1/4 inch of fish per gallon of water

7. *Lymphocystis in pet fish is caused by a:*

a. virus
b. bacterium
c. protozoan
d. sporozoan
e. fungus

8. *Gas-bubble disease of aquarium fish is caused by:*

a. environmental toxins (ammonia, nitrite, chlorine)
b. bacterial infection by gas-forming organisms
c. supersaturation of the water with oxygen
d. excessively high water temperatures
e. encysted protozoan parasites

9. *Copper is often used to treat infection by fungi, algae, bacteria, protozoa and invertebrate parasites in saltwater aquaria. What is the recommended concentration of copper when the saltwater aquarium is to be treated for a minimum of 10 days?*

a. 0.50 parts per million
b. 0.20 parts per million
c. 0.10 parts per million
d. 0.05 parts per million
e. 0.02 parts per million

10. *Live fish are frequently sacrificed so as to identify disease outbreaks in aquarium systems. Which of the following sites is the preferred location to obtain samples for culture and identification of systemic bacterial pathogens in fish?*

a. heart
b. liver
c. kidney
d. stomach
e. gill

Answers

1. **d** Chlorine in municipal water supplies is used to sterilize drinking water for people. Chlorinated water can be fatal to fish, and chlorine should be removed before introduction of fish into the aquarium. Chlorine can be removed by aerating the water for several days or by adding sodium thiosulfate, which immediately inactivates the harmful chlorine by forming sodium chloride. Three grams of sodium thiosulfate can remove chlorine from 250 gallons of water containing chlorine at 20 parts per million.

2. **b** The portion of un-ionized (NH_3) and ionized (NH_4+) ammonia depends primarily on pH and, to a lesser degree, temperature, salinity and pressure. There is a 10-fold increase in un-ionized ammonia nitrogen in aquarium water at pH 8 than at pH 7. Nitrification in the biologic filter removes ammonia from a healthy aquarium. *Nitrosomonas* bacteria use the ammonia (NH_3) excreted from the fish, and heterotrophic bacteria convert it to less harmful nitrite (NO_2^-). *Nitrobacter* bacteria convert the nitrite to the relatively harmless nitrate (NO_3^-).

3. **a** *Ichthyophthirius multifiliis* is the causative organism of "ich," a disease readily identified by small white spots over the fish several days after introduction of carrier fish into the aquarium.

4. **e** Most tropical marine species are best maintained in water with salinity near 35 parts per thousand.

5. **b** Most freshwater tropical fish should ideally be kept in water temperatures between 24 and 27 C (76 and 80 F). Temperatures below this range predispose freshwater tropical fish to a variety of diseases. Temperatures above this range reduce oxygen levels in the water and predispose fish to disease.

6. **c** The rule of thumb is usually 1 inch of fish for each 8-10 square inches of water surface or 1 inch of fish per gallon of water, provided the entire aquarium system is functioning correctly.

7. **a** Lymphocystis was the first viral disease described in fish. The disease is characterized by nodular proliferation on the gills and skin. The cells making up these nodules are grossly enlarged (up to 100,000 times normal).

8. **c** Supersaturation of the water with oxygen may result in gas bubbles in the fins, gill lamellae, eyes and skin. Gas-bubble disease is often caused by cavitating pumps that force oxygen into solution.

9. **b** Concentrations of copper should not exceed the recommended level of 0.20 parts per million when treating copper-tolerant marine fish. Invertebrates and copper-sensitive fish should be removed before water treatment with copper. Copper concentrations above this level may be toxic to the fish. Levels below 0.20 parts per million may be ineffective.

10. **c** The kidney is the site of choice for bacterial culture in fish to detect systemic bacterial disease. It is best to culture from sacrificed live fish rather than from dead fish, as there is rapid postmortem migration of other, normal resident bacteria into these tissues.

Notes

Notes

Section **5**

Care of Cage/Aviary Birds

R.C. Blomquist, B.W. Ritchie

Recommended Reading

Brown AFA: *The Incubation Book.* Wheaton, London, 1985.
Harrison GJ and Harrison LR: *Clinical Avian Medicine and Surgery.* Saunders, Philadelphia, 1986.
Johnston DE: *Exotic Animal Medicine in Practice.* Veterinary Learning Systems, Trenton, NJ, 1991.
Petrak ML: *Diseases of Cage and Aviary Birds.* Lea & Febiger, Philadelphia, 1982.
Journal of the Association of Avian Veterinarians. Published bimonthly.
Journal of Zoo and Wildlife Medicine. Published monthly.
Proceedings of the Association of Avian Veterinarians Annual Conference. Published annually.

Practice answer sheet is on page 353.

Questions

1. *A "tail bob" or "tail jerk" is a sign of:*

   a. central nervous system disease
   b. gastrointestinal disease
   c. ectoparasite infestation
   d. estrus
   e. respiratory difficulty

2. *Pelleted diets are:*

   a. a viable alternative to a seed and table food diet, eliminating problems created by free-choice feeding
   b. complete diets meeting the recommended daily allowances of psittacines
   c. not available for psittacines
   d. a dangerous fad
   e. preferred to seeds by most caged birds

Correct answers are on pages 48-49.

3. *Undigestible grit is:*

   a. probably not necessary and can be dangerous
   b. an essential addition to the diet of pet birds
   c. not consumed by pet birds
   d. never eaten by wild birds
   e. incorporated into pelleted foods

4. *The ear of birds:*

   a. has an external acoustic meatus found caudoventral to the eye
   b. has no external opening
   c. is used to locate ultrasonic vibrations
   d. has a small, primordial pinna
   e. cannot be easily located and need not be examined

5. *Which structure generates the vocalizations of parrots?*

   a. vocal cords
   b. larynx
   c. syrinx
   d. glottis
   e. hyoid apparatus

6. *Air sacs primarily function to:*

   a. provide buoyancy
   b. exchange oxygen and carbon dioxide
   c. clear debris and pathogens from the respiratory tract
   d. pull and push air in and out of the lungs
   e. separate internal organs

7. *Mammals have 2 ovaries. In birds:*

   a. there is only one functional ovary, always located adjacent to the cranial pole of the left kidney
   b. there can be many ovaries adjacent to the cloaca
   c. there are no ovaries but, instead, a unisex gonad producing eggs or sperm, depending on hormonal influences
   d. there is only one functional ovary, always located adjacent to the right kidney
   e. there is only one ovary, either right or left, located adjacent to the cloaca

8. *A young budgerigar has marked beak deformities and crusting of featherless areas of the skin. The most likely cause of these signs is:*

   a. temporomandibular joint abnormalities
   b. candidiasis
   c. hepatopathy
   d. *Knemidokoptes* infestation
   e. dermatophytosis

9. *In general, the feces of psittacine birds should contain:*

   a. almost exclusively Gram-positive bacteria
   b. almost exclusively Gram-negative bacteria
   c. a nearly equal mixture of Gram-positive and Gram-negative bacteria
   d. almost no microorganisms
   e. almost exclusively yeasts, with a few Gram-negative bacteria

10. *The underlying cause of feather picking is usually:*

   a. ectoparasitic infestation
   b. an allergic reaction
   c. psychological in origin
   d. endoparasitic infection
   e. nutritional deficiency

11. *Which treatment is* ***least*** *likely to curtail feather picking?*

   a. placing the bird in isolation
   b. administering parenteral mood-altering drugs
   c. applying an Elizabethan collar
   d. enriching the environment with distractions
   e. administering parenteral progesterone

12. *Psittacine beak and feather disease is caused by:*

   a. feather picking
   b. an immunodeficiency

c. a bacterium
d. a fungus
e. a virus

13. Psittacine beak and feather disease is definitively diagnosed by:

a. Wood's lamp fluorescence of skin and feathers
b. fecal culture
c. serologic tests
d. microscopic examination of skin scrapings
e. histopathologic examination of feathers and bursa

14. Psittacine beak and feather disease is a:

a. progressive disease that is ultimately fatal
b. skin disorder that does not alter life expectancy
c. behavioral problem
d. disorder that is readily treated
e. noncontagious problem

15. A yellow-naped Amazon parrot suddenly develops depression, anorexia and "lime-green" droppings. Laboratory abnormalities include a high white blood cell count, increased serum activity of liver-derived enzymes, and slight anemia. The most appropriate diagnostic test is:

a. serologic examination for Pacheco's disease
b. whole-body radiographs
c. cloacal culture
d. electrocardiogram
e. enzyme-linked immunosorbent assay for *Chlamydia*

16. A psittacine bird was domestically raised and kept in a single-bird household for years. Recently the bird has shown some signs resembling those of psittacosis (chlamydiosis). Concerning the possibility of psittacosis in this bird, which statement is most accurate?

a. Psittacosis is not a concern because the bird has been isolated.
b. Psittacosis should only be considered if the bird has recently been boarded in a pet store.
c. Despite the bird's isolation, psittacosis is still a diagnostic consideration.
d. Psittacosis should only be considered if the bird is manifesting all of the classic clinical signs.
e. Psittacosis is not a consideration because it usually causes peracute and rapidly fatal infection in isolated birds.

17. The parasiticide of choice for treatment of Knemidokoptes *infestation is:*

a. amitraz
b. ivermectin
c. pyrethrin
d. mineral oil
e. fenthion

18. A vaccine is commercially available for prevention of:

a. Newcastle disease
b. macaw wasting syndrome
c. poxviral infection
d. budgerigar fledgling disease
e. reoviral infection

19. Environmental contamination with chlamydial organisms:

a. is of no concern regarding spread to birds
b. is not possible due to the intracellular nature of the parasite
c. affects a small radius of only a few feet from the cage of the infected bird
d. can be minimized by disinfection with quaternary ammonium compounds
e. is of no concern regarding spread to people

20. A vaccine is commercially available for prevention of:

a. Pacheco's disease
b. gout
c. avian leukosis
d. proventricular dilatation
e. psittacine beak and feather disease

Correct answers are on pages 48-49.

21. *In pet psittacine birds, toxicosis most commonly results from ingestion of:*

a. household insecticide strips
b. lead or lead-coated articles
c. excessive fat-soluble vitamins
d. excessive water-soluble vitamins
e. toxic plants

22. *The safest and most easily accessible venipuncture site in psittacine birds is the:*

a. left jugular vein
b. cutaneous ulnar vein
c. right jugular vein
d. heart
e. ocular venous plexus

23. *The largest blood volume that can be safely collected from an adult Amazon parrot is approximately:*

a. 0.1 ml
b. 0.8 ml
c. 3 ml
d. 10 ml
e. 30 ml

24. *Sudden death in pet psittacine birds, without any obvious clinical signs, is most commonly associated with:*

a. electrocution
b. plant toxicities
c. inhalation of fumes from overheated Teflon
d. poxviral infection
e. psittacosis (chlamydiosis)

25. *The recommended volume for a single gavage feeding of a hospitalized Amazon parrot is approximately:*

a. 1-3 ml
b. 3-6 ml
c. 4-12 ml
d. 15-25 ml
e. 35-60 ml

26. *Feather picking related to behavior and not to organic disease is indicated by intact feathers on the:*

a. wings
b. breast
c. legs
d. head
e. tail

27. *The inhalant anesthetic of choice for avian patients is:*

a. ether
b. nitrous oxide
c. isoflurane
d. halothane
e. methoxyflurane

28. *In psittacine birds, fractures of the humerus or femur:*

a. are best repaired by splinting
b. are most commonly repaired by intramedullary pinning
c. cannot be repaired by intramedullary pinning due to their pneumatic bones
d. necessitate amputation
d. are not commonly seen in clinical practice

29. *Surgical determination of a bird's gender is:*

a. usually performed via laparotomy
b. dangerous and unnecessary in most psittacines
c. performed via laparoscopy, with the bird in sternal recumbency
d. performed via laparoscopy, with the bird in right lateral recumbency
e. performed via transcloacal laparoscopy

30. *The average number of young per clutch of Amazon parrots is:*

a. 1
b. 2
c. 5
d. 8
e. 10

31. *Avian erythrocytes are:*

a. oval to elliptic, with a similarly shaped nucleus

b. oval to elliptic, with no nucleus
c. round, with a nucleus containing multiple nucleoli
d. round, with a similarly shaped nucleus
e. bifurcate, with or without a nucleus, depending on the age of the cell

32. *Avian basophils are:*

a. less common in avian blood than basophils are in mammalian blood
b. similar in appearance to mammalian basophils
c. similar in appearance to mammalian eosinophils
d. similar in function to mammalian mast cells
e. absent in avian blood

33. *Avian lymphocytes and monocytes are:*

a. nearly identical in function
b. nearly identical in appearance
c. nearly identical in function and appearance
d. not found in peripheral blood
e. found in greater numbers than any other cell type

34. *The air sacs in birds:*

a. increase surface area for respiratory gas exchange
b. allow gas exchange on inspiration and expiration
c. reduce weight and add lift
d. decrease tidal volume
e. help reduce core body temperature during exercise

35. *In a respiratory emergency involving obstruction of the upper trachea, the most appropriate emergency treatment is:*

a. cardiopulmonary resuscitation
b. tracheostomy
c. high-frequency jet ventilation
d. oxygenation in an oxygen chamber
e. air sac intubation

36. *The best site for blood collection in an anesthetized macaw is the:*

a. saphenous vein
b. cephalic vein
c. left jugular vein
d. right jugular vein
e. femoral vein

37. *Molting cycles in birds generally occur:*

a. after the breeding season
b. before the breeding season
c. after fall migration
d. early in the spring
e. during the breeding season

38. *The avian female reproductive tract consists of:*

a. paired ovaries and oviducts, and a vagina
b. paired ovaries and oviducts, a uterus and a vagina
c. a left ovary and oviduct and a uterus
d. a left ovary, an oviduct and a vagina
e. a left ovary, an oviduct, a uterus and a vagina

39. *The principal type of granulocyte seen in avian blood is the:*

a. heterophil
b. neutrophil
c. basophil
d. eosinophil
e. large lymphocyte

40. *Medication added to drinking water is:*

a. readily consumed by most patients and usually achieves therapeutic blood levels
b. recommended for treatment of most problems because it is a stress-free method of administration
c. usually ineffective
d. only effective in large birds, as small birds consume less liquid
e. very effective for most intestinal problems

Correct answers are on pages 48-49.

41. *The fluid maintenance requirement of birds is generally considered to be:*

a. 10 ml/kg/day
b. 5 ml/kg/hr
c. 25 ml/kg/day
d. 50 ml/kg/day
e. 10 ml/kg/hr

42. *Fluid therapy can be most appropriately provided to a severely dehydrated bird through:*

a. oral administration
b. repeated subcutaneous injections
c. repeated injections into the jugular vein
d. bolus injection into the jugular vein
e. intraosseous cannulation

43. *The commercially available poxvirus vaccine for canaries:*

a. provides lifetime immunity
b. should be used in the face of an outbreak
c. must be given every 6 months to be effective in protecting a flock
d. is a repackaged version of a fowlpox vaccine
e. prevents the cutaneous form but not the systemic form of canary pox

44. *Psittacine beak and feather disease:*

a. does not occur in birds older than 3 years of age
b. is associated with necrosis of the bursa and thymus, which probably causes immunosuppression
c. is a major problem primarily in budgerigars and lovebirds
d. usually affects birds 3-5 years of age
e. does not affect South American psittaciformes

45. *The most common tumor of pet birds is the:*

a. lipoma
b. xanthoma
c. papilloma
d. adenocarcinoma
e. bile duct carcinoma

46. Knemidokoptes:

a. infests only budgerigars and canaries
b. is highly contagious to all exposed psittacine birds
c. is best controlled by removing infested birds
d. infestation probably involves some degree of genetic predisposition
e. is a zoonotic parasitic infestation that should be reported to public health officials

47. *Continuous egg-laying in cockatiels is most practically prevented by:*

a. ovariohysterectomy
b. removing the nest box
c. removing the mate
d. repeated administration of medroxyprogesterone
e. hysterectomy

48. *Mature male eclectus parrots are:*

a. red
b. green
c. the same color as females
d. green or red, depending on recessive genes for color phase
e. red only during the breeding season

49. *A 90-day-old blue and gold macaw that has been housed in an incubator maintained at 88 F develops open-mouth breathing, lethargy and drooping wings. The most likely cause of these signs is:*

a. aspiration pneumonia
b. toxicity from Teflon fumes
c. aspergillosis
d. foreign-body aspiration
e. hyperthermia

50. *A 4-week-old hyacinth macaw has episodes of repeatedly flipping onto its back. Between episodes the bird appears clinically normal. The most likely cause of these signs is:*

a. bacterial encephalitis
b. normal defensive behavior

c. hypoglycemia
d. episodic epilepsy
e. peracute proventricular dilatation syndrome

51. *The blood volume of a bird is generally considered to be:*

a. 15-20% of body weight
b. 5-8% of body weight
c. 6-10% of body weight
d. 25-30% of body weight
e. 6-12 ml/kg

52. *In a peripheral blood smear of avian blood, polychromatic erythrocytes:*

a. are not observed
b. are rarely seen and indicate the need for immediate treatment
c. indicate chronic nonregenerative anemia
d. indicate a hemolytic crisis
e. should be considered normal if they constitute less than 5% of blood cells

53. *Experiments with pigeons indicate that heterologous blood transfusion for acute blood loss is:*

a. effective
b. effective but not as valuable as fluid replacement
c. effective if given with iron dextran
d. not effective
e. effective only for marginal blood loss

54. *Birds are:*

a. more prone to hypovolemic shock than mammals
b. equally prone to hypovolemic shock as compared with mammals
c. more prone to hypovolemic shock than mammals because of limited capability for splenic contraction
d. more prone to hypovolemic shock than mammals because of limited blood volume
e. less prone to hypovolemic shock than mammals because of greater capacity for mobilization of extravascular fluid

55. *Casts in avian urine:*

a. indicate renal disease
b. are common in the meat eaters but rare in psittaciformes
c. are difficult to detect because of the many urate crystals
d. indicate chronic renal failure
e. are common in birds

56. *The most accurate avian white blood cell count can be achieved with:*

a. a Coulter counter
b. the Eosinophil Unopette method
c. a mathematical formula applied to a direct smear estimate
d. a hematoxylin and eosin-stained direct smear that is heat fixed immediately after collection
e. a hematoxylin and eosin-stained direct smear that is not heat fixed

57. *Fertility of a psittacine egg can usually be demonstrated by candling after incubation for:*

a. 1-2 days
b. 3-4 days
c. 5-6 days
d. 7-8 days
e. 9-10 days

58. *The avian heart is:*

a. similar to the reptilian heart and has only 3 chambers
b. similar to a mammalian heart and has 4 chambers
c. more like a reptilian heart than a mammalian heart in that oxygenated blood mixes with unoxygenated blood in the right ventricle
d. unique in being composed primarily of striated muscle
e. able to pump a proportionately greater quantity of blood than a mammalian heart because of its unique valve system

Correct answers are on pages 48-49.

59. *In an Amazon parrot, barium sulfate administered by crop tube usually enters the cloaca within:*

a. 150 minutes
b. 60 minutes
c. 200 minutes
d. 90 minutes
e. 45 minutes

60. *The primary feathers of birds are the:*

a. flight feathers that originate from the ulnar area
b. wing and tail feathers
c. feathers used for flight
d. flight feathers that originate from the carpal area
e. feathers that replace the juvenile down feathers

Answers

1. **e** Because birds have no diaphragm, dyspnea often produces a "tail bob" as part of an exaggerated effort to respire.
2. **a** Most manufacturers claim their pelleted diets are "complete" in all nutrients, but daily requirements have not been established for most nutrients in most species. However, cage birds often favor a particular seed or fruit, making free-choice feeding unreliable.
3. **a** Overeating grit can lead to impactions and death. Omitting grit from the diet has never been shown to be detrimental.
4. **a** The avian ear has an easily located external acoustic meatus in this location. There is no pinna. Sound waves are detected, not ultrasonic vibrations.
5. **c** The syrinx is a muscular structure at the tracheal bifurcation that generates sound.
6. **d** Air sacs function as a bellows to pull and push air in and out of the lungs. Respiration does not take place in the air sacs.
7. **a**
8. **d** Knemidokoptic mange or "scaly leg and face mites" are common in budgerigars.
9. **a**
10. **c**
11. **a** Isolation or boredom is a primary cause of feather picking. All of the other choices listed could be helpful in selected cases of feather picking.
12. **e** Psittacine beak and feather disease is caused by a small DNA circovirus. This progressive, eventually fatal disease is most common in white cockatoos. Histopathologic examination of feather follicles and bursa reveals basophilic granules in macrophages, where the virus can be found by electron microscopy.
13. **e**
14. **a**
15. **e** This is the classic clinical presentation of chlamydial infection.
16. **c** Asymptomatic carriers of psittacosis are possible. Many domestically raised birds are exposed to the disease via imported birds also handled by wholesalers or retailers.
17. **b**
18. **c**
19. **d** Transmission of the disease is possible through contamination of the environment with feces, fecal dust or feather dander. The last 2 can travel some distance on air currents. Thorough disinfection of the environment with quaternary ammonium compounds (*eg*, Roccal) is recommended.
20. **a**
21. **b** Birds are commonly poisoned by oral manipulation and chewing of wine foil wrappers, weights, paint, stained-glass windows and other lead-based metals.

22. **c** The right jugular vein is more prominent in psittacine birds. The cutaneous ulnar or wing vein is a possible venipuncture site, but large hematomas and persistent bleeding are common.
23. **c**
24. **c** Overheating of cookware coated with polytetrafluoroethylene (Teflon) can cause immediate death in pet birds inhaling the fumes.
25. **d**
26. **d** If the feather picking is related to a behavioral problem, the feathers of the head are unaffected because the bird cannot reach this area with its beak.
27. **c**
28. **b**
29. **d** The incision is made or the trocar is inserted caudal to the last rib at approximately midshaft and cranial to the femur.
30. **b**
31. **a**
32. **b** Avian basophils are more common in avian blood than their mammalian counterparts. They serve the same function as mammalian basophils and are nearly identical in appearance.
33. **b** Avian lymphocytes and monocytes are very difficult to distinguish, but they are not functionally related.
34. **b** Air sacs serve as a reservoir of air and allow the lungs to receive oxygen on both inspiration and expiration.
35. **e** Placement of an air sac tube most rapidly ensures that the lungs are ventilated.
36. **d** The right jugular vein is larger than the left and is the best site for collecting blood.
37. **a** Molting cycles in birds generally occur after the breeding season.
38. **e** The avian female reproductive tract consists of a left ovary and oviduct, the uterus and the vagina. Birds do not have a right ovary.
39. **a** Heterophils are the principal granulocyte seen in avian blood.
40. **c** With few exceptions, medications added to the drinking water are poorly accepted, and it is difficult to properly regulate the amount of medication consumed.
41. **d** Maintenance fluid levels for birds are generally considered to be 50 ml/kg/day.
42. **e** Intraosseous catheters provide the best access to the peripheral circulation of severely dehydrated birds.
43. **c** Commercially available canary pox vaccines should be given every 6 months to provide adequate protection.
44. **b** Psittacine beak and feather disease virus commonly causes necrosis of the bursa and thymus.
45. **a** Lipomas are the most common tumors of birds.
46. **d** A genetic predisposition is thought to control susceptibility to *Knemidokoptes* infestation.
47. **e** Hysterectomy is the only way to permanently stop a hen from chronically laying eggs. Ovariohysterectomy is not routinely performed because of the difficulties in removing the ovary.
48. **b** Male eclectus parrots are green.
49. **e** A bird that is 90 days of age would have substantial feather development and could easily become hyperthermic at 88 F.
50. **b** This can be normal behavior for a hyacinth macaw chick.
51. **c**
52. **e** Small numbers of polychromatic erythrocytes are normal in a peripheral blood smear.
53. **b**
54. **e**
55. **a**
56. **b** The Eosinophil Unopette method provides the most consistent white blood cell counts in birds.
57. **c**
58. **b**
59. **a**
60. **d**

Notes

Section 6

Care of Food Animals

T.R. Ames, K.N. Bretzlaff, R.G. Elmore, N.L. Gates, S.C. Henry, T.H. Herdt, L.R. Krcatovich, K.A. Moriello, D.G. Morrical, D.R. Nelson, G.M.H. Shires, B.E. Straw, E.P. Tulleners, D.C. Van Metre, C.E. Wallace

Recommended Reading

Blood DC *et al: Veterinary Medicine.* 7th ed. Bailliere Tindall, London, 1989.
Howard JL: *Current Veterinary Therapy: Food Animal Practice 2.* Saunders, Philadelphia, 1986.
Howard JL: *Current Veterinary Therapy: Food Animal Practice 3.* Saunders, Philadelphia, 1992.
Jennings PB: *The Practice of Large Animal Surgery.* Saunders, Philadelphia, 1984.
Pratt PW: *Medical Nursing for Animal Health Technicians.* American Veterinary Publications, Goleta, CA, 1985.
Smith BP: *Large Animal Internal Medicine.* Mosby, St. Louis, 1991.

Practice answer sheet is on page 355.

Questions

1. *How often does the rumen contract in cattle?*
   a. 0-1 time per minute
   b. 1-2 times per minute
   c. 1-4 times per minute
   d. 2-5 times per minute
   e. 6-8 times per minute

2. *Which set of vital signs is normal in adult cattle?*
   a. temperature 100 F, pulse 80/minute, respiration 55/minute
   b. temperature 101 F, pulse 70/minute, respiration 25/minute
   c. temperature 103.5 F, pulse 70/minute, respiration 20/minute
   d. temperature 99 F, pulse 70/minute, respiration 30/minute
   e. temperature 101.5 F, pulse 30/minute, respiration 40/minute

Correct answers are on pages 66-69.

3. *Which set of vital signs is normal in adult goats?*

   a. temperature 100 F, pulse 90/minute, respiration 25/minute
   b. temperature 99.5 F, pulse 15/minute, respiration 50/minute
   c. temperature 105 F, pulse 70/minute, respiration 30/minute
   d. temperature 102 F, pulse 25/minute, respiration 25/minute
   e. temperature 103 F, pulse 75/minute, respiration 15/minute

4. *Which set of vital signs is normal in adult sheep?*

   a. temperature 100 F, pulse 90/minute, respiration 75/minute
   b. temperature 101 F, pulse 80/minute, respiration 60/minute
   c. temperature 101.5 F, pulse 20/minute, respiration 25/minute
   d. temperature 102 F, pulse 70/minute, respiration 20/minute
   e. temperature 103.5 F, pulse 50/minute, respiration 5/minute

5. *Which set of vital signs is normal in adult pigs?*

   a. temperature 102 F, pulse 65/minute, respiration 10/minute
   b. temperature 101 F, pulse 100/minute, respiration 40/minute
   c. temperature 104 F, pulse 20/minute, respiration 20/minute
   d. temperature 103 F, pulse 80/minute, respiration 5/minute
   e. temperature 99 F, pulse 60/minute, respiration 35/minute

6. *In adult cattle, in what area can the skin be pinched to best determine the state of hydration?*

   a. lateral aspect of forelimb, at the elbow
   b. over the shoulder
   c. lateral aspect of the neck
   d. dorsal to the eye
   e. over the flank

7. *In addition to dehydration, what is another common cause of severely sunken eyes in cattle?*

   a. ocular disease
   b. severe weight loss
   c. depression
   d. cranial edema
   e. bottle jaw (hypoproteinemia)

8. *To determine the number of ruminations per minute in cattle, the stethoscope is applied over the:*

   a. right paralumbar fossa
   b. left cranial paralumbar fossa
   c. left flank
   d. left caudal paralumbar fossa
   e. right ventral abdominal region

9. *In addition to the rate of contraction, what other aspect of rumen contraction should be noted when auscultating ruminants?*

   a. the duration of contraction
   b. the completeness of contraction
   c. the strength or loudness of contraction
   d. on which side it is better heard
   e. rate of eructation

10. *To aid in diagnosing a displaced abomasum, the veterinarian percusses and auscultates the left and right abdominal region. The veterinarian is listening for a resonant tone that indicates a gas-filled organ. The resonance produced by percussion over a gas-filled abomasum or other viscus is commonly called a:*

    a. tinkle
    b. crackle
    c. ping
    d. ring
    e. boom

11. *In what areas is mucous membrane perfusion best checked by visual examination?*

a. tongue, axilla
b. conjunctiva, vulva
c. tongue, nasal passage
d. nasal passage, axilla
e. scrotum, anus

12. *Where is the pulse rate most readily counted in adult cattle?*

a. coccygeal vein, brachiocephalic artery
b. coccygeal artery, femoral artery
c. mandibular artery, axillary artery
d. jugular vein, mammary vein
e. carotid artery, epigastric artery

13. *Why is it difficult to evaluate the mucosal color in certain breeds of sheep?*

a. the mouth is not opened easily
b. excessive handling causes stress
c. the mucosae of sheep normally appear congested
d. many sheep normally have blue-gray mucosae
e. the mucosae of sheep normally look pale or anemic

14. *When examining a lactating dairy cow, the urine or milk should be checked for:*

a. ketones
b. bacteria
c. white blood cells
d. somatic cells
e. red blood cells

15. *What types of restraint are most commonly used to restrain adult cattle for jugular venipuncture?*

a. halter, tail jack
b. stanchion, tail jack
c. halter, nose tongs
d. halter, cinch
e. halter, lip twitch

16. *A client calls the clinic to ask if the veterinarian can examine a cow with milk fever. An important question to ask the owner is:*

a. "When did the cow freshen (calve)?"
b. "When was the cow milked last?"
c. "How much milk does the cow produce?"
d. "What breed is the cow?"
e. "When was the cow bred?"

17. *A client reports that his Hereford cow has prolapsed a large round organ out through the labia. What question would you ask the client to differentiate between a vaginal prolapse and a uterine prolapse?*

a. "Is the cow down?"
b. "Is the cow milking?"
c. "Is the cow eating and drinking normally?"
d. "Has the cow calved?"
e. "Is the cow ruminating normally?"

18. *In lactating dairy cattle, which samples are commonly tested for ketones?*

a. urine, feces
b. saliva, blood
c. urine, saliva
d. urine, milk
e. saliva, feces

19. *What method is most commonly used to restrain adult cattle for coccygeal (tail) venipuncture?*

a. nose tongs
b. skin twitch
c. sedation
d. tail jack
e. halter

20. *In adult cattle, what is the largest volume of injectable solution that should be given intramuscularly at any single site?*

a. 5-10 ml
b. 10-15 ml
c. 15-20 ml
d. 20-25 ml
e. 25-30 ml

Correct answers are on pages 66-69.

21. *In adult goats, what is the largest volume of injectable solution that should be given intramuscularly at any single site?*

a. 1-5 ml
b. 5-10 ml
c. 10-15 ml
d. 15-20 ml
e. 20-25 ml

22. *The sites most commonly used for intramuscular injections in adult cattle are the:*

a. gluteals, semitendinosus/semimembranosus, quadriceps
b. lateral cervicals, pectorals, gluteals
c. lateral cervicals, gluteals, semitendinosus/semimembranosus, quadriceps
d. triceps, gluteals, lateral cervicals
e. pectoral, semitendinosus/semimembranosus, quadriceps

23. *The site recommended for intramuscular injections in adult sheep and goats is the:*

a. semitendinosus/semimembranosus
b. quadriceps
c. gluteals
d. triceps
e. biceps

Questions 24 and 25

24. *What is the best site for intramuscular injections in llamas?*

a. gluteals
b. semitendinosus/semimembranosus
c. triceps
d. quadriceps
e. lumbar

25. *Why would you choose this site for intramuscular injection of llamas?*

a. less chance of being kicked
b. larger muscle mass
c. site readily accessible
d. less hair in this area
e. llamas object less to injection in this area

Questions 26 through 28

26. *What muscle should be* ***avoided*** *for intramuscular injection in market-bound swine?*

a. lateral cervical muscles
b. gluteals and cervical muscles
c. triceps
d. gluteals and semitendinosus/semimembranosus
e. quadriceps

27. *Why would you be concerned about avoiding this site for intramuscular injection in market-bound swine?*

a. more danger for the person giving the injection
b. site not very accessible
c. decreased value of the meat at slaughter
d. insufficient muscle mass
e. very slow absorption of medication

28. *What muscle group should be used for intramuscular injection of market-bound swine?*

a. gluteals
b. semitendinosus/semimembranosus
c. quadriceps
d. lateral/dorsal cervical muscles
e. biceps

29. *Which instrument is* ***not*** *used in administration of oral medications to cattle?*

a. Frick's speculum
b. balling gun
c. dose syringe
d. nasal insufflation tube
e. orogastric tube

30. *Which of the following is **not** a method to verify correct positioning of a gastric tube in adult cattle?*

a. smell rumen gas exiting the end of the tube
b. observe or feel the tube on the lateral aspect of the neck as it moves down the esophagus
c. inject 5 ml of tap water into the tube and see if the animal coughs
d. blow into the end of the tube while another person listens to the rumen with a stethoscope to detect a bubbling sound
e. determine if air exits the tube upon exhalation

31. *The California mastitis test is widely used by the veterinary profession and lay people. This test is based upon detection of:*

a. flakes in milk
b. antibiotics in milk
c. somatic cells in milk
d. clots in milk
e. bacteria in the udder

Questions 32 and 33

32. *The best time of the day to infuse antibacterials into the udder of a cow is:*

a. mid-day
b. after the morning milking
c. before the evening milking
d. after the last milking of the day
e. first thing in the morning

33. *Why is it best to infuse medication at this time?*

a. most convenient time
b. cow is not active at this time
c. less milk is produced at this time
d. cows are less likely to kick at this time
e. drug remains in the udder for a longer period

34. *Before a cow is milked, the udder should be washed with warm soapy water and dried. In addition to removing contaminants from the udder surface, what else does this accomplish?*

a. prevents chapping of teats
b. helps keep teat inflations in place during milking
c. stimulates oxytocin release for milk letdown
d. decreases the bacterial count in milk
e. decreases the severity of mastitis

35. *False positives may occur on the California mastitis test when a cow has gone "off feed" or is drying off. In what other instance are you likely to obtain a false-positive reaction?*

a. when the cow has a yeast infection
b. when the cow has recently freshened and is secreting colostrum (first 3 days postpartum)
c. when the cow is febrile
d. when the cow has metritis
e. when the sample tested is contaminated with debris or dirt

36. *Results of the California mastitis test are interpreted after milk is added to the reagent in cups on the testing "paddle."" What are the possible "scores" for milk sample, in order of least abnormal reaction to most abnormal reaction?*

a. +1, +2, +3
b. trace, +1, +2, +3
c. negative, trace, +1, +2, +3
d. +1, +2, +3 negative
e. +4, +3, +2, +1, trace

37. *Milk samples can be cultured to diagnose the causative agent of mastitis. After washing the teat with warm soapy water, it must be dried to prevent water droplets from contaminating the sample. What is the next step in preparing the teat for collection of milk samples for culture?*

a. dry the teat with a paper towel and spray the teat orifice with chlorhexidine solution
b. wipe the teat orifice with an alcohol-soaked swab
c. air dry the teat and dip in an iodine teat dip
d. dry the teat with a paper towel
e. spray the teat with iodine solution and dry it with a paper towel

Correct answers are on pages 66-69.

Questions 38 and 39

38. Before intramammary infusion of medication, the teat should be prepared as for obtaining milk samples for culture. One important procedure before infusion of medication is to:

a. dip the teat in teat dip
b. give the cow an intramuscular injection of oxytocin to stimulate milk letdown
c. spray iodine solution on the teat
d. "strip" the milk out of the quarter
e. check the milk with a strip cup

39. Why is this procedure necessary before intramammary infusion of medication?

a. decreases the number of bacteria present
b. makes infusion easier
c. prevents dilution of medication with milk
d. medication may react with milk
e. decreases the volume of milk in the udder so a large volume of medication can be infused

40. When testing the milk of goats using the California mastitis test, a sample is not considered mastitic unless the reaction is 2+ or 3+. Why are the results for goats' milk interpreted differently than for cows' milk?

a. goats' milk normally has a higher somatic cell count than cows' milk
b. the reagent reacts differently with goats' milk
c. cows have more bacteria in their milk
d. cows have a lower neutrophil count in their milk
e. cows' milk is more concentrated than goats' milk

41. The veins most often used to collect blood samples from cattle are the:

a. jugular and mammary veins
b. jugular and coccygeal veins
c. jugular and cephalic veins
d. mammary and auricular veins
e. coccygeal and mammary veins

42. Which veins are most commonly used for blood collection in swine?

a. auricular (ear) and coccygeal (tail) veins
b. auricular (ear) jugular veins
c. jugular and coccygeal (tail) veins
d. jugular vein and cranial vena cava
e. jugular and cephalic veins

43. Which vein is most accessible and most commonly used to collect blood from goats, sheep and young calves?

a. coccygeal (tail) vein
b. cephalic vein
c. jugular vein
d. femoral vein
e. mammary vein

Questions 44 through 50

44. Milk fever in dairy cattle is caused by:

a. negative energy balance
b. hypocalcemia
c. overfeeding of corn silage
d. overwhelming septicemia
e. coliform mastitis

45. Milk fever is most likely to occur:

a. 1-3 days after calving
b. 1 week before calving
c. in the last 6 weeks of gestation
d. 3-4 weeks after calving
e. at breeding time

46. Another term for milk fever is:

a. ketosis
b. obturator nerve paralysis
c. parturient paresis
d. grass tetany
e. hypomagnesemia

47. What are the typical clinical signs of milk fever?

a. fever, hyperactivity, swollen udder
b. hypothermia, recumbency, cold extremities
c. abdominal distention, bloody diarrhea, sloughing of the hooves
d. strabismus, seizures, "goose-stepping" gait
e. rumen hypermotility, projectile diarrhea, udder hyperemia

48. *A diagnostic test to confirm milk fever is:*

a. ketone levels in urine
b. serum calcium levels
c. serum magnesium levels
d. complete blood count
e. white blood cell count in urine

49. *A normal serum calcium level for a lactating dairy cow is in the range of:*

a. 8.5 mg/dl
b. 5.0 mg/dl
c. 12.0 mg/dl
d. 3.0 mg/dl
e. 15.0 mg/dl

50. *Treatment for milk fever typically includes:*

a. electrolytes per os
b. milking 6-8 times daily
c. calcium solution intravenously and/or subcutaneously
d. glucose intravenously
e. corticosteroids intramuscularly

Questions 51 through 54

51. *Hardware disease is usually associated with accidental ingestion of nails, bailing wire or other sharp objects with the feed. The organ usually penetrated by these sharp objects is the:*

a. omasum
b. jejunum
c. cecum
d. abomasum
e. reticulum

52. *Hardware disease of cattle is more appropriately called:*

a. pseudotuberculosis
b. traumatic reticuloperitonitis
c. pseudorabies
d. abomasal displacement
e. rumen tympany

53. *Which of the following is* **not** *a typical clinical sign of hardware disease?*

a. acute anorexia
b. abdominal pain
c. decreased rumen motility
d. bloody feces
e. acute drop in milk production

54. *In an effort to prevent hardware disease, many producers give their cattle:*

a. antibiotics intramuscularly
b. a magnet per os
c. a laxative per os
d. antiinflammatories intramuscularly
e. an enema

Questions 55 through 59

55. *What organism causes Johne's disease in cattle?*

a. *Clostridium perfringens*
b. *Cryptosporidium seeberi*
c. *Mycobacterium paratuberculosis*
d. *Corynebacterium pseudotuberculosis*
e. *Escherichia coli*

56. *Which of the following is* **not** *typical of Johne's disease?*

a. normal rectal temperature
b. weight loss
c. persistent or recurrent diarrhea
d. normal appetite
e. urticaria (hives)

Correct answers are on pages 66-69.

57. *What is appropriate management of cattle with Johne's disease?*

a. segregate infected cattle from uninfected cattle
b. administer antidiarrheal medication as needed
c. administer sulfonamides in the feed for 4-6 months
d. cull infected cattle
e. perform fecal examinations on all cattle and deworm infected cattle

58. *Johne's disease is transmitted by:*

a. blood-sucking insects
b. fecal-oral route
c. transplacental infection
d. venereal transmission during breeding
e. contaminated needles, or dehorning or castration instruments

59. *At what age do infected cattle begin showing clinical signs of Johne's disease?*

a. 2-5 years
b. 3-21 days
c. 3-5 months
d. 6-12 months
e. 8-10 years

60. *At what time should a lactating dairy cow be "dried off"?*

a. 2 weeks before calving
b. 1 month before calving
c. 20-30 days after calving
d. 45-60 days before calving
e. 3 months before calving

Questions 61 through 64

61. *Ketosis typically affects high-producing dairy cows, in which dietary energy is insufficient to meet the demands of heavy lactation. In such cows, fat is metabolized for energy, resulting in accumulation of ketone bodies in the blood. An example of a ketone body is:*

a. pindone
b. cortisol
c. secretin
d. bilirubin
e. acetone

62. *Cows with ketosis may show depression, anorexia and decreased milk production. Some cows show hyperexcitability and aggression. These neurologic manifestations of ketosis are commonly referred to as:*

a. hyperactive ketosis
b. nervous ketosis
c. furious ketosis
d. pseudorabies
e. mad itch

63. *Treatment for ketosis may include oral propylene glycol, in an effort to stimulate the cow's appetite, and intravenous infusion of solutions containing:*

a. calcium
b. potassium
c. glucose
d. vitamin E and selenium
e. magnesium

64. *To help prevent ketosis, it is important to:*

a. keep cows as fat as possible in the dry period
b. keep cows as thin as possible during lactation
c. extend the dry period
d. keep cows in good condition in the dry period
e. delay breeding after calving

Questions 65 through 67

65. *Why is bloat considered an emergency situation?*

a. the rumen may rupture
b. the rumen contents may spill over into the reticulum
c. rumen expansion could impair the blood supply to the remainder of the gastrointestinal tract

d. affected cattle stop producing milk
e. gas accumulation can impair respiration

66. What is the most obvious visual sign of bloat?

a. distention of the right paralumbar fossa
b. distention of the left paralumbar fossa
c. jugular vein pulsations
d. edema in the dewlap (ventral cervical) area
e. udder edema

67. Bloat can sometimes be treated nonsurgically by:

a. rolling the cow slowly through a 180-degree arc, from one side to another
b. administration of repeated saline enemas
c. passage of an orogastric tube
d. oral administration of propylene glycol
e. intramuscular injection of neostigmine

Questions 68 through 71

68. Grain overload is a common name for:

a. rumen tympany
b. rumen acidosis
c. septicemia
d. rumen atony
e. vagal indigestion

69. Consumption of excessive grain alters rumen fermentation, resulting in production by rumen microflora of excessive amounts of:

a. lactic acid
b. polyglycolic acid
c. lipoproteins
d. muriatic acid
e. amino acids

70. Cattle with grain overload are most likely to show:

a. anemia
b. respiratory acidosis
c. hypoxemia
d. metabolic acidosis
e. hyperactivity

71. The most important aspect of treating cattle with grain overload is to:

a. administer amino acid solutions intravenously
b. quickly empty the rumen
c. immediately administer aspirin and phenylbutazone per os
d. feed only hay during the next 24-48 hours
e. administer large volumes of water by orogastric tube

Questions 72 through 76

72. In dairy cows, abomasal displacement most commonly occurs:

a. 1-3 weeks after calving
b. 1-3 days before calving
c. 1-3 weeks before calving
d. 6-7 months after breeding
e. in the dry period

73. There are many theories on how abomasal displacement occurs. The abomasum can displace to the left or to the right side. In some cows, the abomasum twists to form a torsion/volvulus. Which form of abomasal displacement is most common?

a. left-displaced abomasum without torsion/volvulus
b. right-displaced abomasum without torsion/volvulus
c. right-displaced abomasum with torsion/volvulus
d. left-displaced abomasum with torsion/volvulus
e. midline abomasal displacement with torsion/volvulus

Correct answers are on pages 66-69.

74. *A displaced abomasum can be corrected using several procedures. Which of the following is* ***not*** *a procedure to correct uncomplicated abomasal displacement?*

   a. rolling the cow
   b. abomasopexy
   c. omentopexy
   d. rolling the cow, followed by percutaneous abomasopexy
   e. rumenotomy

75. *You are asked to prepare a cow for omentopexy to correct left displacement of the abomasum. What area would you prepare for surgical incision?*

   a. right paralumbar fossa
   b. right paracostal area
   c. ventral right abdomen
   d. ventral left abdomen
   e. ventral midline

76. *You are asked to prepare a cow for standing abomasopexy to correct left displacement of the abomasum. The cow's ventral aspect is exceptionally contaminated with caked manure and straw. Which area is most appropriate to prepare for abomasopexy in this case?*

   a. left paralumbar fossa
   b. ventral midline, far cranially
   c. ventral abdomen, left paramedian
   d. ventral abdomen, right paramedian
   e. ventral midline, far caudally

77. *A heifer calf born twin to a bull calf is called a:*

   a. spayed heifer
   b. springing heifer
   c. cryptorchid
   d. freemartin
   e. pseudohermaphrodite

78. *How much milk should a 110-lb neonatal calf be fed?*

   a. 5 pints once daily
   b. 8 pints twice daily
   c. 11 pints once daily
   d. 11 pints twice daily
   e. 12 pints twice daily

79. *Young calves are often raised in separate hutches to decrease the spread of disease. The main* ***disadvantage*** *of using calf hutches is:*

   a. extra labor is required
   b. calves are exposed to the weather
   c. too cold for calves
   d. too windy for calves
   e. calves may become sunburned

80. *The most important procedure performed on newborn calves is to:*

   a. disinfect the umbilical cord
   b. dry the calf off and keep it warm
   c. inject vitamin E and selenium
   d. administer an enema to remove meconium
   e. ensure sufficient intake of good-quality colostrum as soon as possible

81. *The 2 most common causes of mastitis in cattle are:*

   a. *Streptococcus agalactiae* and *Staphylococcus aureus*
   b. *E coli* and *Pasteurella hemolytica*
   c. *Pseudomonas aeruginosa* and *Klebsiella genitalium*
   d. *Staphylococcus dermatitidis* and *Streptococcus pyogenes*
   e. *Proteus vulgaris* and *Enterococcus bovis*

82. *White muscle disease is associated with a deficiency of:*

   a. vitamin A
   b. selenium and/or vitamin E
   c. calcium
   d. sodium bicarbonate
   e. thiamin

83. *Polioencephalomalacia is associated with a deficiency of:*

   a. selenium

b. thiamin
c. vitamin A
d. vitamin D
e. vitamin E

84. The organism most commonly associated with shipping fever in cattle is:

a. *Pasteurella hemolytica*
b. *Chlamydia psittaci*
c. bovine respiratory syncytium-forming virus
d. infectious bovine rhinotracheitis virus
e. *Escherichia coli*

85. Mature bulls should never be vaccinated against:

a. brucellosis
b. infectious bovine rhinotracheitis
c. bovine virus diarrhea
d. bovine respiratory syncytium-forming virus infection
e. parainfluenza-3 virus infection

86. In people, poxviral infection causes a condition known as "orf." In sheep, the infection is commonly known as "sore mouth." What is the scientific name of this disease in sheep?

a. enzootic pneumonia
b. contagious ecthyma
c. pseudocowpox
d. foot and mouth disease
e. anthrax

87. The practice of feeding extra grain to ewes just before breeding is called:

a. hyperalimentation
b. conditioning
c. flushing
d. brooding
e. superovulation

*88. Which of the following is **least** likely to cause tetanus in sheep?*

a. foot punctures
b. castration
c. tail docking
d. shearing
e. contact with infected sheep

Questions 89 and 90

89. Enterotoxemia in feedlot lambs is commonly referred to as:

a. white muscle disease
b. bloat
c. overeating disease
d. blind staggers
e. circling disease

90. Enterotoxemia can be prevented by vaccinating sheep against:

a. *Clostridium perfringens* types C and D
b. enterotoxigenic *E coli*
c. *Pasteurella hemolytica* serovar M12
d. *Clostridium tetani*
e. *Campylobacter fetus* type B

91. Tetanus and infections relating to tail docking and castration may cause similar clinical signs of high fever and stiffness. One method of differentiating tetanus from less serious bacterial infection is to:

a. check for pain at the surgical site
b. check the surgical site for inflammation
c. perform a neurologic examination
d. determine when surgery was performed
e. determine when the animal was last vaccinated against tetanus

*92. Which procedure is **not** normally done on 3- to 10-day-old lambs?*

a. injection of vitamin E/selenium
b. vaccination against enterotoxemia
c. administration of tetanus antitoxin
d. tail docking, castration
e. ear notching

Correct answers are on pages 66-69.

Questions 93 through 98

A 5-year-old female Alpine goat is recumbent and depressed, but has been eating and drinking small amounts. The doe is due to kid in 2 weeks and has had twins the previous 2 years.

93. *After performing a physical examination, the veterinarian decides to examine the doe's abdomen by ultrasonography to:*

 a. determine if goat has multiple fetuses or a single large fetus
 b. look for ovarian cysts
 c. look for abdominal tumors
 d. determine if the goat is really pregnant
 e. determine the stage of gestation

94. *You collect urine from the goat to test for:*

 a. white blood cells
 b. ketones
 c. fat droplets
 d. red blood cells
 e. bacteria

95. *A positive urine test, along with the doe's history and clinical signs, strongly suggests:*

 a. contagious ecthyma
 b. listeriosis
 c. neonatal isoerythrolysis
 d. pregnancy toxemia
 e. hepatic lipidosis

96. *When does this metabolic disorder usually occur in goats and sheep?*

 a. 1-2 months after parturition
 b. 6-12 hours before parturition
 c. 2-4 weeks before parturition
 d. 1-2 months after breeding
 e. any time in the last 12 weeks of gestation

97. *The veterinarian prescribes intravenous infusion of dextrose solution. Using a 3-liter bag of sterile water, how many milliliters of 50% dextrose should you add to make a 5% dextrose solution?*

 a. 50 ml
 b. 150 ml
 c. 300 ml
 d. 3000 ml
 e. 1500 ml

98. *Treatment for this condition typically includes intravenous dextrose solution, oral propylene glycol and general nursing care. In some severely affected does, it may be necessary to:*

 a. place the animal in a sling to prevent decubital ulcers
 b. provide parenteral nutrition until the animal eats voluntarily
 c. induce abortion or perform a cesarean section
 d. administer repeated blood transfusions
 e. infuse dextrose into the uterus

99. *In goats, caseous lymphadenitis is caused by:*

 a. *Cryptosporidium seeberi*
 b. *Mycobacterium paratuberculosis*
 c. *Corynebacterium pyogenes*
 d. *Clostridium perfringens*
 e. *Corynebacterium pseudotuberculosis*

100. *Which organism causes external abscesses in goats?*

 a. *Listeria monocytogenes*
 b. *Pasteurella hemolytica*
 c. *Streptococcus epidermidis*
 d. *Corynebacterium pyogenes*
 e. *E coli*

101. *Goats and sheep should be regularly vaccinated against:*

 a. pneumonia and botulism

b. tetanus and enterotoxemia
c. scours and polioencephalomalacia
d. pregnancy toxemia and encephalomyelitis
e. contagious ecthyma and papillomatosis

102. A client's goat has 6 permanent incisors and 2 deciduous incisors. How old is this animal?

a. 4 years
b. 2 years
c. 3 years
d. 1 year
e. 5 years

103. Goats are normally tattooed in the ear for identification. One breed of goat is not tattooed in this way because these goats have no pinnae. Which breed is this?

a. Angora
b. Saanen
c. Nubian
d. La Mancha
e. French Alpine

104. Procedures routinely performed on 1-day-old pigs include ear notching, clipping of the needle teeth and:

a. collecting blood for pseudorabies testing
b. castration
c. selection for breeding stock
d. trimming the hooves
e. docking the tail

105. From birth until weaning, a young lamoid (llama, alpaca, vicuña, guanaco) is known as a:

a. calf
b. cria
c. cub
d. sloe
e. fawn

For Questions 106 through 110, select the correct answer from the 5 choices below.

a. steer
b. boar
c. buck
d. gilt
e. heifer

106. A young female pig that has not yet given birth.

107. A castrated bovine.

108. An intact (uncastrated) male pig.

109. A young female bovine that has not yet given birth to a calf.

110. An intact male goat.

For Questions 111 through 115, select the correct answer from the 5 choices below.

a. barrow
b. wether
c. weanling
d. freshen
e. farrow

111. A young animal that has recently changed from suckling to another source of food.

112. The act of giving birth in pigs.

113. A castrated pig.

114. The act of a cow's giving birth to a calf, after which lactation begins.

115. A castrated sheep.

Correct answers are on pages 66-69.

For Questions 116 through 120, select the correct answer from the 5 choices below.

a. emasculator
b. emasculatome
c. elastrator
d. electroejaculator
e. artificial vagina

116. *Probe inserted into the rectum of bulls to induce ejaculation.*

117. *Instrument used to apply rubber bands to the base of the scrotum in young calves and lambs, inducing testicular necrosis.*

118. *Instrument to castrate a large animal by simultaneously cutting and crushing the spermatic cord.*

119. *Instrument, also known as a burdizzo, used to castrate large animals by crushing the vessels in the spermatic cord.*

120. *Device into which male animals ejaculate semen for use in artificial insemination.*

For Questions 121 through 125, select the correct answer from the 5 choices below.

a. stiff lamb disease
b. circling disease
c. bottlejaw
d. lockjaw
e. scours

121. *Common name for diarrhea.*

122. *Common name for tetanus.*

123. *Common name for listeriosis.*

124. *Common name for edema in the intermandibular space.*

125. *Common name for muscular dystrophy in lambs and calves, associated with a deficiency of vitamin E or selenium.*

126. *The clinical sign seen most often in cows with cystic ovarian disease is:*

a. nymphomania
b. anestrus
c. vulvar hemorrhage
d. estrus
e. vulvar mucous discharge

127. *After parturition, most cows expel the placenta within:*

a. 8 hours
b. 8-16 hours
c. 16-24 hours
d. 24-48 hours
e. 48-72 hours

128. *Parturient paresis usually occurs:*

a. before calving
b. at calving
c. within 24 hours after calving
d. 24-48 hours after calving
e. more than 48 hours after calving

129. *Which of the following is* **not** *a clinical sign of severe dehydration in cattle?*

a. urine specific gravity of 1.009
b. eyes sunken into the orbits
c. sticky, viscous saliva
d. skin over neck and eyelids remains tented after being lifted with the fingers
e. cold ears and tail

130. *Which clinical sign is* **not** *consistent with milk fever?*

a. cold extremities
b. heart rate greater than 110/minute
c. paralysis
d. hypothermia

e. sluggish or incomplete pupillary light response

131. *Capillary refill time in cattle can be assessed by pressing firmly on the animal's gingivae with a finger and noting how long it takes for color to reenter the area after pressure is removed. Normal capillary refill time in cattle is:*

a. 5-10 seconds
b. less than 1 second
c. less than 3 seconds
d. 15-20 seconds
e. 4-5 seconds

132. *Intravenous fluids used to treat severely diarrheic, dehydrated calves should include:*

a. ammonium chloride
b. glucose
c. sodium bicarbonate
d. sodium chloride
e. calcium borogluconate

133. *The normal pH range of rumen fluid is:*

a. 2.5-3.5
b. 7.0-8.5
c. 3.5-8.5
d. 5.5-7.0
e. 6.8-7.4

134. *In cattle with urolithiasis, urinary obstruction:*

a. occurs primarily in castrated males
b. occurs only in grain-fed cattle
c. occurs equally in male and female cattle
d. never occurs in pastured animals
e. occurs primarily in bulls

135. *The parasite, and its associated lesion, of greatest impact on the swine industry is:*

a. *Ascaris suum* and pneumonia
b. *Hyostrongylus rubidis* and gastric ulcers
c. *Stephanurus dentatus* and pyelonephritis
d. *Oesophagostomum dentatum* and proliferative adenomatosis
e. *Balantidium coli* and typhlitis

136. *As you stand in a wet, hot, poorly ventilated nursery barn, you recall that environmental conditions may markedly affect the transmission and expression of swine respiratory conditions. Considering the poor ventilation, you tell the owner that he should install several fans to:*

a. remove animal-generated heat from the barn
b. remove toxic gases, especially ammonia, from the barn
c. pull needed oxygen into the barn
d. remove water-laden air from the barn
e. prevent accumulation of carbon dioxide and carbon monoxide in the barn

137. *Which disease is most common in newborn piglets?*

a. hypoglycemia
b. iron deficiency
c. streptococcal meningitis
d. middle ear infection
e. congenital tremors

138. *Agitation of an under-floor pit in a confinement swine facility can quickly release a high concentration of:*

a. ammonia
b. nitrogen
c. hydrogen sulfide
d. methane
e. carbon dioxide

139. *Recommended management practices to control contagious footrot in sheep include all of the following* ***except:***

a. foot trimming
b. disinfectant foot baths
c. parenteral antibiotics
d. culling
e. vaccination

Correct answers are on pages 66-69.

140. Nutritional flushing of ewes is accomplished by feeding:

a. higher levels of protein
b. higher levels of energy
c. lower levels of fat
d. higher levels of minerals
e. lower levels of vitamin E

141. The primary clinical sign of iodine deficiency in goats is:

a. goiter in the majority of goats in the herd
b. small mature size of adults
c. inappetance and diarrhea
d. parakeratosis
e. birth of dead, weak or premature kids with a scant haircoat and goiter

*142. Oral electrolyte replacement formulas for diarrheic calves should contain all of the following **except**:*

a. sodium chloride
b. sucrose
c. an alkalinizing agent
d. glycine and glucose
e. potassium salts

143. What is the most specific sign of gastrointestinal dysfunction in a cow?

a. anorexia
b. decreased milk production
c. ketosis
d. abnormal rumination
e. dehydration

144. An instrument useful for crushing the spermatic cord in castration of calves, without cutting the skin, is called an:

a. ecraseur
b. emasculator
c. emasculatome
d. effeminator
e. elastrator

145. The Burley method for casting cattle involves application of pressure to the:

a. trachea
b. penis
c. udder
d. mammary veins
e. dorsal spinal area

146. In a goat that is lame on the left hind limb, you can flex the stifle and extend the hock. This indicates damage to the:

a. check ligament
b. medial patellar ligament
c. cruciate ligament
d. gastrocnemius tendon
e. peroneus tertius muscle

147. Goats should ideally be:

a. dehorned at about 6 months of age so that the musk glands can also be removed simultaneously
b. dehorned at about 30 days of age with a caustic dehorning paste
c. disbudded at less than 10 days of age with elastrator bands
d. dehorned at about 30 days of age with a Barnes dehorner
e. disbudded at less than 10 days of age using a heated dehorning iron with a sized copper ring on the applicator end

---

Answers

1. **b**
2. **b**
3. **e**
4. **d**
5. **a**
6. **d**

7. **b**
8. **b**
9. **b**
10. **c**
11. **b**
12. **b**
13. **d**
14. **a** The presence of ketones indicates a negative energy balance, typically in a high-producing dairy cow.
15. **c**
16. **a** Milk fever is most common in cows that have recently calved.
17. **d** Cows that have calved can prolapse the vagina. Cows that have not yet calved cannot prolapse the uterus.
18. **d**
19. **d**
20. **c**
21. **b**
22. **c**
23. **a**
24. **b**
25. **d**
26. **d**
27. **c**
28. **d**
29. **d** This is used to administer oxygen.
30. **c** Not all animals cough if the tube has entered the trachea.
31. **c** More specifically, the test detects the DNA in white blood cells and epithelial cells.
32. **d**
33. **e**
34. **c**
35. **b** The reagent used in the California mastitis test reacts with colostral antibodies.
36. **c**
37. **b**
38. **d**
39. **c**
40. **a**
41. **b**
42. **d**
43. **c**
44. **b** It is usually seen in heavily lactating cows soon after calving.
45. **a**
46. **c**
47. **b**
48. **b** Cows with a serum calcium level below 7.5 mg/dl are considered hypocalcemic.
49. **a**
50. **c** Calcium solutions must be infused cautiously so as to avoid adverse cardiac effects.
51. **e**
52. **b** Perforation of the reticulum typically causes localized periotonitis.
53. **d** The feces of affected cattle is not bloody.
54. **b** In theory, the magnet remains in the reticulum and attracts metal objects, preventing reticular perforation.
55. **c**
56. **e** Urticaria are not a feature of this disease.
57. **d** This is a reportable disease. All infected animals should be culled. Check the regulations in your state.
58. **b**
59. **a**
60. **d**
61. **e** Other ketone bodies include acetoacetate and betahydroxybutyrate.
62. **b**
63. **c** Glucose is given in an effort to curtail production of ketone bodies.
64. **d**
65. **e**
66. **b** The rumen is located on the left side.
67. **c** In some affected cattle, gas can be released from the rumen in this way.
68. **b**
69. **a**
70. **d** Overproduction of lactic acid leads to acidosis.
71. **b** Emptying the rumen removes the source of lactic acid overproduction.
72. **a**

73. **a** This is by far the most common form. Right-sided displacement occurs at about 10-15% of the frequency of left-sided displacement, and right-sided displacement with torsion/volvulus is even less common.

74. **e** Rumenotomy cannot help correct abomasal displacement.

75. **a** This is the preferred area for incision.

76. **a** This is the preferred area for incision in standing abomasopexy. A ventral site is nearly impossible to disinfect for abomasopexy in very dirty recumbent cows.

77. **d**

78. **c** A rule of thumb is 1 pint of milk for every 10 lb of body weight.

79. **a**

80. **e** It is important because this ensures sufficient levels of antibodies to prevent infection.

81. **a**

82. **b**

83. **b**

84. **a**

85. **a** Brucellosis vaccine is a modified-live bacterin that can cause orchitis and decrease a bull's fertility.

86. **b**

87. **c**

88. **e**

89. **c**

90. **a**

91. **a** With a dock infection, the surgery site is painful. With tetanus, the dock site is not painful.

92. **e** The ears of lambs are not notched.

93. **a**

94. **b**

95. **d** This condition is caused by a negative energy balance resulting from rapid fetal growth in late gestation.

96. **c**

97. **c** Concentration$_1$ x volume$_1$ = concentration$_2$ x volume$_2$. 5% x 3 L = 50% x X. $X = \frac{5\% \times 3\text{ L}}{50\%} = \frac{15}{50} = 0.3\text{ L} = 300\text{ ml}$.

98. **c**

99. **e**

100. **d**

101. **b**

102. **c** One set of 2 permanent incisors appears with each year of age. Goats have all 4 sets of permanent incisors (8) by 4 years of age. Age in years = number of permanent incisors ÷ 2. This goat has 6 permanent incisors. 6 ÷ 2 = 3 years old.

103. **d**

104. **e**

105. **b**

106. **d**

107. **a**

108. **b**

109. **e**

110. **c**

111. **c**

112. **e**

113. **a**

114. **d**

115. **b**

116. **d**

117. **c**

118. **a**

119. **b**

120. **e**

121. **e**

122. **d**

123. **b**

124. **c**

125. **a**

126. **b** Approximately 80% of all cows with cystic ovarian disease are anestrous. About 20% exhibit nymphomania. Vulvar hemorrhage is seen during metestrus, and a mucous vulvar discharge is seen during estrus.

127. **a** The placenta is normally expelled within 8 hours after calving. However, many cows not passing their placenta until later do not exhibit signs of illness.

128. **c** Though parturient paresis can occur anytime near parturition, it usually occurs within the first 24 hours following calving.

129. **a** Severely dehydrated animals usually have concentrated urine with a specific gravity well above 1.009.

130. **b** Most cows with milk fever have a slightly elevated heart rate, usually in the range of 70-90/minute, and seldom over 100/minute.

131. **c** Normal capillary refill time in cattle is less than 3 seconds.

132. **c** Oral and intravenous fluids for replacement therapy in calves with diarrhea usually include sodium bicarbonate.

133. **d** Rumen fluid has a normal pH range of 5.5-7.0.

134. **a** Obstruction of the urinary tract by calculi occurs primarily in steers.

135. **a** The other parasites listed are not associated with the lesion shown or cause relatively low economic losses.

136. **d** The primary purpose of exhaust fans is to remove water-laden air.

137. **e** The other conditions listed require time to develop.

138. **c**

139. **c** Parenteral antibiotics have very limited efficacy in contagious footrot in sheep.

140. **b**

141. **e**

142. **b**

143. **d**

144. **c** The emasculatome is the correct choice. The elastrator does not cause crushing, but places a rubber band tightly around the scrotum to cut off all blood supply to the tissues.

145. **e**

146. **e**

147. **e** Goats are disbudded at this age before horn growth. At this age the procedure is much less difficult and less traumatic to the animal, and has a higher success rate than if it is delayed until the animal is older and the horns have erupted.

Notes

Notes

Section 7

Care of Horses

A.N. Baird, J.P. Caron, B.J. Darien, S. Clark Eades, A. Lamar, J.N. Moore, K.A. Moriello, M.R. Paradis

Recommended Reading

Colahan PT *et al: Equine Medicine and Surgery.* 4th ed. American Veterinary Publications, Goleta, CA, 1991.

Pratt PW: *Medical Nursing for Animal Health Technicians.* 1st ed. American Veterinary Publication, Goleta, CA, 1985.

Robinson NE: *Current Therapy in Equine Medicine 3.* Saunders, Philadelphia, 1992.

Stashak T: *Adams' Lameness in Horses.* Lea & Febiger, Philadelphia, 1986.

Varner DD *et al: Diseases and Management of Breeding Stallions.* American Veterinary Publications, Goleta, CA, 1991.

Practice answer sheet is on page 357.

Questions

1. *Which type of horse should **not** be handled from the left side?*

   a. a mare whose foal is walking on her right side
   b. any normal horse
   c. a fractious yearling
   d. a gelding that is blind in the left eye
   e. a breeding stallion approaching a mare to be bred

2. *When removing a horse from a trailer, what is the **first** thing to be done to ensure safety?*

   a. move the trailer partition over to one side
   b. open the back door
   c. let down the ramp
   d. let down the chain or bar located behind the horse
   e. untie the horse's head and attach a lead shank

Correct answers are on pages 84-87.

3. *When tying a horse for examination,:*

   a. always tie the animal loosely so it does not feel restrained
   b. always tie the horse to a solid, stationary object, using a quick-release knot
   c. tie the horse with a double half-hitch knot
   d. if the horse is fractious, tie it with the chain shank placed over the nose
   e. tie the animal to an object so the lead can slide down in case the horse lowers its head

4. *A drug commonly used to sedate or tranquilize horses is:*

   a. chloral hydrate
   b. flunixin meglumine
   c. pentazocine
   d. xylazine
   e. ketamine

5. *The most effective way to restrain neonatal foals is the:*

   a. ear twitch
   b. tailjack
   c. lip twitch
   d. lifting a leg
   e. chain shank over the nose

6. *Which set of values is considered normal in an adult horse?*

   a. temperature 101.5 F, pulse 40/minute, respiration 36/minute
   b. temperature 100.5 F, pulse 36/minute, packed cell volume 58%
   c. pulse 36/minute, respiration 20/minute, total plasma protein 9.5 g/dl
   d. respiration 20/minute, packed cell volume 32%, total plasma protein 7.0 g/dl
   e. temperature 99 F, packed cell volume 32%, respiration 68/minute.

7. *Which set of serum chemistry values is considered normal in an adult horse?*

   a. urea nitrogen 15 mg/dl, sodium 135 mEq/L, pH 7.5
   b. pH 6.5, potassium 3.6 mEq/L, glucose 100 mg/dl
   c. fibrinogen 280 mg/dl, urea nitrogen 25 mg/dl, sodium 120 mEq/L
   d. potassium 2.5 mEq/L, pH 8.0, fibrinogen 280 mg/dl
   e. sodium 135 mEq/L, fibrinogen 150 mg/dl, urea nitrogen 5 mg/dl

8. *Which muscle group should be avoided when administering intramuscular injections to neonatal foals?*

   a. gluteals
   b. lateral neck muscles
   c. semimembranosus
   d. pectorals
   e. semitendinosus

9. *Which 3 muscle groups are commonly used for intramuscular injections in adult horses?*

   a. semimembranosus, gluteals, lateral neck muscles
   b. semitendinosus, gluteals, pectorals
   c. gluteals, lateral neck muscles, triceps
   d. lateral neck muscles, triceps, pectorals
   e. semimembranosus, triceps, gluteals

10. *Which structures delineate the area on the lateral side of the neck used for intramuscular injections?*

   a. withers, crest, jugular furrow
   b. scapula, jugular furrow, crest
   c. scapula, cervical vertebrae, crest
   d. scapula, cervical vertebrae, ligamentum nuchae
   e. shoulder, jugular furrow, ligamentum nuchae

11. *When administering intravenous medication to a horse, precautions are taken to avoid perivascular or intracarotid injection. Which of the following is **not** one of these precautions?*

   a. perform the injection in a well-lit area
   b. apply proper restraint to prevent excessive movement

c. visualize the vein by obstructing blood flow with digital pressure
d. insert the needle smoothly and gently at a 90-degree angle to the vein to ensure proper entry into its lumen
e. aspirate during injection to ensure proper location of the needle

12. *The most suitable location for subcutaneous injection of medication in horses is:*

a. over the withers
b. caudal to the elbow
c. on the lateral side of the neck
d. over the chest
e. on the back

13. *Which of the following is* **not** *a consideration when administering oral medication via dose syringe?*

a. deliver the medication quickly before the horse objects to the procedure
b. introduce the dose syringe at the corner of the mouth
c. avoid placing the dose syringe between the cheek teeth by directing it toward the center of the mouth
d. thicken the medication with molasses or another palatable thick medium for ease of administration
e. administer the medication slowly, allowing the horse to swallow as it is given

14. *When administering anthelmintics, what is the most reliable way to ensure that the patient receives all of the drug intended?*

a. give the medication in the feed
b. give the medication by nasogastric intubation
c. use a dose syringe
d. give the medication in the water
e. use a balling gun

15. *Which of the following is* **not** *a good indicator of proper or improper placement of a nasogastric tube?*

a. the tube is visualized while passing down the esophagus, which in most horses is located near the left jugular furrow
b. the horse coughs during passage of the nasogastric tube if it has entered the trachea
c. resistance is felt as the tube passes down the esophagus
d. during exhalation, air can be felt exiting the nasogastric tube if it is in the trachea
e. gurgling can be heard and a distinct gastric odor may be detected once the tube has entered the stomach

16. *Which of the following is* **not** *a procedure to follow when maintaining intravenous catheters for long-term use?*

a. withdraw any required blood samples from the catheter to preserve other veins for future use
b. flush the catheter with heparinized saline every 4 hours
c. change the catheter every 3 days
d. keep the dressing clean and dry
e. use aseptic technique for catheter placement, administration of drugs or fluids, and changing of infusion lines

17. *The teeth of horses tend to wear unevenly. On the cheek teeth, this uneven wear results in formation of:*

a. points
b. caps
c. hooks
d. wolf teeth
e. cups

18. *Floating of the teeth is routinely performed on most horses. Based upon the conformation and wearing patterns of the normal horse's mouth, which portions of the occlusal surfaces of the premolars and molars require floating?*

a. lingual maxillary, buccal mandibular
b. lingual maxillary, lingual mandibular
c. buccal maxillary, lingual mandibular
d. buccal maxillary, buccal mandibular
e. lingual maxillary, buccal maxillary

Correct answers are on pages 84-87.

For Questions 19 through 23, select the correct answer from the 5 choices below.

a. deep digital flexor tendon
b. intermediate carpal bone
c. palmar digital nerve
d. coronary band
e. second metatarsal bone

19. A bone located in the first row of carpal bones.

20. A structure providing nourishment to the hoof.

21. This structure inserts on the palmar surface of the third phalanx.

22. "Splints" are often associated with this structure.

23. A portion of this structure may be removed to relieve navicular disease.

For Questions 24 through 28, select the correct answer from the 5 choices below.

a. digital cushion
b. tibiotarsal joint
c. collateral cartilages
d. check ligament
e. first phalanx

24. A fibroelastic structure in the hoof that comprises the bulk of the bulbs of the heel.

25. Sidebone results when these structures ossify.

26. The longest of the phalanges.

27. This structure is frequently incised to correct flexural deformities.

28. Distention of this structure is called "bog spavin."

For Questions 29 through 33, select the correct answer from the 5 choices below.

a. coffin bone
b. suspensory ligament
c. third metatarsal bone
d. extensor process of the third phalanx
e. navicular bone

29. The distal sesamoid bone.

30. This structure acts as a sling for the fetlock and prevents it from sinking to the ground.

31. This structure may rotate downward and away from the hoof wall when the laminae become inflamed.

32. The common digital extensor inserts on this structure.

33. The hind limb cannon bone.

For Questions 34 through 38, select the correct answer from the 5 choices below.

a. medial patellar ligament
b. bars
c. fourth metacarpal bone
d. frog
e. white line

34. The junction between the hoof wall and sole.

35. This triangular structure provides traction and shock absorption, and assists venous return from the hoof.

36. This portion of the hoof walls bears weight and allows the foot to expand.

37. The lateral splint bone.

38. This structure is often incised to relieve upward fixation of the patella.

For Questions 39 through 43, select the correct answer from the 5 choices below.

a. second phalanx
b. suprascapular nerve
c. proximal sesamoid bone
d. plantar ligament
e. cunean tendon

39. *Paired osseous structures associated with each metacarpophalangeal and metatarsal-phalangeal joint.*

40. *Inflammation of this structure is termed "curb."*

41. *One-half of this structure is located within the hoof and one-half outside the hoof.*

42. *A portion of this structure may be removed to relieve bone spavin.*

43. *Damage to this structure results in atrophy of scapular muscles, known as "sweeny."*

Questions 44 and 45

A distraught client telephones and asks to have the veterinarian out right away to see her old gelding. The owner says her horse is reluctant to move, and is leaning way back on its front feet, with the back feet up under its body. The horse is sweating and breathing hard.

44. *Which question is **least** appropriate in attempting to gain more information about this horse?*

a. "Has the horse had this problem previously?"
b. "Does the horse have a draining wound at the top of a front coronary band?"
c. "Are the horse's feet warm to the touch?"
d. "Can you feel a pulse on the back of the foreleg pasterns, immediately above the bulbs of the heels?"
e. "Has the horse recently been put onto a lush pasture, or could the animal have gotten into your grain storage area?"

*The client answers yes to all of your questions. To prepare for the farm call, you ensure that all of the necessary items are packed in the truck. Which of the following is **not** a necessity?*

a. surgery pack
b. mineral oil
c. local anesthetics
d. padding to tape to the feet
e. phenylbutazone

Questions 46 through 48

A client calls and is extremely upset because she thinks her horse has fractured its right front leg.

46. *A positive response to which of the following questions you ask would have the most profound impact on the prognosis of this case?*

a. "Is the horse bearing weight on the affected limb?"
b. "Can you see a deviation in the limb, indicating a fracture?"
c. "Is there a lot of swelling present?"
d. "Is the affected area below the knee?"
e. "Is there an open skin wound over the affected area?"

47. *The owner reports that the area involved is below the knee, there is minimal swelling, the leg deviates slightly medially, the horse is not bearing weight on it, and there is a skin wound on the medial aspect of the metacarpus. Which type of emergency care should you recommend to the owner until the veterinarian arrives in 1 hour?*

a. hose the leg with cold water and walk the horse slowly in a soft paddock
b. move the horse to a well-bedded stall and encourage it to lie down
c. find some sort of padding material (pillow), a broom handle and strips of sheeting, and immobilize the leg from the ground to above the knee
d. tranquilize the horse and keep it quiet until the veterinarian arrives
e. apply an antibacterial ointment to the wound and bandage that area only

Correct answers are on pages 84-87.

*48. The veterinarian repairs a compound fracture of the right metacarpus. The horse recovers well, with a cast from the ground to the elbow. You are responsible for postoperative care of this horse. Which procedure is **not** indicated in care of this horse?*

a. monitor the cast for heat and odor
b. monitor the horse's temperature, pulse rate and respiratory rate daily
c. monitor feed and water intake and fecal output
d. exercise the horse daily to stimulate circulation to the fracture site
e. observe the horse's attitude and the way it uses the affected limb

For Questions 49 through 53, select the correct answer from the 5 choices below.

a. stringhalt
b. ringbone
c. winging
d. corns
e. laminitis

49. A cause of chronic lameness resulting from repeated injury to the hoof, such as from an ill-fitting shoe.

50. Inflammation of the laminae of the foot, which may be chronic or acute and can cause severe lameness.

51. Characterized by involuntary hyperflexion of the hock with each step taken.

52. Inward deviation of a foot in flight, caused by a toe-out conformation.

53. New bone growth on the phalanges, due to periostitis, that may lead to osteoarthritis or ankylosis.

For Questions 54 through 58, select the correct answer from the 5 choices below.

a. arthrodesis
b. ankylosis
c. navicular disease
d. thoroughpin
e. thrush

54. A natural process that results in fusion of a joint.

55. Synovial distention of the deep digital flexor tendor sheath at the point of the hock.

56. A progressive and incurable condition that begins as bursitis and affects regional tendons and bones, causing moderate to severe lameness.

57. A degenerative condition of the frog, characterized by black, necrotic material.

58. A surgical procedure used to fuse a diseased joint.

For Questions 59 through 63, select the correct answer from the 5 choices below.

a. bog spavin
b. bucked shins
c. sidebone
d. windpuff
e. paddling

59. Synovial swelling of joints or tendon sheaths caused by injury; a cosmetic blemish but not a cause of lameness.

60. Synovial distention of the tibiotarsal joint.

61. Outward deviation of a foot in flight due to a toe-in conformation.

62. Inflammation of the periosteum of the dorsal (cranial) surface of the third metacarpal bone that occurs frequently in young race horses.

63. *Ossification of the collateral cartilages of the third phalanx.*

64. *A retained deciduous cheek tooth is called a:*

   a. point
   b. cap
   c. cup
   d. wolf tooth
   e. dental star

65. *Most female horses have 36 teeth, while most males have 40. Concerning the teeth of male and female horses, which statement is most accurate?*

   a. Males have 4 extra wolf teeth.
   b. Males have 4 more canine teeth than females.
   c. Females have 4 fewer premolars than males.
   d. Males have 4 more molars than females.
   e. Females have 4 fewer incisors than males.

66. *Fecal flotation can be used to diagnose infection with any of the following parasites* ***except:***

   a. *Gasterophilus intestinalis*
   b. *Strongylus vulgaris*
   c. *Strongyloides westeri*
   d. *Parascaris equorum*
   e. *Anoplocephala perfoliata*

67. *In its migratory stage,* Parascaris equorum *can cause damage to the:*

   a. cranial mesenteric artery
   b. stomach
   c. lungs
   d. cecum
   e. large colon

68. *Which parasite can be detected by microscopic examination of cellophane tape that has been applied to hair around the anal area?*

   a. *Strongylus vulgaris*
   b. *Parascaris equorum*
   c. *Gasterophilus intestinalis*
   d. *Oxyuris equi*
   e. *Anoplocephala perfoliata*

69. *The most common parasite involved in thromboembolic colic is:*

   a. *Strongylus vulgaris*
   b. *Parascaris equorum*
   c. *Gasterophilus intestinalis*
   d. *Oxyuris equi*
   e. *Anoplocephala perfoliata*

70. *Which parasite may cause intestinal obstruction in a young horse dewormed with a large, single dose of anthelmintic?*

   a. *Strongylus vulgaris*
   b. *Parascaris equorum*
   c. *Gasterophilus intestinalis*
   d. *Oxyuris equi*
   e. *Anoplocephala perfoliata*

71. *The larval form of* Gasterophilus intestinalis *attaches itself to the mucosa of the:*

   a. small intestine
   b. large intestine
   c. rectum
   d. stomach
   e. anus

72. *Eggs of* Gasterophilus intestinalis *are deposited:*

   a. in the mucosa of the stomach
   b. in the tissues of the tongue
   c. on the hair of the horse's legs
   d. on the hair around the horse's anus
   e. in the mucosa of the large intestine

Correct answers are on pages 84-87.

For Questions 73 through 77, select the correct answer from the 5 choices below.

a. torsion/volvulus
b. ileus
c. intussusception
d. tympany
e. impaction

73. *Accumulation of hardened ingesta in the bowel or stomach.*

74. *Invagination of a portion of intestine into an adjacent portion.*

75. *Accumulation of gas in a hollow organ.*

76. *Twisting of a section of bowel at its mesenteric attachment or on its long axis.*

77. *Cessation of intestinal motility.*

78. *A worried owner calls and says her 10-day-old foal has rather watery, yellow diarrhea. You ask her about its attitude and she responds that the foal is nursing and acting completely normal. The most appropriate advice for this client is to:*

a. submit a fecal sample for parasite evaluation
b. give the foal a kaolin-pectin preparation (*eg*, Kaopectate)
c. bring the foal to your clinic so that fluid and antibiotic therapy may be initiated
d. not allow the foal to nurse for 24 hours so that the intestinal tract can rest
e. monitor the foal's temperature daily, watch its appetite, and keep its tail and buttock area clean

Questions 79 through 84

The owner of a boarding stable calls to tell you that one of the horses at the barn is exhibiting signs of colic. The horse seemed fine at feeding time in the morning. In fact, it ate all of its grain. Now, at about 2 PM, the horse is very painful. Your employer will be back shortly and it sounds as though the horse is in serious condition, so you tell the gentleman to bring the horse in to the clinic.

79. *When the horse arrives, you gather some initial diagnostic information. Which of the following is normal?*

a. temperature 100.6 F
b. pulse 88/minute
c. respiration 48/minute
d. packed cell volume 65%
e. total plasma protein 8.0 g/dl

80. *Which of the following is* ***least*** *appropriate in the initial diagnostic workup and treatment of this horse?*

a. abdominocentesis
b. nasogastric intubation
c. gastrointestinal endoscopy
d. intravenous fluid therapy
e. rectal examination

81. *Rectal examination reveals that the spleen has been displaced toward the midline. You are preparing to obtain a peritoneal fluid sample. How might this information on splenic displacement assist you?*

a. you would prepare a location more to the left of the midline than is customary
b. you would not perform abdominocentesis due to the findings of rectal examination
c. it would not affect your preparation for abdominocentesis
d. you would prepare an area more caudal and to the right of the midline than is customary
e. you would use different instruments, such as a longer needle than is customary

82. *The peritoneal fluid sample you collect appears serosanguineous. What is the color of normal peritoneal fluid in horses?*

a. slightly pink
b. yellow
c. transparent (resembling water)
d. dark red
e. light brown

83. *The veterinarian decides to perform an exploratory laparotomy. Which of the following is **not** a necessary part of presurgical preparation for any exploratory abdominal surgery?*

a. rinse out the horse's mouth
b. clip and scrub the surgical site
c. stabilize the horse's metabolic state (fluid therapy)
d. begin antibiotic therapy
e. administer an enema

84. *The doctor resects 15 feet of necrotic bowel from the horse. Which of the following complications is **least** likely to occur in this horse during its recovery period?*

a. pneumonitis
b. laminitis
c. peritonitis
d. thrombophlebitis
e. incisional dehiscence

85. *The organism involved in strangles is:*

a. *Clostridium tetani*
b. equine herpesvirus type 1
c. myxovirus
d. *E coli*
e. *Streptococcus equi*

86. *The organism that commonly causes respiratory disease in the first 2 years of life is:*

a. *Mycoplasma pneumoniae*
b. *Clostridium perfringens*
c. equine herpesvirus type 4
d. encephalomyelitis virus
e. *Ehrlichia risticii*

87. *The organism that causes rhinopneumonitis in mares is:*

a. *Streptococcus equi*
b. *E coli*
c. myxovirus
d. equine herpesvirus type 1
e. *Clostridium tetani*

88. *Which of the following is **not** a common clinical sign in horses with strangles?*

a. fever
b. abortion of a fetus in late gestation
c. abscessed lymph nodes
d. coughing
e. purulent nasal discharge

89. *If a pregnant mare is not vaccinated 1 month before parturition, the newborn foal should be vaccinated with:*

a. rabies vaccine
b. blackleg vaccine
c. leptospirosis bacterin
d. tetanus antitoxin
e. tetanus toxoid

90. *Equine infectious anemia is commonly known as:*

a. swamp fever
b. sleeping sickness
c. Coggins' disease
d. quittor
e. blind staggers

91. *Which of the following is **not** a type of encephalomyelitis known to affect horses?*

a. Venezuelan
b. Near Eastern
c. Western
d. Eastern
e. Chinese

92. *The recommended treatment for a horse clinically ill with equine infectious anemia is:*

a. isolation and stall rest
b. antibiotics
c. corticosteroids
d. blood transfusions
e. euthanasia

Correct answers are on pages 84-87.

93. Equine encephalomyelitis is commonly known as:

a. swamp fever
b. sleeping sickness
c. Potomac horse fever
d. blind staggers
e. rhinopneumonitis

94. The Coggins' test is used to diagnose:

a. Potomac horse fever
b. Eastern equine encephalomyelitis
c. rhinopneumonitis
d. influenza
e. equine infectious anemia

Questions 95 and 96

A frantic owner calls to say her horse is acting very strangely. She says the horse does not appear to be able to eat or drink. The horse is sweating and moves very stiffly. There is something pink covering the inside corner of the eye. Loud noises or quick movements cause an exaggerated response.

95. Considering the client's description, this horse appears to be exhibiting signs of:

a. equine encephalomyelitis
b. equine infectious anemia
c. rhinopneumonitis
d. tetanus
e. Potomac horse fever

96. You tell the client that the veterinarian will come out immediately. What is the most appropriate advice for the client while waiting for the veterinarian to arrive?

a. walk the horse to work out some of the stiffness
b. put the horse in a quiet, dark, well-bedded stall
c. bathe the horse with cold water to cool it
d. tranquilize the horse
e. encourage the horse to drink water

97. The horseman's term used to describe laryngeal hemiplegia is:

a. heaves
b. roaring
c. laryngitis
d. pharyngitis
e. fistulous withers

98. A disease characterized by expiratory dyspnea is:

a. chronic obstructive pulmonary disease
b. laryngeal hemiplegia
c. lymphoid hyperplasia
d. guttural pouch empyema
e. displaced soft palate

*99. Which diagnostic procedure is **not** routinely done on horses with chronic respiratory disease?*

a. transtracheal aspiration
b. respiratory endoscopy
c. thoracic radiography
d. lung biopsy
e. complete blood count

100. Which of the following has the most impact on the onset of reproductive cycling in mares?

a. increasingly warm weather
b. increasing length of daylight
c. increased amount of grain
d. increased amount of exercise
e. increased amount of green grass available

101. You analyze the semen of a breeding stallion. Which of these findings is normal?

a. transparent appearance
b. volume 25 ml
c. 75% motile sperm
d. sperm concentration 25×10^6/ml
e. pH 6.5

102. Concerning foaling, which statement is most accurate?

a. The amnion appears at the labia as a dark red, velvety membrane.
b. The escape of allantoic fluid marks the beginning of the first stage of parturition.
c. The nose is the first part of the foal seen as delivery begins.
d. It is not uncommon for the mare to get up and lie down a few times during delivery.
e. Once the foal is delivered, the placenta should be removed by applying gentle pressure downward.

Questions 103 through 106

An ecstatic owner calls to tell you that her mare just foaled a beautiful bay filly. This is the owner's first experience with a foal, and she wants to know if there is anything she should do.

*103. Which of the following is **not** appropriate advice for this client?*

a. encourage the foal to stand within the first hour of life
b. make sure that the foal nurses from the mare shortly after it stands and continues nursing at intervals of 30-60 minutes
c. give the foal a soapy-water enema as soon as possible after it nurses
d. dip the foal's umbilical stump in tincture of iodine several times during the first few hours of life
e. make certain the foal starts passing its meconium within the first few hours of life

104. You also tell the client that the veterinarian will be out the following day to collect a blood sample from the foal. What is routinely checked in blood samples from newborn foals?

a. monocyte count
b. immunoglobulin G level
c. serum urea nitrogen level
d. immunoglobulin E level
e. serum glucose level

*105. The results of this blood test indicate that the foal did not achieve the desired level of antibodies for a foal of this age. This could have resulted from any of the following **except**:*

a. premature lactation in the mare, which reduced the amount of colostrum available for the foal
b. poor quality of colostrum
c. foal did not nurse from the mare
d. the blood sample was taken prematurely, as newborn foals do not begin absorbing colostral antibodies until 24 hours old
e. the foal's intestine did not absorb colostral antibodies

106. What is the most appropriate treatment for such neonatal foals deficient in maternal antibodies?

a. intravenous plasma transfusion
b. administration of at least 1 liter of plasma via nasogastric tube
c. feeding colostrum from another source
d. wait until the foal starts producing its own antibodies
e. administer prophylactic broad-spectrum antibiotics

107. Which horse breed is most commonly affected by combined immunodeficiency?

a. Thoroughbred
b. Arabian
c. Quarter Horse
d. Morgan
e. Appaloosa

108. In blood samples collected before a newborn foal has suckled, combined immunodeficiency is strongly suggested by a lack of:

a. immunoglobulin R (IgR)
b. immunoglobulin E (IgE)
c. immunoglobulin T (IgT)
d. immunoglobulin L (IgL)
e. immunoglobulin M (IgM)

Correct answers are on pages 84-87.

109. Which disease of newborn foals is very similar to the "blue baby" syndrome in human infants involving Rh factor?

a. neonatal isoerythrolysis
b. combined immunodeficiency
c. failure of passive transfer of maternal antibodies
d. neonatal maladjustment syndrome
e. agammaglobulinemia

*110. Which of the following is **not** usually indicated in a foal with neonatal maladjustment syndrome?*

a. feeding via nasogastric tube
b. administration of colostrum or plasma to ensure sufficient passive antibodies
c. placement of a urinary catheter
d. prevention of self-inflicted trauma with padding and restraint
e. intravenous fluid therapy via a catheter

111. Which clinical sign is most likely to be seen in a newborn foal with a patent urachus?

a. distended abdomen
b. failure to urinate
c. anorexia and lethargy
d. colic
e. urine dripping from the umbilicus

*112. Which of the following is **not** a consideration when a mare has previously produced foals that develop neonatal isoerythrolysis?*

a. determine the foal's serum level of IgM before it nurses
b. do not allow the foal to ingest that mare's colostrum
c. provide colostrum from another source before the foal is 24 hours old
d. determine the blood type of the mare and the stallion
e. crossmatch the foal's erythrocytes with the mare's colostrum before allowing the foal to nurse

*113. Which of the following is **not** a likely cause of tail rubbing in horses?*

a. behavioral problem (vice)
b. food allergy
c. *Oxyuris equi* infection
d. *Culicoides* hypersensitivity
e. straw itch mite infestation

114. The average quantity of colostrum ingested by healthy, active foals by sucking the dam in the first day of life is:

a. 500 ml
b. 1 L
c. 2 L
d. 4 L
e. 6 L

115. After a foal's birth, maternal immunoglobulins are no longer present in the mare's milk by:

a. 12 hours
b. 24 hours
c. 48 hours
d. 72 hours
e. 96 hours

116. After birth, the intestine of the foal loses the ability to absorb immunoglobulins by:

a. 12 hours
b. 24 hours
c. 48 hours
d. 72 hours
e. 96 hours

*117. Concerning management practices used in equine parasite control, which statement is **least** accurate?*

a. Frequent removal of feces from pastures and paddocks reduces the number of infective larvae.

b. Manure removed from a pasture should be composted for 3 months to kill cyathostome larvae before spreading the manure on a pasture to be grazed by horses.
c. Parasite transmission can be minimized by deworming all horses on a farm at one time.
d. Deworming horses and moving them to a pasture that has not been grazed for some time is an effective means of breaking the parasite life cycle.
e. Because third-stage larvae may persist in pastures for more than 20 weeks in northern temperate climates, pasture rotation may not be completely beneficial.

118. *Concerning evaluation of the efficacy of parasite control programs, which statement is **least** accurate?*

a. At 1-2 weeks after anthelmintic therapy, 20% of the horses should be evaluated for nematode ova.
b. Tapeworm ova are best detected using the Wisconsin technique.
c. Fecal egg counts should be performed on all fecal samples that show eggs on fecal flotation.
d. Fecal egg counts cannot predict the number of parasites a horse harbors.
e. Pasture contamination can be considered low if fecal egg counts are below 50 eggs per gram.

119. *Which of the following is **not** associated with wolf teeth?*

a. behavioral problems in young horses
b. abnormal head carriage
c. head shaking
d. refusing to take a bit
e. snorting while working with a bit

120. *Nutritional support is very important in management of neonatal foals. Each day, a normal 40-kg foal requires approximately how much mare's milk?*

a. 1 L
b. 2 L
c. 4 L
d. 6 L
e. 8 L

121. *The fluid of choice for treatment of foals in shock is:*

a. 0.45% saline
b. 0.9% saline plus 20% dextrose
c. lactated Ringer's solution plus 5% dextrose
d. 5% dextrose
e. 50% dextrose plus amino acid solution

122. *After a mare has foaled, the placenta is normally passed within:*

a. 3 hours
b. 6 hours
c. 9 hours
d. 12 hours
e. 24 hours

123. *"Founder" is a colloquial term for:*

a. proximal enteritis
b. anterior uveitis
c. laminitis
d. penile prolapse
e. rectal prolapse

124. *Anhidrosis in horses is manifested as:*

a. urticaria
b. decreased water intake
c. increased ingestion of salt
d. inability to sweat
e. vesicle formation on the dorsum

125. *Which of the following is **not** a property of fiberglass casting material?*

a. porous
b. stronger than plaster
c. cures quicker than plaster
d. lighter weight than plaster
e. more radiopaque than plaster

Correct answers are on pages 84-87.

126. *After castration of his yearling colt, the owner, a neophyte equestrian, is concerned about postoperative problems. You would be correct to inform him that the most common complication after equine castration is:*

a. serious hemorrhage
b. evisceration
c. peritonitis
d. scirrhous cord
e. preputial swelling

127. *The cryogen most commonly used in equine practice is:*

a. nitrous oxide
b. nitric oxide
c. carbon dioxide
d. liquid nitrogen
e. liquid propane

128. *Sutures that lose their tensile strength within 60 days after implantation are termed "absorbable." Which absorbable suture material persists in the tissues for the longest time?*

a. polyglycolic acid
b. chromic catgut
c. polyglactin 910
d. polydioxanone
e. plain catgut

Answers

1. **d** A partially blind horse is much more comfortable if it can see you and where you are leading it.
2. **e** Many horses can perceive when the back of the trailer is open, and they try to exit. If they are still tied when attempting to back out, they panic and often break their halter and get away from you.
3. **b** Always tie the horse to a sturdy object so that they do not hurt themselves.
4. **d**
5. **b** Foals can be restrained by lifting the tail up and over the back.
6. **d**
7. **a**
8. **b** The muscles on the lateral side of the neck are rather underdeveloped in neonates. Also, if repeated injections are given in this area, it may become painful and the foal may stop nursing.
9. **a** The pectorals and triceps can be used in horses requiring prolonged therapy but only as a last resort.
10. **d**
11. **d** The needle should be inserted at an angle of approximately 30 degrees. Inserting the needle at an angle more steep than that risks the possibility of entering the carotid artery. The jugular vein is usually located just under the skin in horses.
12. **c** The skin is most pliable in the region of the neck.
13. **a** If the medication is administered rapidly, the horse often loses most of the medication out of the side of the mouth because it cannot swallow quickly.
14. **b** Nasogastric intubation allows the medication to be deposited directly into the horse's stomach.
15. **b** Coughing is not a reliable indicator that the nasogastric tube is in the trachea. Some horses cough no matter where the tube is located.
16. **a** Withdrawal of blood from the catheter shortens its life.
17. **a**
18. **c** Because of the way the teeth meet, points form on the outside (cheek side) of the upper

molars and premolars and the inside (tongue side) of the lower molars and premolars.

19. **b**
20. **d**
21. **a**
22. **e**
23. **c**
24. **a**
25. **c**
26. **e**
27. **d**
28. **b**
29. **e**
30. **b**
31. **a**
32. **d**
33. **c**
34. **e**
35. **d**
36. **b**
37. **c**
38. **a**
39. **c**
40. **d**
41. **a**
42. **e**
43. **b**
44. **b** The signs described by the owner clearly indicate laminitis. Draining wounds at the coronary band indicate an abscess associated with "gravel," which breaks out at that location.
45. **a** Surgery is not indicated at this stage in a case of laminitis.
46. **e** Compound fractures always warrant a poor prognosis because of possible bone infection.
47. **c** Immobilization of a fracture is extremely important, especially if it is compound. Always apply padding and a rigid object acting as a splint, and immobilize the joint above and below the fracture.
48. **d** Exercise is contraindicated. The horse must remain in its stall for several weeks, with minimal movement so that healing can take place.
49. **d**
50. **e**
51. **a**
52. **c**
53. **b**
54. **b**
55. **d**
56. **c**
57. **e**
58. **a**
59. **d**
60. **a**
61. **e**
62. **b**
63. **c**
64. **b**
65. **b** Usually only males have canine teeth.
66. **a** The bot fly lays its eggs on the hair of the horse. The larvae are located in the stomach.
67. **c**
68. **d**
69. **a** This parasite causes damage to the arteries that supply the intestinal tract. If these vessels become thrombosed, the blood supply is cut off to portions of the intestine, leading to bowel necrosis.
70. **b** If a young horse with large numbers of this parasite is given a large single dose of anthelmintic, all of the parasites die at the same time and could cause an impaction.
71. **d**
72. **c** The bot fly lays its eggs on the hair of the horse. They are often seen as small white dots over the distal limbs, neck and shoulders.
73. **e**
74. **c**
75. **d**
76. **a**
77. **b**
78. **e** If the foal is normal in all other aspects, this is probably "foal heat diarrhea," which is usually self-limiting in a matter of days. Simply watching the foal's progress and keeping the area clean and dry are sufficient.
79. **a**

80. **c** This may or may not be appropriate at a later time, but it is unlikely to be productive initially.

81. **d** When the spleen is displaced, it usually drifts from its normal location on the left side of the body wall toward the center of the body. In this case, the tip of the spleen can become located directly above (dorsal to) where you would normally insert the needle. Moving caudally and toward the right often allows you to avoid this structure when advancing your cannula.

82. **b**

83. **e** Enemas are seldom done on horses exhibiting signs of colic unless an impaction can be felt in the terminal section of the small colon or rectum.

84. **a**

85. **e**

86. **c**

87. **d**

88. **b** Late-term abortion may occur in mares with rhinopneumonitis.

89. **d** The mare will not secrete sufficient antibodies against this disease in her colostrum if she has not been vaccinated. Therefore, the foal should receive immediate protection with tetanus antitoxin.

90. **a**

91. **e**

92. **e** Because this animal is clinically ill, it can spread the disease to other horses. It would be dangerous to allow this animal to reside near others for this reason.

93. **b**

94. **e**

95. **d**

96. **b** Because these horses have an exaggerated response to external stimuli, they should be housed in a quiet, dark stall.

97. **b**

98. **a**

99. **d** While lung biopsy may be warranted in some horses, it is not routinely done on the initial diagnostic examination.

100. **b** As the length of daylight increases in the spring, the anterior pituitary begins to secrete hormones that stimulate the reproductive system to again become active.

101. **c** Immediately after ejaculation, at least 60% motility is considered normal.

102. **d** Mares often rise and lie down again during the foaling process. It is said that this repositions the fetus and allows the process to proceed more rapidly.

103. **c** One should wait to see if the foal can expel the meconium on its own. Colostrum contains an intestinal lubricant that assists in this process.

104. **b** Foal blood samples are routinely checked for IgG to ensure absorption of sufficient maternal antibodies in colostrum.

105. **d** Antibody absorption in the foal's intestinal tract continues until the foal is 18-24 hours old, with peak absorption at 6 hours. After this, these macromolecules are no longer absorbed in this fashion.

106. **a** The only way to ensure that the foal receives these passive antibodies is through intravenous administration of equine plasma rich in antibodies.

107. **b**

108. **e** Normal foals are usually born with some IgM. If these foals have no IgM before nursing from the mare, it strongly suggests combined immunodeficiency.

109. **a** In this disease, the mare's colostrum contains antibodies against the foal's red blood cells. When the foal nurses, its red cells are attacked and broken down, which gives the foal an icteric appearance. If left untreated, the foal will die.

110. **c** These foals must be protected from self-inflicted injury and supported medically. They seldom have difficulty urinating unless there is another disease present at the same time.

111. **e** Most of these foals appear completely normal, except that urine drips from the umbilicus.

112. **a** The level of IgM present in the foal's blood has nothing to do with this disease.

113. **e** Straw itch mites eat the larvae of grain insects. Horses become infested while eating contaminated hay from overhead racks. The lesions are nonpruritic and consist of crusted papules on the dorsum.

114. **d**
115. **b**
116. **b**
117. **b** Before manure is spread on a pasture, it should be composted for 1 year to kill cyathostome laevae.
118. **b** Tapeworms are best detected using a sedimentation technique.
119. **e** Snorting and upper airway sounds are not associated with wolf teeth problems.
120. **e** Foals generally ingest a volume of milk approximating 20% of their body weight in kg.
121. **c** Because lactated Ringer's solution is a crystalloid fluid, it stays in the vascular space better than 5% dextrose alone. Foals in shock are often hypoglycemic and acidotic; this solution helps correct these problems.
122. **a** Most mares expel their placenta within 3 hours after foaling. If the placenta has not been expelled by this time, it is considered retained.
123. **c**
124. **d** Anhidrosis is the inability to sweat.
125. **e** Fiberglass is more radiolucent than plaster.
126. **e** Incisional and preputial swelling is minimized by postoperative exercise.
127. **d** Liquid nitrogen is used in commercially available cryosurgical units.
128. **d** Polydioxanone suture material can be identified in tissues up to 210 days after implantation.

Notes

Notes

Section 8

Care of Laboratory Animals

W.S. Bivin

Recommended Reading

Guide for the Care and Use of Laboratory Animals. US Dept of Health & Human Services, National Institutes of Health, Bethesda, MD, 1985.

Harkness and Wagner: *Biology and Medicine of Rabbits and Rodents.* 3rd ed. Lea & Febiger, Philadelphia, 1988.

Laboratory Animal Science. Published bi-monthly. Am Assn Lab Anim Science, Joliet, IL.

Poole: *UFAW Handbook on the Care & Management of Laboratory Animals.* Churchill Livingstone, New York, 1987.

Segal: *Housing, Care and Psychological Well-Being of Captive and Laboratory Primates.* Noyes Publications, Park Ridge, NJ, 1989.

Practice answer sheet is on page 359.

Questions

1. *The common names of 6 species of animals, excluding aquatic animals, specifically covered by the Animal Welfare Act are:*
   a. mice, rats, gerbils, hamsters, guinea pigs, armadillos
   b. rats, gerbils, hamsters, opossums, cats, dogs
   c. gerbils, hamsters, guinea pigs, rabbits, cats, cattle
   d. hamsters, guinea pigs, rabbits, cats, dogs, monkeys
   e. guinea pigs, rabbits, cats, dogs, monkeys, cattle

2. *Of the animals used in biomedical research, 90% are:*
   a. mice
   b. mice and rats
   c. mice, rats and gerbils
   d. mice, rats, gerbils and hamsters
   e. mice, rats, hamsters and guinea pigs

Correct answers are on page 94.

3. *Which drug is toxic to ferrets, even when used at the accepted therapeutic dosage?*

   a. trimethoprim-sulfa
   b. penicillin
   c. sulfaquinoxaline
   d. amoxicillin
   e. erythromycin

4. *A laboratory animal with large cheek pouches is the:*

   a. guinea pig
   b. mouse
   c. rat
   d. rabbit
   e. hamster

5. *The species with a high prevalence of spontaneous seizures is the:*

   a. gerbil
   b. hamster
   c. guinea pig
   d. rabbit
   e. chinchilla

6. *The species most susceptible to penicillin toxicity are the:*

   a. gerbil and hamster
   b. hamster and guinea pig
   c. guinea pig and rabbit
   d. rabbit and mouse
   e. mouse and rat

7. *Ich is a disease of:*

   a. rabbits
   b. monkeys
   c. gerbils
   d. lions
   e. fish

8. *Approximately how long can a python go without food before suffering severe effects of malnutrition?*

   a. 1 week
   b. 1 month
   c. 6 months
   d. 1 year
   e. 2 years

9. *Concerning skin testing of primates for tuberculosis, which statement is most accurate?*

   a. All primates should be tested for bovine, avian and human strains of tuberculosis.
   b. A dose of 0.1 ml of tuberculin is required for accurate intradermal tuberculosis testing.
   c. Small nonhuman primates can be safely restrained for tuberculosis testing using only physical restraint.
   d. The intradermal injection site is examined at 24, 48 and 96 hours postinoculation for signs of reaction to the tuberculin.
   e. In the event of a severe hypersensitivity reaction, the eye may become infected and require prolonged treatment to prevent permanent damage.

10. *Large nonhuman primates are most commonly bled by venipuncture of the:*

   a. saphenous vein
   b. cepahlic vein
   c. jugular vein
   d. femoral vein
   e. auricular vein

11. *An ammoniacal odor in a poorly ventilated mouse or rat room indicates that:*

   a. a special inbred strain of rats or mice is housed in the room
   b. the mouse population housed in the room has some degree of kidney damage
   c. the tap water supply is contaminated and must be replaced with filtered water
   d. the sanitation program for cleaning cages must be improved
   e. the room temperature is too high for the number of animals housed in the room

12. *The laboratory species that is* **not** *a rodent is the:*

   a. guinea pig
   b. rat

c. rabbit
d. mouse
e. hamster

13. Cavy is another name for a:

a. hamster
b. gerbil
c. mouse
d. guinea pig
e. rabbit

14. Vitamin C deficiency in guinea pigs is characterized by:

a. widespread hemorrhage of muscles and joints
b. loss of incisor teeth
c. hepatic necrosis
d. myocardial necrosis
e. blindness

*15. Concerning the musk odor of ferrets, which statement is **least** accurate?*

a. The odor is natural and the result of an improper diet.
b. The odor is related to sex hormones to some degree.
c. Removal of the anal sacs only prevents release of musk when the animal is excited.
d. The odor is produced by the anal sacs and by the cutaneous sebaceous glands.
e. Removal of the gonads and anal sacs does not completely remove the odor but reduces it considerably.

16. Observations that most accurately reflect the depth of anesthesia in fish are:

a. anal reflex, rate of opercular movement and palpebral reflex
b. deep tail pain, rate of opercular movement and loss of equilibrium
c. pupil size, corneal reflex and anal reflex
d. rate of opercular movement, anal reflex and loss of equilibrium
e. digital pain, pupil size and lacrimation

17. The most common cause of respiratory disease in rabbits is:

a. *Bordetella*
b. *Pasteurella*
c. *Salmonella*
d. *Moraxella*
e. *Mycoplasma*

18. The preferred agent for anesthetizing amphibians is:

a. ketamine
b. xylazine
c. pentobarbital
d. ether
e. MS-222

*19. Concerning skin shedding in snakes, which statement is **least** accurate?*

a. It is a normal process and is called ecdysis.
b. Ideally the skin should not adhere to the body as it is shed, and it often comes off as one piece.
c. The corneas become cloudy and bluish, but the corneal epithelium is not shed.
d. Snakes often become anorectic and aggressive during this process.
e. Shedding of the skin in small patches indicates a serious health problem.

20. The species most likely to experience dystocia is the:

a. guinea pig
b. rabbit
c. miniature pig
d. hamster
e. gerbil

21. The species in which malocclusion of the premolars and molars is most commonly a serious problem is the:

a. rat
b. guinea pig
c. hamster
d. gerbil
e. mouse

Correct answers are on page 94.

22. *Which species of turtle, native to the United States, is considered threatened and is protected by law?*

a. box turtle
b. red-eared slider
c. musk turtle
d. snapping turtle
e. gopher turtle

23. *Concerning alligators, which statement is **least** accurate?*

a. High ambient temperatures during egg incubation can be used to control the sex of hatchlings.
b. Male alligators grow to a larger adult size than females.
c. Adult alligators provide no parental care after their eggs hatch.
d. They have a 4-chambered heart.
e. They have an extremely small brain in relation to their body size.

24. *The substrate that is **not** an appropriate bedding for reptiles is:*

a. newspaper
b. paper towels
c. aspen shavings
d. cedar shavings
e. sphagnum moss

25. *Laboratory animal medicine is best defined as:*

a. the body of scientific and technical information, knowledge and skills that applies to laboratory animals
b. a specialty field of veterinary medicine concerned with diagnosis, treatment and prevention of diseases of laboratory animals
c. the study of animals for the purpose of gaining new information about normal and abnormal processes in people and animals
d. the application of animal science and veterinary medicine to the procurement and management of laboratory animals
e. the use of animals for any purpose, as long as it is done in a humane and caring manner

26. *Desirable characteristics of contact bedding for laboratory animals include all of the following **except**:*

a. absorbent
b. edible
c. nonabrasive
d. free of pathogens
e. dust free

27. *Concerning salmonellosis in mice, which statement is **least** accurate?*

a. It is a zoonosis and can be transmitted to people.
b. It is characterized by necrotic foci in the liver and spleen.
c. It occurs in acute, subacute and chronic forms.
d. It can be eliminated from a mouse colony by reducing the pH of the drinking water.
e. It is more prevalent and serious in weanlings.

28. *Concerning "ring tail" in rats, which statement is most accurate?*

a. It is a genetic disease.
b. It is caused by *Mycoplasma pulmonis*.
c. It is a new disease, thought to be caused by a virus.
d. It is associated with low humidity and high ambient temperatures.
e. It affects only certain strains of rats and does not occur in other strains.

29. *A rabbit doe typically nurses her young:*

a. every hour
b. every 4 hours
c. every 6 hours
d. every 8 hours
e. once a day

30. *The **least** likely cause of profuse diarrhea in a rabbit is:*

a. mucoid enteropathy
b. Tyzzer's disease
c. coccidiosis
d. excessive lettuce and greens in the diet
e. high ambient temperature and insufficient fiber in the diet

31. *How much blood can be safely drawn from a 350-gram bird?*

    a. 35 ml
    b. 3.5 ml
    c. 0.35 ml
    d. 0.7 ml
    e. 7 ml

32. *The United States Department of Agriculture quarantine period for psittacine birds arriving in the United States from another country is:*

    a. 20 days
    b. 30 days
    c. 40 days
    d. 50 days
    e. 60 days

33. *The best indication of an avian patient's progress in recovering from illness is:*

    a. weight gain or loss
    b. isolates found in cloacal cultures
    c. capillary refill time
    d. body temperature
    e. pupillary light reflex

34. *The injectable anesthetic most commonly used in nonhuman primates is:*

    a. pentobarbital
    b. thiamylal sodium
    c. droperidol-fentanyl
    d. ketamine
    e. tiletamine-zolazepam

35. *The rhesus monkey is a nonhuman primate commonly used in research. It is considered a member of which group?*

    a. prosimians
    b. New World monkeys
    c. Old World monkeys
    d. great apes
    e. hominids

36. *"Kindling" is the term used to describe:*

    a. the maternal behavior of mice
    b. the burrowing instinct of rodents
    c. the estrous cycle of rodents
    d. parturition in rabbits
    e. euthanasia of rodents

37. *Concerning the regulations governing shipment of dogs, cats and nonhuman primates by commercial airlines, which statement is* ***least*** *accurate?*

    a. All animals shipped must have been bred by a commercial vendor.
    b. All animals shipped must be accompanied by a health certificate from a veterinarian accredited by the United States Department of Agriculture.
    c. The ambient temperature in the commercial airplane must be between 45 F and 85 F.
    d. Animals must be housed in a cage of adequate size to allow the animal to stand comfortably and turn around.
    e. Food must be provided every 24 hours and water must be provided every 12 hours after shipment is initiated.

38. *Which species has a life span of 18-24 months, estrous cycle of 4 days and gestation period of 16 days, with adult males weighing 85-130 grams?*

    a. gerbil
    b. rat
    c. mouse
    d. hamster
    e. guinea pig

39. *Concerning animals used in biomedical research, which statement is* ***least*** *accurate?*

    a. Over 90% of the animals are rodents.
    b. About 1-2% of the animals are dogs and cats.
    c. About 17-22 million animals are used annually.
    d. The total number of animals used is increasing annually because of a lack of adequate alternative research models.
    e. Most of the major medical advances in this century have involved use of animals in research.

Correct answers are on page 94.

40. *Concerning the Animal Welfare Act in the United States, which statement is **least** accurate?*

   a. The United States Department of Agriculture may exempt from registration research facilities that do not use dogs or cats, and that only use rodents.
   b. Each registered research facility must have an Institutional Animal Care and Use Committee.
   c. Animals considered in the Act are dogs, cats, birds, hamsters, guinea pigs, rabbits, nonhuman primates and cattle.
   d. The Act does not pertain to retail pet stores and veterinary clinics.
   e. The Act does not pertain to slaughterhouses (abattoirs).

Answers

1. **d**
2. **b**
3. **c**
4. **e**
5. **a**
6. **b**
7. **e**
8. **c**
9. **a**
10. **d**
11. **d**
12. **c**
13. **d**
14. **a**
15. **a**
16. **b**
17. **b**
18. **e**
19. **c**
20. **a**
21. **b**
22. **e**
23. **c**
24. **d**
25. **b**
26. **b**
27. **d**
28. **d**
29. **e**
30. **e**
31. **b**
32. **b**
33. **a**
34. **d**
35. **c**
36. **d**
37. **a**
38. **d**
39. **d**
40. **c**

Section 9

Care of Marine Mammals

R. Aguilar, T.W. Campbell, L.A. Dierauf, T. Gemeinhardt, D. Huff, J.D. Letcher

Recommended Reading

Dierauf LA: *CRC Handbook of Marine Mammal Medicine: Health, Disease and Rehabilitation.* CRC Press, Boca Raton, FL, 1990.

Fowler ME: *Zoo and Wildlife Medicine.* 2nd ed. Saunders. Philadelphia, 1986.

Geraci JR: *Marine Mammal Care.* 2nd ed. University of Guelph, Ontario, 1981.

Harrison RJ: *Functional Anatomy of Marine Mammals.* Academic Press, New York, 1977.

Howard EB: *Pathobiology of Marine Mammal Diseases.* CRC Press, Boca Raton, FL, 1983.

Kinne O: *Diseases of Marine Animals: Reptilia, Aves, Mammalia.* Biolog Anstalt Helgoland, Hamburg, Germany, 1985.

Ridgway SH: *Mammals of the Sea: Biology and Medicine.* Charles C Thomas, Springfield, IL, 1972.

Practice answer sheet is on page 361.

Questions

1. *The best site for collection of venous blood from a cetacean (whale, dolphin) is the:*

   a. caudal gluteal vein
   b. caudal peduncle
   c. interdigital veins
   d. extradural intravertebral vein
   e. brachial venous plexus

2. *While continuing to nurse, young cetaceans (whales, dolphins) in captivity begin to eat some fish at:*

   a. 3-4 months of age
   b. 12-14 months of age
   c. 6-8 months of age
   d. 18 months of age
   e. 24 months of age

Correct answers are on page 97.

3. *Concerning anesthesia of dolphins, which statement is* ***least*** *accurate?*

   a. When cetaceans are under anesthesia, they do not spontaneously breathe, and require ventilatory support.
   b. Inhalation anesthesia may be induced by applying a mask over the dolphin's blowhole.
   c. A high-frequency jet ventilation anesthetic system is required for dolphins.
   d. Barbiturates are contraindicated for anesthesia of dolphins.
   e. During anesthesia, the body of even small dolphins must be properly supported to ensure that organ function is not compromised by ventral compression.

4. *What is the best way to thaw frozen saltwater fish, so as to minimize loss of nutrients and avoid spoilage?*

   a. gradually in tepid water
   b. in cold, running freshwater
   c. in cold, running saltwater
   d. quickly in hot water
   e. gradually at room temperature without immersion in water

5. *Sea otters differ from most other marine mammals in which way?*

   a. Sea otters have very poor eyesight above water.
   b. Sea otters do not have a thick subcutaneous fat layer.
   c. Sea otters cannot dive to depths greater than 20 meters.
   d. Sea otters have a low metabolic rate as compared with most other marine mammals.
   e. Sea otters eat a diet consisting of 25% vegetable and 75% animal protein.

6. *Scombroid fish poisoning may occur when such species as mackerel or tuna are stored frozen for longer than 4 months. It is caused by:*

   a. oxidation of vitamin E in the fish
   b. conversion of histidine to histamine in the fish
   c. the thiaminase content of the fish
   d. the growth of fungal contaminants
   e. marked depletion of vitamin K levels in the fish

7. *Which of the following marine mammals species is susceptible to infection with the canine heartworm,* Dirofilaria immitis*?*

   a. dolphins (*Tursiops*)
   b. California sea lion (*Zalophus californianus*)
   c. harbor seal (*Phoca vitulina*)
   d. sea otter (*Enhydra lutris*)
   e. polar bear (*Ursus maritimus*)

8. *Which of the following is a common site for blood collection in phocid seals, such as the harbor seal (*Phoca vitulina*)?*

   a. jugular vein
   b. caudal or tail vein
   c. cephalic vein
   d. blood vessels in the plantar aspect of the pelvic flipper
   e. caudal gluteal vein

9. *Pinnipeds frequently exhibit a diving reflex when being anesthetized. The reflex can be recognized by:*

   a. exhalation, followed by apnea, bradycardia and peripheral vasoconstriction
   b. exhalation, followed by apnea, tachycardia and peripheral vasoconstriction
   c. apnea, with no change in heart rate
   d. inhalation, followed by apnea, bradycardia and peripheral vasoconstriction
   e. inhalation, followed by apnea, tachycardia and peripheral vasodilatation

10. *Female, young and adult male cetaceans (whales or dolphins) are traditionally termed, respectively, as:*

   a. doe, fawn and stag
   b. sow, young and boar
   c. cow, calf and bull
   d. female, young and male
   e. ewe, ram and lamb

Answers

1. **b** Blood can be collected from the caudal gluteal vein of otariids, the interdigital veins of pinnipeds, the extradural intravertebral vein of phocids, and the brachial venous plexus of manatees.
2. **a**
3. **d** Barbiturates are routinely used (particularly intravenous sodium thiopental) for anesthetic induction in dolphins.
4. **c** The goal is to minimize loss of nutrients and avoid spoilage.
5. **b**
6. **b**
7. **b** Captive California sea lions are susceptible to the canine heartworm in enzootic areas and must be given preventive therapy. The only filarid recognized in harbor seals is *Dipetalonema spirocauda. Dirofilaria* infection has not been reported in any other marine mammal.
8. **d** Phocid seals are easily sampled from the plantar aspect of the pelvic flipper. A needle is directed at a 10- to 20-degree angle directly over the second digit or medial to the fourth digit at the origin of the interdigital webbing. Blood is collected from a main vessel or a vascular rete, often resulting in a mixed venous and arterial sample.
9. **a** Diving mammals exhale before diving so as to allow for nearly total lung collapse. Bradycardia and peripheral vasoconstriction allow efficient use of stored oxygen by the brain and heart.
10. **c**

Notes

Notes

Section 10

Care of Poultry and Wild Fowl

E.M. Odor

Recommended Reading

A Laboratory Manual for the Isolation and Identification of Avian Pathogens. 3rd ed. American Assn of Avian Pathologists, Kennett Square, PA.

Avian Disease Manual. 3rd ed. American Assn of Avian Pathologists, Kennett Square, PA.

Calnek BW: *Diseases of Poultry.* 9th ed. Iowa State University Press, Ames, IA, 1991.

Field Guide to Wildlife Diseases. Resource Publication 167, United States Department of the Interior, Fish and Wildlife Service, Washington DC.

Schwartz LD: *Poultry Health Handbook.* 3rd ed. College of Agriculture, Pennsylvania State University, University Park, PA.

Practice answer sheet is on page 363.

Questions

1. *Which respiratory disease is **not** caused by a virus?*

   a. infectious bronchitis
   b. fowl pox
   c. laryngotracheitis
   d. infectious coryza
   e. quail bronchitis

2. *Another name commonly applied to chlamydiosis in turkeys is:*

   a. hemorrhagic enteritis
   b. psittacosis
   c. black head
   d. ornithosis
   e. coryza

Correct answers are on page 101.

3. *Reoviral infection in broiler chicks is most often associated with:*
   a. abnormal bone and feather development
   b. impaired egg production
   c. increased respiratory disease
   d. *Salmonella* infection
   e. immunosuppression

4. *The sample of choice to isolate the virus of Marek's disease is:*
   a. tracheal swab
   b. buffy coat
   c. tendon tissue
   d. skin section
   e. peripheral nerve section

5. *"Vent gleet" can cause significant losses in turkeys. This condition primarily involves the:*
   a. circulatory system
   b. respiratory system
   c. muscular system
   d. skeletal system
   e. urinary system

6. *Infectious bursal disease virus is generally considered to be most pathogenic in:*
   a. broiler chickens
   b. layer chickens
   c. turkeys
   d. commercial ducks
   e. Cornish game birds

7. *Consumption of improperly handled or improperly prepared poultry meat and eggs have raised public health concerns centered around:*
   a. *Pseudomonas* and coliform bacteria
   b. *Staphylococcus* and *Streptococcus*
   c. *Chlamydia* and *Histomonas*
   d. *Salmonella* and *Campylobacter*
   e. *Bacillus* and *Cryptococcus*

Questions 8 through 10

8. *A common insect pest of poultry houses that transmits diseases to chickens and causes structural damage to the poultry house is the:*
   a. common house fly
   b. poultry louse
   c. army worm larva
   d. darkling beetle
   e. mosquito

9. *A common intestinal parasite of chickens that is transmitted by the insect pest in the preceding question is:*
   a. *Echinococcus granulosus*
   b. *Raillietina cesticillus*
   c. *Cryptosporidium*
   d. *Davainea meleagridia*
   e. *Eimeria acervulina*

10. *The common name for the intestinal parasite mentioned in the preceding question is the:*
    a. cecal worm
    b. capworm
    c. roundworm
    d. hookworm
    e. tapeworm

11. *Coccidian oocysts are:*
    a. immediately infective when passed in the feces
    b. infective only after desiccation and rehydration
    c. infective after sporulation in a warm, moist environment
    d. not infective until passed by an intermediate host
    e. not infective until frozen and thawed

12. *Which class of commercial poultry is most susceptible to aflatoxicosis?*
    a. broiler chicks
    b. broiler breeders

c. commercial egg layers
d. turkey poults
e. commercial ducklings

13. *Migratory waterfowl become infected with avian cholera:*

a. only through contact with domestic poultry
b. only through contact with resident nonmigrating waterfowl
c. through vertical transmission from chronically infected parent stock
d. through contact with a contaminated environment
e. through various sources, such as domestic poultry, waterfowl, domestic mammals, wild carnivores and rodents

14. *Botulinus toxin is most likely to be produced in:*

a. deep, cold, stagnant bodies of water with a rocky bottom and little organic matter
b. shallow bodies of water covered by ice, with anaerobic conditions under the ice
c. deep, warm, fast-moving bodies of water with a rocky bottom and little organic matter
d. shallow, warm, fast-moving bodies of water containing considerable organic matter
e. shallow, warm, stagnant bodies of water containing considerable organic matter

15. *Oil toxicity of waterfowl causes death by:*

a. ingestion of toxic hydrocarbons
b. loss of insulation and buoyancy, with resultant hypothermia, starvation or drowning
c. absorption of toxic hydrocarbons through the skin
d. paralysis of neck muscles, with resultant drowning
e. wasting of skeletal muscle tissue

Answers

1. **d** This is the only nonviral disease listed. It is caused by a bacterium.
2. **d** In turkeys, the term ornithosis is used. Psittacosis is used when the disease occurs in psittacine birds.
3. **a** Reoviral infection is referred to as brittle bone disease because it adversely affects bone development.
4. **b** The buffy coat includes the lymphocytes that contain the virus.
5. **e** Urate "flushing" causes the vent region to become coated and often infected. This can be quite a problem, especially in turkey breeder flocks.
6. **b** Though bursal disease is a problem in many different types of poultry, commercial egg layers are quite susceptible.
7. **d** Both pathogens pose a public health risk that is real but not fully defined.
8. **d** Darkling beetles (Order: Coleoptera) are a big problem for poultry producers.
9. **b** *Raillietina cesticillus* is most easily controlled by reducing populations of darkling beetles.
10. **e**
11. **c** This is a very important consideration in control of these parasites.
12. **e** Though all of the others listed are affected, commercial ducklings are especially susceptible.
13. **e**
14. **e** *Clostridium botulinum* requires warm, anaerobic conditions with organic matter, such as in slow-moving or stagnant water, to produce enough toxin to be a threat to birds.
15. **b** The other factors listed may be involved, but this is usually the cause of death.

Notes

Section 11

Care of Small Animals

K.C. Bovée, R.M. Bright, D.E. Brooks, P.A. Bushby, S.M. Cotter, S.K. Fooshee, J. Harari, E.T. Keller, J.N. Kornegay, D.W. Macy, N.S. Moise, K.A. Moriello, J.K. Roush, F.W. Scott, R.G. Sherding, C.B. Waters, M.D. Willard

Recommended Reading

Intravartolo CS and Richardson RC: *The Veterinary Technician in Small Animal Practice: Patient Management and Client Instructions.* Burgess Publishing, Minneapolis, 1983.

Pratt PW: *Medical Nursing for Animal Health Technicians.* American Veterinary Publications, Goleta, CA, 1985.

Practice answer sheet is on page 365.

Questions

1. *An 8-year-old female Labrador Retriever is presented because of polyuria and polydipsia. In obtaining the history, it is appropriate to ask the owner about all of the following* ***except:***

   a. appetite
   b. general attitude and activity level
   c. reproductive history
   d. dental history
   e. drugs given recently and currently

2. *A dog is hit by a car and presented to your clinic 10 minutes later, in shock. The illness in this dog is classified as:*

   a. acute
   b. peracute
   c. subacute
   d. chronic
   e. subchronic

Correct answers are on pages 117-119.

3. *A cat has been coughing intermittently for 4 months. The illness in this cat is classified as:*

   a. acute
   b. peracute
   c. subacute
   d. chronic
   e. subchronic

4. *A dog with lameness for 1 day is presented for treatment. The illness in this dog is classified as:*

   a. acute
   b. peracute
   c. subacute
   d. chronic
   e. subchronic

5. *A dog has had diarrhea for 4 days. The illness in this dog is classified as:*

   a. acute
   b. peracute
   c. subacute
   d. chronic
   e. subchronic

6. *In obtaining an animal's history, routine questions concerning vaccination should include all of the following* ***except****:*

   a. dates of most recent vaccination
   b. date and type of initial vaccinations
   c. if a cat, date and result of feline leukemia virus test
   d. dates and types of annual vaccinations
   e. if a dog, date and result of canine parvovirus test

7. *A client complains that his dog has had diarrhea for 4 weeks. To determine if the diarrhea is of small bowel or large bowel origin, questions should include all of the following* ***except****:*

   a. "Does the dog strain to defecate?"
   b. "Does the stool appear bloody?"
   c. "Does the dog eat with a hearty appetite?"
   d. "Is there any mucus on the stools?"
   e. "How many times per day does the dog defecate?"

8. *Clients are asked to provide information on their pet's history so you can:*

   a. get to know the client better and develop rapport
   b. become acquainted with the pet's personality and advise the veterinarian if the animal is fractious
   c. obtain pertinent information that may help define the animal's presenting problem
   d. learn what the cat or dog likes to eat in the event it must be hospitalized
   e. occupy the client until the doctor enters the examination room

For Questions 9 through 14, select the correct answer from the 6 choices below.

   a. ascites
   b. melena
   c. hematochezia
   d. hematuria
   e. icterus/jaundice
   f. dyspnea

9. *Frank (red) blood in the stool.*

10. *Dark, tarry stools containing occult (digested) blood.*

11. *Accumulation of serous fluid in the abdominal cavity.*

12. *Bloody urine.*

13. *Difficulty in breathing.*

14. *Yellow discoloration of the mucosae and sclerae.*

Questions 15 and 16

A 6-year-old male Corgi is rushed to your clinic after the owner finds the dog prostrate at home. You quickly evaluate the dog and observe that the mucous membranes are pale and capillary refill time is 4 seconds. The dog is unable to stand and the abdomen is markedly distended. The dog appears alert.

15. *Which of the following best describes this dog's condition?*

   a. comatose and overhydrated
   b. demented and cyanotic
   c. weak and in shock
   d. psychotic and polycythemic
   e. semicomatose and dyspneic

16. *The dog has a rectal temperature of 37.2 C, a respiratory rate of 45 breaths per minute, a heart rate of 200 beats per minute, and 80 pulses palpated per minute. Which of the following best describes this dog's condition?*

   a. hypothermic and eupneic, with pulse deficits
   b. normothermic and eupneic, with pulse deficits
   c. hypothermic and tachypneic, with appropriate pulses
   d. hyperthermic and tachypneic, with pulse deficits
   e. hypothermic and tachypneic, with pulse deficits

17. *Epiphora is a term describing:*

   a. excessive tearing
   b. difficult breathing
   c. uncontrollable hemorrhage
   d. excessive urination
   e. difficulty in passing stools

18. *A 13-year-old cat is presented because of lethargy and anorexia. You notice that the skin remains tented when you pinch it away from the body. The cat's mucous membranes feel very dry. In regard to hydration status, this cat is most likely:*

   a. not dehydrated but very emaciated
   b. 2% dehydrated
   c. 4% dehydrated
   d. 6% dehydrated
   e. 8% or more dehydrated

19. *Damage to the spinal cord is* ***least*** *likely to cause:*

   a. paresis
   b. paralysis
   c. loss of proprioception
   d. head tilt
   e. urinary or fecal incontinence

20. *Glaucoma is an ocular disease characterized by:*

   a. inflammation of the conjunctiva
   b. increased intraocular pressure
   c. inflammation of the retina
   d. corneal edema
   e. corneal and conjunctival dryness

Questions 21 and 22

A client brings his 6-month-old Labrador Retriever to your clinic. The dog vomited twice this morning, but now appears alert and normal.

21. *Relevant questions you should ask include all of the following* ***except****:*

   a "What is the dog's current diet?"
   b. "Does the dog receive any table scraps or treats?"
   c. "Does the dog have access to garbage?"
   d. "Has the dog ever limped or exhibited pain in its limbs?"
   e. "What is the dog's deworming history?"

Correct answers are on pages 117-119.

22. *The veterinarian examines this dog and finds no abnormalities. The most appropriate course of action is to:*

 a. administer metoclopramide until the vomiting stops
 b. admit the dog to the hospital, perform a complete blood count, serum chemistry assays and urinalysis, administer intravenous fluid therapy, and withhold food and water
 c. advise the owner to withhold food and water for 24 hours and gradually reintroduce water and then foods if the vomiting ceases; if vomiting persists, bring the dog back for reevaluation
 d. make abdominal radiographs to look for a possible foreign body
 e. administer Pepto-Bismol until the vomiting stops

23. *In female dogs, the entire estrous cycle spans:*

 a. 2-4 months
 b. 4-7 months
 c. 7-9 months
 d. 8-12 months
 e. 10-14 months

24. *In female cats, the entire estrous cycle spans:*

 a. 18 days
 b. 21 days
 c. 24 days
 d. 28 days
 e. 32 days

25. *Though there may be considerable individual variation, the average gestation length in cats and dogs is:*

 a. 58 days
 b. 54 days
 c. 63 days
 d. 66 days
 e. 69 days

26. *Signs of proestrus in the bitch include all of the following* ***except:***

 a. vulvar swelling
 b. bloody vulvar discharge
 c. attraction of males
 d. courtship play
 e. standing to be mounted

27. *Normal puppies are characterized by all of the following* ***except:***

 a. crawl and right themselves at birth
 b. open eyelids by 1-3 weeks of age
 c. regulate their body temperature by 4 days of age
 d. ear canals open by 13-17 days of age
 e. suckle at birth

28. *Distichiasis is characterized by:*

 a. ingrown eyelashes
 b. a double row of eyelashes, one or both of which contact the eyeball
 c. lack of eyelashes
 d. increased intraocular pressure
 e. opacification of the lens

29. *A client presents a 3-year-old Basset Hound with a 1-week history of a bloody nasal discharge. The clinical sign this dog is displaying is termed:*

 a. hematemesis
 b. hemoperitoneum
 c. hemonasum
 d. epistaxis
 e. hemostaxis

30. *The hematocrit (packed cell volume) is the:*

 a. volume percentage of red blood cells in plasma
 b. volume percentage of red blood cells in whole blood
 c. concentration of hemoglobin in whole blood
 d. number of red blood cells per 100 white blood cells
 e. volume percentage of all blood cells in whole blood

31. *Leukocytosis refers to:*

a. an increased number of neutrophils
b. an increased total number of white blood cells
c. an increased number of monocytes
d. a decreased number of neutrophils
e. a decreased number of leukocytes

32. *In dogs and cats, acceptable sites for venipuncture include all of the following* ***except*** *the:*

a. jugular vein
b. cephalic vein
c. coccygeal (tail) vein
d. lateral saphenous vein (dog)
e. medial saphenous vein (cat)

33. *Serum values of which constituents are most likely to be increased in an azotemic dog?*

a. alanine aminotransferase and alkaline phosphatase
b. aspartate aminotransferase and creatine phosphokinase
c. urea nitrogen and creatinine
d. unconjugated bilirubin and cholesterol
e. gamma glutamyltransferase and glucose

34. *A 10-year-old dog with chronic renal failure has a blood urea nitrogen level of 90 mg/dl and a serum creatinine level of 4.0 mg/dl. The specific gravity of urine from this dog is most likely to be:*

a. between 1.020 and 1.040
b. between 1.006 and 1.025
c. less than 1.006
d. between 1.030 and 1.055
e. greater than 1.050

35. *The most sensitive laboratory test for detecting heartworm infection in dogs is:*

a. a direct blood smear
b. a modified Knott's test
c. a filter test
d. an antigen test
e. an antibody test

36. *After a dog is determined to be infected with heartworms, the most appropriate additional diagnostic tests before starting treatment include:*

a. thoracic radiographs and a serum biochemistry panel
b. abdominal radiographs and ultrasonographic examination
c. direct blood pressure measurements and blood gas analysis
d. pulmonary function tests and a liver biopsy
e. ophthalmologic examination and pelvic radiographs

37. *When performing cystocentesis, it is important to:*

a. direct the needle cranially before inserting it into the abdomen
b. aspirate as you withdraw the needle through the bladder and abdominal walls
c. insert the needle to the hub
d. stabilize the bladder before inserting the needle
e. use an 18-gauge, 1 1/2-inch needle

38. *An electrocardiogram measures:*

a. mechanical activity of the heart
b. electrical activity of the heart
c. volume of heart chambers
d. cardiac contractility
e. pulse conduction

39. *The most common risk associated with bladder catheterization via the urethra is:*

a. damage to the urethra
b. damage to the bladder
c. bacterial infection
d. overinserting the catheter, causing the catheter to knot in the urinary bladder
e. damage to the ureters

Correct answers are on pages 117-119.

40. The earliest time in gestation that radiographs can be used to diagnose pregnancy in dogs and cats is:

a. 20 days
b. 25 days
c. 35 days
d. 45 days
e. 55 days

Questions 41 and 42

41. A cat is presented with pinpoint hemorrhages on the skin and mucous membranes. This condition is called:

a. anemia
b. cyanosis
c. icterus
d. purpura
e. petechiation

42. In this cat showing hemorrhages, what is the most likely hematologic abnormality?

a. increased packed cell volume
b. decreased packed cell volume
c. increased platelet count
d. decreased platelet count
e. decreased bleeding time

43. Another term for false pregnancy is:

a. pseudogestation
b. nymphomania
c. pseudocyesis
d. pseudoestrogenism
e. feminization

*44. Concerning shock, which statement is **least** accurate?*

a. Shock is a maldistribution of blood flow, causing decreased delivery of oxygen to tissues.
b. Shock should be considered an emergency situation, warranting immediate treatment.
c. Shock causes a marked parasympathetic response.
d. Shock can be caused by hemorrhage, severe stress, infection or anaphylaxis.
e. An animal in shock can develop tachypnea and tachycardia.

For Questions 45 through 50, select the correct answer from the 6 choices below.

a. calculus
b. stomatitis
c. enteritis
d. colitis
e. coprophagy
f. anorexia

45. Inflammation of the oral mucosa.

46. An abnormal concretion, usually composed of mineral salts.

47. Inflammation of the large intestine.

48. Inflammation of the small intestine.

49. Ingestion of feces.

50. Loss of appetite.

For Questions 51 through 55, select the correct answer from the 5 choices below.

a. constipation
b. obstipation
c. anal sac impaction
d. perianal fistulae
e. rectal prolapse

51. Eversion of the rectum out through the anus.

52. Infected draining tracts around the anal region.

53. Difficult evacuation of feces.

54. Inability to pass a stool because of long-standing failure to evacuate feces.

55. Common cause of "scooting" or rubbing the anal area along the ground.

56. Regurgitation is:

a. commonly associated with hookworm infection
b. preceded by retching
c. the expulsion of undigested food
d. a definitive sign of lead toxicity
e. almost always seen in old dogs

*57. Pruritus is **least** likely to be seen in an animal with:*

a. flea-allergy dermatitis
b. demodicosis
c. sarcoptic mange
d. bacterial pyoderma
e. endocrine alopecia

*58. Common signs of congestive heart failure include all of the following **except**:*

a. ascites
b. dyspnea
c. exercise intolerance
d. jugular distention
e. muscle pain

59. Keratitis is an inflammation of the:

a. skin
b. liver
c. brain
d. cornea
e. lips

*60. Common cutaneous and subcutaneous tumors of dogs include all of the following **except**:*

a. lipoma
b. mast-cell tumor
c. malignant melanoma
d. malignant fibrous histiocytoma
e. histiocytoma

61. Hip dysplasia:

a. most often affects small breeds of dogs
b. is not hereditary
c. resolves with age
d. is diagnosed by ventrodorsal radiographs of the pelvis
e. is common in cats

*62. Concerning osteomyelitis, which statement is **least** accurate?*

a. Osteomyelitis is a bacterial or fungal infection of the bone.
b. Osteomyelitis may require surgery and long-term medical therapy.
c. Pain, fever and lameness are frequently associated with osteomyelitis.
d. The best way to determine which antibiotic is appropriate for treatment is usually with a Gram-stained preparation.
e. Radiographs can be helpful in making a definitive diagnosis.

63. Many vaccines are available for use in dogs, in many different combinations. In addition to appropriate rabies prophylaxis, dogs are typically vaccinated annually with DHLPP. This vaccine contains preparations of:

a. distemper virus, *Leptospira*, parvovirus, hepatitis virus and parainfluenza virus
b. distemper virus, *Leptospira*, coronavirus, hepatitis virus and *Bordetella*
c. distemper virus, hepatitis virus, *Borrelia*, parvovirus and *Bordetella*
d. *Leptospira*, parvovirus, hepatitis virus and coronavirus
e. parvovirus, *Leptospira*, hepatitis virus and distemper virus

Correct answers are on pages 117-119.

64. In addition to appropriate rabies prophylaxis, cats are typically vaccinated annually with FVRCP. This vaccine contains preparations of:

a. feline leukemia virus, feline infectious peritonitis virus and *Chlamydia*
b. rhinotracheitis virus, calicivirus and panleukopenia virus
c. rhinotracheitis virus, panleukopenia virus and *Chlamydia*
d. feline leukemia virus, panleukopenia virus and rotavirus
e. *Chlamydia,* herpesvirus and calicivirus

*65. An 8-week-old Collie puppy has had diarrhea for 3 days and you suspect a parasite infection. Gastrointestinal parasites this puppy is most likely to have include all of the following **except**:*

a. coccidia
b. roundworms
c. whipworms
d. hookworms
e. tapeworms

66. You perform a fecal flotation on a dog's stool and observe whipworm eggs in the sample. The most appropriate anthelmintic for use in treating this dog is:

a. pyrantel pamoate (Nemex, Strongid-T)
b. piperazine citrate
c. praziquantel (Droncit)
d. fenbendazole (Panacur)
e. bunamidine hydrochloride (Scolaban)

67. Enzyme-linked immunosorbent assay (ELISA) on serum from an apparently healthy cat is positive for feline leukemia virus infection. The most appropriate course of action is to:

a. euthanize the cat immediately
b. retest the cat by ELISA in 1 week
c. retest the cat by ELISA or indirect fluorescent antibody test in 1 month or later
d. permanently isolate the cat to prevent infection of other cats
e. administer a broad-spectrum antibiotic at low levels for 6 months

*68. All of the following are Gram-negative bacteria **except**:*

a. *Pseudomonas*
b. *Staphylococcus*
c. *Escherichia coli*
d. *Salmonella*
e. *Pasteurella*

69. A common yeast that often causes otitis in dogs is:

a. *Candida albicans*
b. *Malassezia pachydermatis*
c. *Sporothrix schenckii*
d. *Blastomyces dermatitidis*
e. *Aspergillus flavus*

70. The most common coccidial parasite of the gastrointestinal tract of dogs and cats is:

a. *Eimeria*
b. *Isospora*
c. *Toxoplasma*
d. *Sarcocystis*
e. *Neospora*

*71. All of the following are gastrointestinal parasites **except**:*

a. *Ancylostoma caninum*
b. *Trichuris vulpis*
c. *Toxocara canis*
d. *Dipylidium caninum*
e. *Paragonimus kellicotti*

72. The vector that transmits infectious microfilariae of heartworms is the:

a. fly
b. tick
c. mosquito
d. flea
e. sandfly

73. *All of the following are caused solely by a virus* ***except:***

a. feline infectious peritonitis
b. canine distemper
c. kennel cough
d. rabies
e. feline panleukopenia

74. *Of the following agents, which is the only one that can destroy parvovirus?*

a. phenol
b. detergents
c. formaldehyde
d. chlorine bleach
e. alcohol

75. *Zoonoses are diseases that:*

a. occur only in wild animals
b. are transmitted between many different animal species
c. are transmitted from animals to people
d. are transmitted only by arthropods, such as insects
e. always have an intermediate host

76. *Of the following sets of diseases, which set consists only of zoonotic diseases?*

a. leptospirosis, ringworm, salmonellosis, toxoplasmosis
b. leptospirosis, Rocky Mountain spotted fever, feline immunodeficiency virus infection, sarcoptic mange
c. leptospirosis, canine parvovirus infection, salmonellosis, giardiasis
d. rabies, brucellosis, canine adenovirus infection, cryptosporidiosis
e. rabies, salmonellosis, toxoplasmosis, feline immunodeficiency virus infection

77. *Concerning demodectic mange in dogs, which statement is* ***least*** *accurate?*

a. It is caused by the mite, *Demodex canis.*
b. Occasional mites may be seen on skin scrapings of normal dogs.
c. The dam transmits the mite to her puppies by direct contact.
d. This is primarily a disease of mixed-breed dogs.
e. Generalized demodicosis can be a sign of immunodeficiency.

78. *Dermatophytosis (ringworm) in dogs and cats can be caused by* Microsporum *and* Trichophyton. *Concerning dermatophytosis, which statement is* ***least*** *accurate?*

a. Approximately 50% of *Microsporum* species cause fluorescence of lesions on exposure to a Wood's lamp.
b. Lesions caused by *Trichophyton* species do not fluoresce on exposure to a Wood's lamp.
c. *Microsporum canis* is the most common genus in dogs and cats.
d. *Microsporum canis* is more common in dogs than in cats.
e. Systemic treatment may be necessary with generalized dermatophytosis.

79. *If a puppy is infected with heartworm (*Dirofilaria immitis*) microfilariae on the second day of life, what is the earliest time at which the animal will test positive for microfilariae?*

a. 2 months of age
b. 3 months of age
c. 6 months of age
d. 8 months of age
e. 9 months of age

80. *Heartworm infection can be prevented by use of any of the following* ***except:***

a. ivermectin
b. milbemycin
c. fenbendazole
d. diethylcarbamazine
e. diethylcarbamazine with oxibendazole

Correct answers are on pages 117-119.

Questions 81 and 82

81. *A drug given to dogs by careful intravenous injection to kill adult heartworms is:*

a. thiobenzamine
b. thiacetarsamide
c. ivermectin
d. diethylcarbamazine
e. levamisole

82. *Major side effects of this drug are:*

a. hepatic and renal toxicity
b. cardiac and otic toxicity
c. anaphylaxis and shock
d. hematuria and melena
e. lymphadenopathy and uveitis

83. *In cats, all of the following diseases may* ***directly*** *cause upper respiratory disease* ***except:***

a. rhinotracheitis
b. calicivirus infection
c. chlamydial infection
d. feline leukemia virus infection
e. bacterial rhinitis

84. *A 3-year-old Golden Retriever is receiving 1 grain of phenobarbital every 12 hours for epilepsy. One grain is equivalent to:*

a. 100 mg
b. 65 mg
c. 10 mg
d. 1000 mg
e. 50 mg

85. *A 28-lb Cocker Spaniel has congestive heart failure and requires furosemide per os at 2 mg/kg of body weight BID. At this dosage, this dog should be given:*

a. 50 mg every 4 hours
b. 25 mg every 12 hours
c. 12.5 mg every 24 hours
d. 100 mg every 12 hours
e. 10 mg every 8 hours

86. *A 55-lb dog develops acute pulmonary edema. The veterinarian orders treatment with 5% furosemide intravenously at 2 mg/kg of body weight. What quantity of furosemide should you give?*

a. 1 ml
b. 0.5 ml
c. 1.5 ml
d. 5 ml
e. 10 ml

87. *A 28-lb mongrel has been vomiting for 3 days and is estimated to be 8% dehydrated. What approximate fluid volume should you give to rehydrate this dog?*

a. 500 ml
b. 1000 ml
c. 2000 ml
d. 2240 ml
e. 1500 ml

88. *When administering intravenous fluids to a cat or dog, care must be taken to monitor for overhydration. The best initial indicator of overhydration is:*

a. edematous skin
b. pulmonary edema
c. polyuria
d. continued weight gain after the animal has been rehydrated appropriately
e. tachypnea

89. *You are using a microdrip to administer intravenous fluids to a cat. The cat must receive 360 ml of fluid during a 24-hour period. At what rate should the fluid be infused?*

a. 15 drops/minute
b. 15 drops/second
c. 150 drops/hour
d. 15 ml/minute
e. 36 ml/hour

*90. You are attempting to infuse intravenous fluids in a cat, but the fluid is not flowing well. What is the **least** likely cause of this problem?*

a. the infusion line is kinked
b. the vein is obstructed
c. the bottle is held above the level of the vein
d. the needle or catheter has become dislodged from the vein
e. the air vent is obstructed

*91. In addition to intravenous administration, routes of fluid administration in small animals include all of the following **except**:*

a. per os
b. intraperitoneal
c. subcutaneous
d. intrathoracic
e. intraosseous

92. An example of an isotonic fluid is:

a. 50% dextrose
b. distilled water
c. 0.9% saline
d. 10% calcium gluconate
e. lactated Ringer's solution with 2.5% dextrose

*93. Nutritional support can be provided to anorectic animals by any of the following **except**:*

a. pharyngostomy tube
b. nasoesophageal tube
c. gastrostomy tube
d. jejunostomy tube
e. duodenostomy tube

94. Concerning total parenteral nutrition (intravenous feeding), which statement is most accurate?

a. The solution usually contains equal volumes of B vitamins and dextrose.
b. If a dextrose solution in a concentration of 10% or higher is used, the fluid should be infused into the jugular vein.
c. The catheter should be flushed thoroughly with saline before administering any intravenous medications.
d. Laboratory tests are seldom necessary, as long as asepsis is strictly observed.
e. Solutions can be mixed in a bowl that has been sterilized in a dishwasher.

95. An owner telephones and says her adult Irish Setter had been fine until an hour ago, when the dog began retching. The owner thinks the dog is becoming progressively more uncomfortable. Additionally, she mentions that the dog's abdomen looks markedly distended. What is the most appropriate advice for this client?

a. withhold food and water overnight and bring the dog to the clinic in the morning if the problem persists
b. the veterinarian will telephone you when she's finished with appointments in 2 hours
c. this could be a life-threatening emergency and she should bring the dog to the clinic immediately
d. induce emesis with syrup of ipecac
e. apply gentle pressure to the abdomen to help relieve the distention

96. The preferred enema solution for cats and dogs is:

a. sodium phosphate
b. soapy water
c. warm tap water
d. mineral oil
e. vegetable oil

*97. Complications of enema administration may include all of the following **except**:*

a. hypothermia
b. vomiting
c. anemia
d. constipation
e. diarrhea

Correct answers are on pages 117-119.

98. *The most concentrated source of red blood cells is:*

a. fresh plasma
b. packed red blood cells
c. whole blood
d. platelet-enriched plasma
e. fresh-frozen plasma

99. *First aid for a limb fracture should include all of the following* ***except:***

a. controlling hemorrhage
b. covering open wounds with a sterile dressing to prevent contamination
c. realigning the bone fragments
d. immobilizing the limb
e. treating for shock, if necessary

100. *When preparing a cutaneous site for surgery, all of the following procedures are recommended* ***except:***

a. clip and then prepare the area 3 times, alternating with a surgical scrub and alcohol
b. prepare the area centripetally, progressively moving toward the site of the incision
c. remove all clipped hair before beginning preparation of the site
d. use one hand to prepare the site ("dirty hand") and one hand to obtain the scrub materials ("clean hand")
e. remove all surface dirt before beginning the surgical scrub

101. *It is important to check a cutaneous incision line postoperatively for dehiscence. Potential causes of dehiscence include all of the following* ***except:***

a. strenuous exercise
b. infection
c. starvation
d. licking at the incision
e. simple-interrupted suture pattern with nonabsorbable material

102. *The main reason for surgically repairing an umbilical, perineal or diaphragmatic hernia is to:*

a. improve the animal's appearance
b. prevent entrapment of internal organs
c. prevent progressive enlargement of the abdomen
d. increase the practice's profits
e. improve the surgeon's surgical technique

103. *Which of the following is* ***not*** *associated with heartworm infection?*

a. pulmonary hypertension
b. no clinical signs
c. dilatation of the pulmonary arteries
d. right ventricular hypertrophy
e. systemic hypertension

104. *Concerning dermatophyte cultures, which statement is* ***least*** *accurate?*

a. Cultures of samples obtained by haircoat brushing with a toothbrush are the most reliable method for cats, especially suspected asymptomatic carriers.
b. When culturing isolated lesions from dogs, it is best to swab the area with alcohol to minimize the number of contaminant fungi.
c. A red color change on dermatophyte test medium is diagnostic for a dermatophyte.
d. Dermatophyte test medium contains Sabouraud's dextrose agar, a pH indicator (phenol red), and antibacterial and antifungal agents.
e. Fungal pathogens are never heavily pigmented, either macroscopically or microscopically.

105. *The anticonvulsant preferred for long-term seizure control in dogs is:*

a. primidone
b. diphenylhydantoin (phenytoin)
c. phenobarbital
d. diazepam
e. valproic acid

106. In cats, a deficiency of which nutrient can cause central retinal degeneration?

a. tryptophan
b. taurine
c. vitamin A
d. proline
e. methionine

107. Which species normally has the highest urine specific gravity (1.065)?

a. horses
b. cattle
c. pigs
d. dogs
e. cats

108. Ovariohysterectomy can help reduce the frequency of mammary neoplasia if performed before the:

a. first estrous cycle
b. second estrous cycle
c. third estrous cycle
d. fourth estrous cycle
e. fifth estrous cycle

109. An owner says that her only cat died a month ago from feline leukemia virus (FeLV) infection, and she now would like to get a new kitten. The most appropriate advice for her is:

a. to wait at least 6 months before obtaining a new kitten
b. to adopt an adult cat rather than a kitten because kittens are more susceptible to FeLV infection
c. it is safe to adopt a new kitten with no special precautions
d. it is safe to adopt a kitten now if it is first vaccinated against FeLV infection
e. to first clean the floors with sodium hypochlorite solution (Clorox) and destroy any dishes used by the previous cat

110. Which of the following is ***not*** *a common part of the history of dogs with cranial cruciate ligament rupture?*

a. obese dog
b. injured while actively playing
c. 8 months old
d. overactive dog, always jumping and running
e. large-breed dog

111. Careless application of a tourniquet to the limb during onychectomy in a cat may result in:

a. ulnar neuropraxis
b. temporary radial nerve paralysis
c. permanent radial nerve paralysis
d. permanent median nerve paralysis
e. severance of the ulnar nerve

112. The most common and serious complication following perineal urethrostomy in male cats is:

a. urethral stricture
b. urinary incontinence
c. fecal incontinence
d. rectal prolapse
e. urine scalding

113. A large dog with sudden, gaseous abdominal distention associated with exercise after eating most likely has:

a. rectal prolapse
b. infectious hepatitis
c. splenic rupture
d. esophageal neoplasia
e. gastric dilatation-volvulus

114. For ovariohysterectomy in a dog, the skin incision is made:

a. caudally from the umbilicus
b. from the umbilicus to the pubis
c. cranially from the umbilicus
d. midway between the umbilicus and pubis
e. midway between the xyphoid and umbilicus

Correct answers are on pages 117-119.

115. Cryosurgery has been advocated as treatment for perianal fistulas, superficial tumors and other lesions in small animals. The most common cryogenic agent used in veterinary medicine is:

a. nitrous oxide
b. freon
c. liquid nitrogen
d. liquid helium
e. carbon dioxide

116. A mixed-breed dog has had a relatively severe, dry cough for the past 10 days. The cough began 4-5 days after the animal was housed at a kennel. The most likely cause of this dog's disease is:

a. herpesvirus
b. *Streptococcus pneumoniae*
c. *Klebsiella pneumoniae*
d. *Pasteurella multocida*
e. *Bordetella bronchiseptica*

117. The most appropriate treatment for a 5-month-old dog with mild, acute diarrhea of 2 days' duration and of unknown origin is:

a. oral rehydration solution
b. a bland, easily digested diet
c. oral neomycin
d. loperamide
e. methscopolamine

*118. Which type of enema should **not** be administered to a constipated Maltese dog?*

a. warm soapy water
b. warm water
c. hypertonic phosphate
d. mineral oil
e. warm water with dioctyl sodium sulfosuccinate

119. Transfusion reactions are rare in cats. What is the most common manifestation of transfusion with incompatible blood?

a. hemolytic anemia
b. respiratory arrest
c. vomiting
d. hemoglobinuria
e. seizures

*120. Which of the following is the **least** appropriate method of resolving hypothermia in the postoperative period?*

a. recirculating warm-water blanket
b. warm inspired air
c. intravenous fluids at normal body temperature
d. warm blankets
e. electric heating pad

121. The anticonvulsant of choice for long-term control of seizures in cats is:

a. phenobarbital
b. phenytoin
c. diazepam
d. acepromazine
e. valproic acid

122. Bilirubinuria is:

a. an abnormal finding in both male and female cats
b. an abnormal finding in male cats only
c. an abnormal finding in female cats only
d. a normal finding in both male and female cats
e. only normal in cats under 4 months of age

123. Concerning polydactylism in cats, which statement is most accurate?

a. Affected cats should have any extra toes removed.
b. Owners should be advised that it is an inherited autosomal dominant disorder.
c. It is a random congenital defect; no genetic information is available.
d. It is seen most often in Siamese.
e. It is seen most often in Rex cats.

124. *Which of the following is the **least** commonly documented result of spaying in dogs?*

a. reduced incidence of mammary tumors if done before 2 1/2 years of age
b. possible urinary incontinence
c. reduced incidence of pyometra
d. no attraction of male dogs
e. obesity

125. *A client's kitten has just died from feline panleukopenia (feline parvovirus) and she wants to replace it with an unvaccinated 14-week-old kitten from a neighbor. How long after vaccination of the kitten should she wait before taking it home?*

a. she can take the kitten home immediately
b. 3 days
c. 1 week
d. 2 weeks
e. 1 year

Answers

1. **d** Dental disease is not directly related to diseases causing polyuria and polydipsia.
2. **b**
3. **d**
4. **a**
5. **c**
6. **e** The test for parvovirus infection is used on sick dogs, not as a screening test.
7. **c** Appetite is not necessarily a good indicator of small bowel versus large bowel disease.
8. **c**
9. **c**
10. **b**
11. **a**
12. **d**
13. **f**
14. **e**
15. **c**
16. **e**
17. **a**
18. **e** This cat is at least 8% dehydrated.
19. **d** A head tilt could be due to damage to the vestibular system, not the spinal cord.
20. **b**
21. **d** Lameness is not pertinent to this case.
22. **c** The vast majority of gastroenteritis is self-limiting.
23. **b**
24. **b**
25. **c**
26. **e** Standing to be mounted is characteristic of estrus.
27. **c** Ability to regulate body temperature takes several weeks to develop.
28. **b**
29. **d**
30. **b**
31. **b**
32. **c**
33. **c**
34. **b**
35. **d**
36. **a** Thoracic radiographs are useful to assess the degree of disease. Serum chemistry assays are useful to assess liver and kidney function before starting treatment.
37. **d**
38. **b**
39. **c**
40. **d**
41. **e**
42. **d**
43. **c**

44. **c** Shock causes a marked sympathetic response.

45. **b**

46. **a**

47. **d**

48. **c**

49. **e**

50. **f**

51. **e**

52. **d**

53. **a**

54. **b**

55. **c**

56. **c**

57. **e**

58. **e**

59. **d**

60. **d** The other tumors listed are relatively common skin tumors.

61. **d**

62. **d** Culture and sensitivity tests are the best way to determine which antibiotic is appropriate for treatment.

63. **a**

64. **b**

65. **c** This 8-week-old puppy is not old enough to develop problems from whipworm infection, as the prepatent period is 3 months.

66. **d**

67. **c**

68. **b**

69. **b**

70. **a**

71. **e** This is a lungworm.

72. **c**

73. **c** Parainfluenza virus, adenovirus or herpesvirus may act in concert with the bacterium *Bordetella bronchiseptica*.

74. **d**

75. **c**

76. **a**

77. **d** Demodicosis is more common in purebred dogs.

78. **d** *Microsporum canis* is more common in cats than in dogs.

79. **c** It takes approximately 6 months after infection for microfilariae to appear in the blood.

80. **c**

81. **b**

82. **a**

83. **d** Feline leukemia virus infection may indirectly cause upper respiratory disease through immunosuppression, allowing secondary bacterial infection.

84. **b**

85. **b** BID indicates twice daily or every 12 hours. 28 lb = approximately 12.5 kg. A dosage of 2 mg/kg = 2 x 12.5 = 25 mg, given every 12 hours.

86. **a** 55 lb = 25 kg. A dosage of 2 mg/kg = 2 x 25 = 50 mg. A 5% solution contains 5000 mg/dl, or 50 mg/ml. Therefore, the dog should receive 1 ml of the 5% furosemide solution.

87. **b** 28 lb = approximately 12.5 kg. 0.08 x 12.5 = approximately 1 kg, which, in fluid weight, is equivalent to 1 L (1000 ml). Not mentioned in the question, but also necessary to consider when treating with fluids, are maintenance needs and continuing losses (vomiting, diarrhea).

88. **d** Weight gain in the face of rehydration indicates overhydration. This is the earliest clinical sign. By the time other signs develop, life-threatening overhydration may be occurring.

89. **a** 360 ml ÷ 24 hours = 15 ml/hour. 60 drops = 1 ml. 60 drops x 15 ml = 900 drops. 900 drops ÷ 60 minutes = 15 drops/minute.

90. **c** If the bottle were below the level of the vein, flow would cease.

91. **d** This could lead to such complications as pneumothorax, hydrothorax or collapsed lungs.

92. **c**

93. **e** A duodenostomy tube is not used because a gastrostomy tube would be easier to place and use. If the animal were vomiting, a jejunostomy tube may be an option, as a gastrostomy tube would be a poor choice.

94. **b** The solution contains very small amounts of B vitamins, but a major percentage is dextrose. Dextrose solutions of greater than 10% are too hyperosmolar for safe infusion into peripheral veins. The catheter should be a dedicated line and *never* used for intravenous medication. Frequent monitoring, particularly of blood glucose, PCV, total protein and electrolytes, is vital to successful total parenteral nutrition. Strict asepsis must be used; ideally a vented hood should be used to mix solutions in sterile containers not exposed to room air.

95. **c** This dog may have gastric dilatation-volvulus, an emergency situation that frequently requires surgery.

96. **c**

97. **c**

98. **b** Though less readily available than whole blood, packed red blood cells provide a higher concentration of red blood cells. They are useful for treatment of animals with acute blood loss, after fluid volume has already been replaced.

99. **c** This is done during fracture repair, but is not typically part of first aid.

100. **b** The site should be prepared by moving centrifugally, moving away from the incision site.

101. **e** Assuming tissues are correctly apposed, this type of suture pattern is unlikely to break down.

102. **b**

103. **e**

104. **c** The red color indicator in dermatophyte test medium is not diagnostic for a pathogen. It only indicates that the organism is using the protein in the agar. Definitive diagnosis of a dermatophyte infection requires microscopic examination of the specimen.

105. **c**

106. **b** Taurine deficiency is associated with development of retinal degeneration and blindness in cats.

107. **e**

108. **d** Studies have shown that before the fourth estrous cycle, the risk of mammary tumors is reduced significantly by ovariohysterectomy.

109. **c** The virus only lives a few hours to a few days in a household after an infected cate leaves the premises.

110. **c** Cranial cruciate ligament ruptures are rare in dogs less than 1 year of age. Ligaments are generally stronger than the bone in young dogs, so injuries in young dogs are more commonly physeal fractures.

111. **b**

112. **a**

113. **e** Gastric dilatation-volvulus occurs most frequently in large dogs that have exercised after eating.

114. **a** The skin incision for ovariohysterectomy in dogs is started at the umbilicus and continued caudally. The anatomic structure that is most difficult to exteriorize is the right ovary; therefore, the incision must be made more cranially (as compared with the incision for ovariohysterectomy in cats) to allow exposure of the ovaries.

115. **c** Liquid nitrogen is the most commonly used cryogen in veterinary medicine because of its temperature, availability and cost.

116. **e** *Bordetella bronchiseptica* is the most common bacterial cause of infectious tracheobronchitis in dogs. Herpesvirus is a rare cause.

117. **b** The dog is not dehydrated and is unlikely to become so; therefore, fluid therapy is not warranted. Most acute diarrhea is caused by the diet, parasites and/or infections. Oral neomycin is rarely useful in acute diarrhea.

118. **c** Hypertonic enemas should not be administered to cats or small dogs, especially if the animal is obstipated.

119. **b** Respiration may cease with an incompatible transfusion; vomiting may occur when the rate of blood administration is excessively rapid.

120. **e** Electric heating pads may cause thermal burns. These are particularly dangerous for the unconscious or immobile patient. These have no place in clinical practice and their use only invites a lawsuit.

121. **a**

122. **a** Bilirubinuria is abnormal in any cat and is an important indicator of liver disease.

123. **b**

124. **e**

125. **d** The general recommendation is to wait 2 weeks after vaccination, even though immunity may be generated before this time.

Notes

Section 12

Care of Zoo and Exotic Animals

R. Aguilar, F.L. Frye, K. Hudelson, J.D. Letcher, D.H. Nielsen, G. Ranglack, D. Schaeffer, S.K. Wells-Mikota, P. Wolff

Recommended Reading

Amlacher E: *Textbook of Fish Diseases.* TFH Publications, Jersey City, NJ, 1970.

Compendium of Animal Rabies Control, 1992. *JAVMA* 200:145-149, 1992.

Davis J *et al: Infectious Diseases of Wild Mammals.* Iowa State University Press, Ames, 1981.

Davis JW and Anderson RC: *Parasitic Diseases of Wild Mammals.* Iowa State University Press, Ames, 1973.

Flecknell PA: *Laboratory Animal Anesthesia.* Academic Press, San Diego, 1987.

Fowler ME: *Medicine and Surgery of South American Camelids.* Iowa State University Press, Ames, 1989.

Fowler ME: *Zoo and Wild Animal Medicine.* 2nd ed. Saunders, Philadelphia, 1986.

Fox JG: *Biology and Diseases of the Ferret.* Lea & Febiger, Philadelphia, 1986.

Fraser CM and Mays A: *The Merck Veterinary Manual.* 7th ed. Merck, Rahway, NJ, 1991.

Frye FL: *Biomedical and Surgical Aspects of Captive Reptile Husbandry.* Krieger Publishing, Malabar, FL, 1991.

Hafez ES: *Comparative Reproduction of Nonhuman Primates.* Charles C Thomas, Springfield, IL, 1971.

Harkness JE: Exotic pet medicine. *Vet Clin No Am* (Small Anim Pract) 17:981-1233, 1987.

Harkness JE and Wagner JE: *The Biology and Medicine of Rabbits and Rodents.* 3rd ed. Lea & Febiger, Philadelphia, 1989.

Jacobson ER *et al: Diseases of Amphibians and Reptiles.* Plenum Press, New York, 1988.

Jacobson ER: Reptiles. *Vet Clin No Am* (Small Anim Pract) 17:1203-1225, 1987.

Jacobson ER and Kollias GV: *Exotic Animals.* Churchill Livingstone, New York, 1988.

Journal of Zoo and Wildlife Medicine. AAZV, 810 E. 10th St, Lawrence, KS.Published quarterly.

Laboratory Animal Management: Nonhuman Primates. National Academy Press, Washington, DC, 1980.

Poole T: *The UFAW Handbook on the Care and Management of Laboratory Animals.* Churchill Livingstone, New York, 1987.

Porter K: *Herpetology.* Saunders, Philadelphia, 1972.

Proceedings of American Association of Zoo Veterinarians. Published annually.

Stoskopf MK: Tropical fish medicine. *Vet Clin No Am* (Small Anim Pract) 18:283-474, 1988.

Vaughan T: *Mammalogy.* Saunders, Philadelphia, 1972.

Wallach JD and Boever WJ: *Diseases of Exotic Animals: Medical and Surgical Management.* Saunders, Philadelphia, 1983.

Practice answer sheet is on page 367.

Questions

1. *Ferrets are highly susceptible to:*

   a. canine parvovirus infection
   b. feline panleukopenia
   c. mink viral enteritis
   d. canine distemper
   e. feline rhinotracheitis

For Questions 2 through 4, select the correct answer from the 5 choices below.

   a. bitch
   b. jill
   c. pup
   d. kit
   e. hob

2. *A male ferret.*

3. *A female ferret.*

4. *A baby ferret.*

5. *Ferrets have an average litter size of 8 (range, 2-17). The deaf, blind infants are born after an average gestation of:*

   a. 21 days
   b. 32 days
   c. 42 days
   d. 50 days
   e. 64 days

6. *Though somewhat variable, gestation in llamas normally lasts approximately:*

   a. 113-125 days
   b. 140-155 days
   c. 260-280 days
   d. 330-360 days
   e. 390-450 days

7. *Except boas and pythons, most snakes have only a single functional:*

   a. kidney
   b. lung
   c. gonad
   d. hemipenis
   e. diaphragm

For Questions 8 through 12, select the correct answer from the 5 choices below.

   a. all nonmammalian vertebrates
   b. elephants
   c. deer
   d. camels and llamas
   e. rabbits

8. *They normally have a large number of bilobed monocytes in peripheral blood.*

9. *Their erythrocytes develop "sickle cell" appearance very shortly after collection.*

10. *They normally have large elliptic erythrocytes in peripheral blood.*

11. *They normally have nucleated erythrocytes in peripheral blood.*

12. *They have heterophil-type leukocytes in peripheral blood.*

13. *When collecting a blood sample from a turtle or tortoise for hematologic analysis,:*

   a. EDTA should be used as an anticoagulant because it allows for excellent preservation of cellular morphology
   b. slides must be made immediately because no commercial anticoagulant prevents clotting of samples
   c. heparin should be avoided as an anticoagulant because it lyses the erythrocytes
   d. EDTA should be avoided as an anticoagulant because it lyses the erythrocytes
   e. the only effective anticoagulant is acid citrate dextrose

14. *What type of gastrointestinal system do giraffes have?*

   a. simple monogastric, similar to pigs
   b. hindgut fermentation, similar to horses
   c. foregut fermentation with 4 forestomachs, similar to cattle
   d. foregut fermentation with 3 forestomachs, similar to llamas
   e. hindgut fermentation, similar to elephants

15. *In most snake species, what is the approximate location of the heart?*

   a. at 10-20% of the distance from its snout to vent
   b. at 20-30% of the distance from its snout to vent
   c. at 30-40% of the distance from its snout to vent
   d. at 40-50% of the distance from its snout to vent
   e. the distance varies widely between individuals and species

16. *Which camelid is considered an endangered species?*

   a. llama
   b. alpaca
   c. vicuna
   d. guanaco
   e. dromedary

17. *From birth to weaning, a young llama is called a:*

   a. calf
   b. kid
   c. cria
   d. kit
   e. lamb

18. *The most reliable site for intradermal injection of tuberculin for tuberculosis testing in a llama is the:*

   a. caudal tail fold
   b. cervical skin
   c. axillary skin
   d. vulvar skin
   e. skin of the eyelid

19. *The normal body temperature for an adult llama is:*

   a. 101.5-104.5 F
   b. 94.5-96.8 F
   c. 96.8-100 F
   d. 102-104 F
   e. 99.5-102 F

20. *Blood is easily collected from llamas at any of the following veins* ***except*** *one. At which site is venipuncture particularly difficult?*

   a. jugular vein, high on the lateral surface of the neck, approximately 4-6 cm ventral to the corner of the jaw
   b. jugular vein, low on the neck, near the thoracic inlet
   c. saphenous vein, on the lateral aspect of the stifle
   d. middle coccygeal vein, on the ventral aspect of the tail
   e. jugular vein, at mid-level on the lateral surface of the neck, lateral to the esophagus on the left side

Correct answers are on pages 128-129.

21. A peculiarity of llama blood is that the:

a. hemoglobin level is lower than in horses and cattle
b. erythrocytes are thin and ellipsoid
c. erythrocytes are nucleated
d. mean corpuscular volume is greater than in other livestock
e. erythrocytes are thick, resulting in high blood viscosity

22. Concerning camelids, which statement is ***least*** *accurate?*

a. Male llamas have an incisor tooth in the maxillary dental arcade.
b. The stomach consists of 4 compartments.
c. All compartments of the stomach are glandular.
d. The cheek teeth are selenodont in nature.
e. The permanent incisor teeth erupt at 2-2.5 years of age.

23. All of the following are considered normal food for an iguana ***except:***

a. small mammals
b. birds
c. insects
d. fruits and vegetables
e. mollusks and gastropods

*24. All of the following are probably normal food items for a gopher tortoise (*Gopherus polyphemus*)* ***except:***

a. miscellaneous meats
b. fish
c. flowers
d. fruit
e. insects

25. Which of the following is ***not*** *a characteristic of a monotreme?*

a. lays eggs
b. may have a pouch
c. has a cloaca
d. males have undescended testicles
e. the adult teeth lack cusps

26. Concerning marsupials, which statement is ***least*** *accurate?*

a. All marsupials are herbivores.
b. Pouches are found on all females.
c. All marsupials have epipubic bones that articulate with the pubis.
d. Their usual dentition includes 4 molars and 3 premolars in each dental arcade.
e. Marsupial milk has a low lactose content.

27. Concerning lagomorphs, which statement is most accurate?

a. Coprophagy is common in rabbits.
b. Prevention of coprophagy has no effect on the nutritional state of rabbits.
c. All domestic rabbits are descended from wild specimens of *Sylvilagus* (cottontails).
d. All rabbits have 2 upper and 2 lower incisor teeth.
e. Myxomatosis vaccine should be used on all wild lagomorphs in captivity.

28. An anorectic elephant has a rectal temperature of 38 C (100 F). This temperature is appropriately considered:

a. normal
b. slightly elevated but not significant
c. elevated and quite significant
d. below normal but not significant
e. extremely low and quite significant

29. In reptiles, infection with the protozoan Isospora *is confined to the:*

a. gallbladder
b. kidneys
c. intestines
d. bile ducts
e. brain

30. To maintain a functional and comfortable body temperature, the preferred optimum ambient temperature range for housing most tortoises is:

a. 26-32 C (79-90 F)
b. 21-26 C (70-79 F)

c. 16-20 C (60-69 F)
d. 32-35 C (90-95 F)
e. not critical because tortoises have excellent thermoregulatory capacity

31. *Normal, mature reptilian erythrocytes are:*

a. elliptic and nucleated
b. elliptic with no nucleus
c. oval and nucleated
d. oval with no nucleus
e. nucleated and irregularly shaped

32. *Chinchillas in captivity are predisposed to a variety of skin problems. To avoid these problems, chinchillas should be:*

a. provided with rocks and branches for rubbing so as to facilitate shedding and stimulate hair regrowth
b. misted with water daily
c. kept at 90-100 F, with a relative humidity of 80-90%
d. provided with dust baths and a cool, dry environment
e. brushed daily with a soft brush

33. *If guinea pigs are to be allowed to produce young, females should be bred before 6-9 months of age so as to prevent:*

a. permanent fusion of the pelvic symphysis
b. cannibalism of the young
c. attacks on the male by the female
d. dystocia due to large fetuses
e. abandonment of the young

34. *The Bactrian camel has 2 prominent dorsal humps that:*

a. are easily damaged if weight is placed between them; riders or packs should be placed caudal to the second hump
b. are filled with spongiose tissue capable of storing fluid for use during periods of water restriction
c. are primarily used in heat exchange to help maintain homeostatic body temperatures in extremely hot climates
d. are depots of subcutaneous fat used during periods of food deprivation
e. secrete a musk-like substance during rut, which flows ventrally over the body

35. *When a deer's antlers are covered by velvet, the antlers:*

a. are covered with a thick, strong, cornified material firmly attached to the antler
b. are shed within 3-4 days
c. should be covered with a thin layer of adhesive tape to prevent discoloration of the outer layer of velvet
d. are highly vascular, and damage can cause profuse hemorrhage and attract flies, with resultant infestation of maggots
e. can be easily removed from the deer by slight pressure, and any hemorrhage can be easily controlled with digital pressure

36. *The male dromedary has a structure called the gula, which is used to make a sound when the animal is excited or angered. This structure arises from the:*

a. cheek pouches
b. syrinx
c. soft palate
d. arytenoid cartilages
e. laryngeal folds

37. *Because of their unique anatomy and physiology, a major concern when restraining bears is:*

a. the danger of hyperthermia because of their thick layer of subcutaneous fat
b. their characteristically short neck and thick muzzle, making them especially difficult to snare
c. cardiac failure from increase of their normally high blood pressure by stress
d. extreme acidosis stemming from rapid production of lactic acid
e. cyanosis because bears cannot adequately oxygenate blood during acute periods of stress

Correct answers are on pages 128-129.

38. *In an established wolf pack, dominant females often do **not**:*

a. mate but continue to hunt throughout the year
b. allow other females to mate
c. mate but go through a false pregnancy
d. produce offspring, though they mate frequently
e. enter into estrus until late in the season and mate only if no other litters have been produced

39. *The digestive system of elephants is similar to that of:*

a. mice
b. cattle
c. pigs
d. people
e. horses

40. *In ferrets, venous blood is most easily collected from the:*

a. cephalic vein
b. saphenous vein
c. jugular vein
d. tarsal vein
e. median vein

41. *How often do female rabbits normally nurse their young?*

a. once a day
b. 4 times a day
c. 6 times a day
d. every 2 hours
e. hourly

42. *Rabbits should be picked up:*

a. by the ears using one hand
b. by the scruff using one hand
c. behind the shoulders using both hands
d. by the scruff using one hand while supporting the hind end with the other hand
e. by the ears using one hand while supporting the hind end with the other hand

43. *What is the preferred ambient temperature range for housing domestic rabbits?*

a. 60-70 F
b. 70-80 F
c. 90-90 F
d. 72-75 F
e. 75-80 F

44. *The gestation length of guinea pigs is:*

a. 21 days
b. 28 days
c. 42 days
d. 45 days
e. 63 days

45. *Which species normally produces scant amounts of highly concentrated urine?*

a. mouse
b. rat
c. hamster
d. gerbil
e. guinea pig

46. *Which species has open-rooted molars that may lead to malocclusion?*

a. rat
b. mouse
c. gerbil
d. hamster
e. guinea pig

47. *In which species is dystocia a major problem?*

a. rat
b. hamster
c. gerbil
d. rabbit
e. guinea pig

48. In which species is it absolutely necessary to remove the male before parturition?

a. rat
b. mouse
c. gerbil
d. hamster
e. guinea pig

49. Which species bears young that are precocial (fully furred, eyes open)?

a. mouse
b. rat
c. hamster
d. gerbil
e. guinea pig

50. The average life span of mice, rats and hamsters is:

a. 6 months
b. 1 year
c. 2 years
d. 4 years
e. 6 years

51. Which species has cheek pouches?

a. mouse
b. rat
c. chinchilla
d. guinea pig
e. hamster

*52. Which species has the **shortest** gestation period?*

a. mouse
b. rat
c. guinea pig
d. hamster
e. chinchilla

*53. Which species has the **longest** gestation period?*

a. mouse
b. rat
c. guinea pig
d. hamster
e. chinchilla

54. Which species hibernates at ambient temperatures of 40-60 F?

a. rabbit
b. rat
c. guinea pig
d. hamster
e. chinchilla

55. As you enter an ostrich enclosure, a male develops a spiral appearance to the neck. This is a sign of:

a. sexual attraction
b. surprise
c. illness
d. aggression
e. submission

56. The most common chronic disease problem in managing captive elephants is related to:

a. the skin
b. diet
c. weight
d. the teeth
e. foot care

57. In elephants, gestation lasts for:

a. 11 months
b. 24 months
c. 22 months
d. 16 months
e. 18 months

58. In nonhuman primates, venous blood is most easily collected from the:

a. jugular vein
b. saphenous vein
c. femoral vein
d. cephalic vein
e. tail vein

Correct answers are on pages 128-129.

59. *Penicillin and other penicillin-like antibiotics are **not** recommended for use in rodents and lagomorphs (rabbits, hares) because:*

a. these drugs are ineffective in those species
b. rodents and lagomorphs are allergic to these antibiotics
c. rodents and lagomorphs possess Gram-positive gut microorganisms; elimination of these organisms may result in fatal colibacillosis
d. rodents and lagomorphs possess Gram-negative gut microorganisms; elimination of these organisms may result in fatal colibacillosis
e. rodents and lagomorphs are not prone to infection with microorganisms that are likely to be sensitive to penicillin-like antibiotics

60. *Many reptiles have moveable eyelids. Which reptiles **lack** these structures?*

a. turtles, tortoises and terrapins
b. alligators, caimans, crocodiles and gharials
c. snakes and some lizards
d. the tuatara, a sole survivor of the Mesozoic era, native to some small islands off the coast of New Zealand
e. frogs and toads

61. *Rapidly growing juvenile lizards, such as green iguanas, often develop metabolic bone disease as a result of which dietary imbalance?*

a. vitamin A deficiency and vitamin D excess
b. vitamin C excess and vitamin E deficiency
c. vitamin B_1 deficiency and vitamin D excess
d. vitamin D deficiency and calcium deficiency
e. vitamin D deficiency and phosphorus deficiency

62. *Metabolic bone disease is relatively common in herbivorous or insectivorous lizards kept in captivity. The most likely cause of this disorder of osseous mineralization is:*

a. deficiency of vitamin D and phosphorus
b. deficiency of vitamin D, an imbalance or deficiency of calcium and excessive phosphorus
c. deficiency of vitamin D and beta carotene
d. deficiency of vitamin D , excessive vitamin A
e. deficiency of vitamin D, excessive pyridoxine

63. *Which nutrient is **not** synthesized by guinea pigs?*

a. lipids
b. vitamin C
c. sulfur-containing amino acids
d. vitamin B_1
e. vitamin K

Answers

1. **d** Ferrets are exquisitely sensitive to canine distemper virus. Modified-live-virus canine distemper vaccines are frequently produced from ferret cell lines.
2. **e**
3. **b** Female dogs are bitches, foxes are vixens and ferrets are jills.
4. **d** Juvenile dogs are pups; young ferrets and foxes are kits.
5. **c** Gestation in ferrets lasts 42 days.
6. **d** Old World camels have a longer gestation (approximately 390 days).
7. **b** Boas and pythons have a small left lung; other snakes have only a functional right lung. Reptiles do not have a functional diaphragm. The other listed organs are paired.
8. **b**
9. **c** The red blood cells of deer are disk shaped *in vivo* but rapidly assume a sickle shape *in*

vitro. This is usually due to the high pH of diluting fluids or to elevated oxygen tension.

10. **d** The size and shape of camelid red blood cells may make the cells resistant to osmotic lysis during rapid expansion of vascular volume when the animal ingests large amounts of water.
11. **a**
12. **e**
13. **d** EDTA often lyses tortoise erythrocytes. Heparin works well as an anticoagulant.
14. **c** Giraffes are true ruminants.
15. **b** Viperidae are an exception, and have a heart farther caudal than in other snakes.
16. **c**
17. **c**
18. **c** This site is currently recommended, but this may change in the near future, when only a blood test may be accepted.
19. **e**
20. **e** Jugular venipuncture is almost impossible in this area because of the muscle mass covering the vein.
21. **b** This apparently is an adaptation to high altitudes.
22. **b** The stomach of camelids consists of only 3 compartments.
23. **e**
24. **b**
25. **e** Adult monotremes rarely have teeth.
26. **a** Some marsupials are omnivores and a few are carnivores.
27. **a**
28. **c**
29. **c**
30. **a** 26-32 C represents the ambient temperature that most tortoises encounter in their natural habitat.
31. **c**
32. **d**
33. **a**
34. **d**
35. **d**
36. **c**
37. **a**
38. **b**
39. **e**
40. **c**
41. **a** Female rabbits nurse their young in the morning or evening, but spend most of the time away from the nest.
42. **d** The rear end must be supported or the rabbit can kick out and cause vertebral fractures and paralysis. Rabbits should *never* be picked up by the ears.
43. **a** Rabbits prefer relatively cool ambient temperatures.
44. **e** This is the same gestation length as in dogs and cats.
45. **d** Gerbils are desert dwellers that drink little and produce small amounts of urine.
46. **e**
47. **e** If a guinea pig is bred for the first time after 8 months of age, the pelvic bones cannot separate adequately at parturition and dystocia is likely.
48. **d** Female hamsters should be housed alone after breeding because they may attack and kill the male. They should not be disturbed for at least a week following parturition, as any disturbance could cause them to cannibalize their young. In all of the other species listed, the male helps care for the young.
49. **e**
50. **c**
51. **e**
52. **d** Gestation lasts only 16 days in hamsters.
53. **e** Gestation lasts 3-4 months in chinchillas.
54. **d**
55. **d**
56. **e**
57. **c**
58. **c**
59. **c**
60. **c** Snakes and some lizards lack moveable eyelids.
61. **d** Deficiency of vitamin D and calcium often leads to metabolic bone disease.
62. **b** Deficiency of vitamin D, an imbalance of deficiency of calcium, and excessive phosphorus often lead to metabolic bone disease.
63. **b** Vitamin C is not synthesized by guinea pigs; it must be present in their diet.

Notes

Section **13**

Clinic Administration and Client Relations

A.H. Bush, J.B. McCarthy, P.M. Newman, P.K. Stockner

Recommended Reading

Lawson JG and McConnell JW: *Starting and Managing Your Practice.* Oelgeschlager, Gunn & Hain, Cambridge, MA.

McCarthy JB: *Basic Guide to Veterinary Hospital Management.* American Animal Hospital Association, Denver, CO, 1992.

McCurnin DM: *Veterinary Practice Management.* Lippincott, Philadelphia, 1988.

Musselman VA and Jackson JH: *Introduction to Modern Business.* 10th ed. Prentice-Hall, Englewood Cliffs, NJ.

Pratt PW: *Veterinary Practice Management.* American Veterinary Publications, Goleta, CA, 1979.

Stockner PK: *A Practice Management Manual for Veterinarians.* Available from the author, 1992.

Successful Financial Management for the Veterinary Practice. Am Animal Hosp Assn, Denver, CO.

Thomas JM and Gustafson M: *Valuing Your Business.* Holt Rinehart & Winston, New York.

Veterinary Economics. Published monthly by Veterinary Medicine Publishing, Lenexa, KS.

Wilson JF: *Business Guide for Veterinary Practice.* Squibb, Vet Learning Systems, Trenton, NJ.

Wilson JF: *Law and Ethics in the Veterinary Profession.* Priority Press, Yardley, PA, 1988.

Practice answer sheet is on page 369.

Correct answers are on pages 139-140.

Questions

1. *The most important skill that the successful clinic administrator (manager) can have is the ability to:*

   a. diagnose diseases over the telephone
   b. hire new employees
   c. communicate with other people
   d. organize hospital open houses
   e. use a computer

2. *Successful administrators (managers) should:*

   a. be aware of their own values and management style
   b. be unwilling to listen to concerns about their management style
   c. never criticize or reprimand anyone they are managing
   d. try to intimidate staff members
   e. avoid being assertive

3. *Which of the following is **not** an effective means of communication between management and staff in a well-managed animal hospital?*

   a. personnel policy manual
   b. staff meetings
   c. handwritten notes
   d. verbal messages
   e. bulletin boards

4. *Job descriptions:*

   a. are unnecessary
   b. are written once and never changed
   c. state the essential functions of various jobs
   d. are not written for the hospital manager
   e. can legally state that a disability would make a job candidate unacceptable

5. *Which of the following questions should **not** be asked on a job application or in a job interview?*

   a. "Tell me about yourself."
   b. "Why are you leaving your present position?"
   c. "How does this position fit your long-term goals?"
   d. "Is there any medical reason that would affect your doing this job?"
   e. "What jobs have you held?"

6. *Which of the following questions can be legally asked on a job application or in an interview?*

   a. "Are you married?"
   b. "What ages are your children?"
   c. "What church do you attend?"
   d. "Can you perform the essential functions of this job?"
   e. "Do you have a disability?"

7. *The best person on a hospital staff to train a new receptionist is:*

   a. the doctor
   b. a recently fired receptionist
   c. the hospital administrator (manager)
   d. the hospital accountant
   e. a recently hired receptionist

8. *As a hospital administrator (manager), you are required to fire an employee. Concerning termination of employment, which statement is **least** accurate?*

   a. Firing an employee should be done with dignity and your emotions should be controlled.
   b. The reasons for the firing must be documented in writing and explained to the employee, and a record of the meeting placed in the employee's personnel file.
   c. The fired employee should be asked to stay until a replacement can be found.
   d. The firing should not be done when you are angry or in haste at the time of transgression.
   e. The fired employee should be told what your intentions are with regard to giving him or her a reference for a future job.

*9. Which aspect of personnel management is **not** covered by a federal or state law or regulation?*

a. paid holidays and sick leave
b. employment of noncitizens
c. occupational hazards
d. minimum wage scale
e. sexual harassment

10. When answering the ABC Animal Hospital telephone, which of the following is the most appropriate greeting?

a. "Hello."
b. "ABC Animal Hospital."
c. "ABC Animal Hospital, this is Mary. How may I help you?"
d. "ABC Animal Hospital, hold please." CLICK
e. "Animal Hospital."

*11. Which of the following is the **least** effective means of communicating with clients?*

a. hospital information brochure
b. pamphlets and brochures on various diseases
c. hospital newsletters
d. verbal explanations
e. client satisfaction surveys

12. When handling a client who is annoyed about a hospital charge, the receptionist should:

a. argue with the client
b. tell the client to leave and not return
c. refer the client to the doctor or hospital manager
d. tell the client that the bill will be sent to a collection agency
e. tell the client to sue the hospital

*13. Financial transactions should be recorded for all of the following reasons **except**:*

a. provide the client with an itemized list of charges
b. provide the client with a diagnosis of the patient's condition
c. provide the client with a statement of charges to be paid
d. provide the hospital with necessary information for its financial records
e. provide the hospital with information required by law

14. Accounts receivable are:

a. usually written off as uncollectable after 15 days
b. revenue earned but not received at the time the service was rendered
c. credit card charges received for services rendered
d. personal checks received for services rendered
e. a good way to receive payment for services rendered

15. When calling a client about an overdue bill, you should:

a. threaten to distribute bad credit information about the client
b. call at midnight to make sure they are home
c. threaten physical harm if the bill is not paid
d. have all of the information available about the overdue account in front of you
e. start the conversation by asking how the patient is

*16. Concerning internal control, which statement is **least** accurate?*

a. Internal control is all measures used by a business to prevent errors, waste, fraud and loss so as to ensure the reliability of the hospital's financial data.
b. Internal control generally concerns itself with loss of revenue because of the action of some staff member.
c. Internal control includes collection of overdue accounts receivable.
d. Internal control dictates that staff members handling money be carefully selected and bonded.
e. Internal control includes serially numbered charge slips, and approval of any discounts and writeoffs by the hospital manager or doctor.

Correct answers are on pages 139-140.

17. If a hospital administrator (manager) suspects employee embezzlement, s/he should:

a. confront the employee and tell him or her how much money is missing
b. say nothing because the suspected employee is probably doing a good job otherwise
c. notify the hospital owners and ask the hospital accountant and lawyer for advice
d. call the police
e. allow the employee to resolve the problem by promising to repay the embezzled money

For Questions 18 through 22, select the correct answer from the 5 choices below.

a. assets
b. liabilities
c. equity
d. balance sheet
e. income statement

18. Report used to evaluate the performance of a business by comparing or matching revenue with related expenses during a particular period.

19. Resources owned by a business, including buildings, land, supplies, cash on hand and accounts receivable.

20. The amount invested in a business, plus the amount of profit retained in the business.

21. A financial statement that shows the financial position of a business by summarizing the assets, liabilities and owners' equity as of a particular date.

22. The debts or obligations of a business, including accounts payable, mortgages payable and taxes due.

23. Which of the following most accurately describes the cash basis of accounting?

a. accounts receivable are declared as income
b. revenue is recorded when received and expenses are recorded when paid
c. cost of an inventory item is not considered an expense until it is sold
d. expenses are deferred for payment during a period of higher tax obligations
e. income and expense are matched in the same period in which they are earned and spent

24. Medical records:

a. are the property of the client and must be sent to any client leaving the area
b. can be shared with any party requesting copies
c. can be thrown away if the client moves away
d. are essential for the defense of civil or criminal suits for malpractice
e. do not include radiographs and lab reports

25. Medical records that are considered legally valid include all of the following ***except:***

a. computerized records
b. handwritten records
c. records that have been altered
d. problem-oriented records
e. source-oriented records

26. Which of the following is normally ***not*** *a part of a problem-oriented medical record?*

a. subjective information, including the presenting complaint and history
b. objective information, including examination and laboratory findings
c. financial information, including credit references
d. assessment of clinical data, including a provisional diagnosis
e. plans for further diagnostic studies, medical treatment and possible surgery

27. For which of the following is maintenance of a written record/log required by federal law?

a. radiographic procedures
b. laboratory tests
c. surgical procedures

d. dispensing of controlled substances
e. necropsy reports

*28. Concerning computerized patient records, which statement is **least** accurate?*

a. They may become inaccessible in the event of computer failure without backup copies.
b. They may be used to "target" selected parts of the patient database for promotional mailings.
c. They are relatively easily maintained, using commercially available practice management computer programs.
d. Once information is entered into a patient's record, it cannot be altered.
e. Patient records usually can be rapidly located by the pet's name, owner's name or other owner information.

*29. Concerning an effective inventory control system, which statement is **least** accurate?*

a. It ensures that patients and clients have the necessary medications and supplies when they need them.
b. It allows all doctors in the practice to order drugs and supplies at any time.
c. It allows accurate assessment of the value of the inventory on hand at any time.
d. It allows the hospital to do cost-effective purchasing.
e. It ensures that controlled substances are properly monitored and dispensed.

Questions 30 through 33

An owner reluctantly agrees to take the doctor's advice and have her beloved pet euthanized after several days of unsuccessful treatment. Personally, you disagree with the doctor's recommendation and think that more time should be allowed for treatment.

30. As a staff member, what is the most appropriate course of action?

a. reinforce the doctor's recommendation or remove yourself from the case
b. confide to the client that you disagree with the doctor's recommendation
c. display no concern to the client because "it is only an animal"
d. let the owner go home with unresolved feelings of guilt
e. discourage the owner from seeing the pet and being present during euthanasia

*31. The owner insists on being present during euthanasia. Which of the following is **least** appropriate in this situation?*

a. explain the procedure of euthanasia to the client, and possible reactions of the animal
b. allow the client to spend some time alone with the animal before euthanasia
c. educate the owner on normal grieving responses
d. schedule euthanasia during a very busy period so the client will be distracted and not display grief
e. discuss involved fees and disposition of the animal's remains before euthanasia is performed

32. A week after euthanasia is performed, the owner calls, accusing the doctor of unnecessarily killing her pet. What is the most appropriate course of action?

a. agree with her
b. tell her that she is experiencing normal grieving and that those feelings will subside
c. suggest that the owner consult a grief counselor (have a name to suggest) or a trusted clergy person
d. defend the doctor's decision, even if an argument results
e. tell the owner that she needs a new pet to resolve her feelings of grief

*33. Which of the following is **not** a normal reaction to loss of a beloved pet?*

a. denial
b. anger
c. guilt
d. ritual
e. depression

Correct answers are on pages 139-140.

34. *Marketing of veterinary services:*

a. is illegal and an indication of a highly unethical veterinarian
b. is legal but unethical
c. is another name for advertising, which should be avoided by any professional
d. includes client relations, appearance of the hospital, speaking with clients, sending newsletters, and giving career talks at schools
e. should only be done by veterinary associations

35. *Which of the following is **not** a consideration of marketing (the "4 Ps")?*

a. people
b. place
c. price
d. product
e. promotion

For Questions 36 through 39, select the correct answer from the 4 choices below.

a. segmentation
b. frequency
c. target marketing
d. message

36. *Identifying a group of clients by specific characteristics, such as age, income, zip code, or breed or age of pet.*

37. *Information presented to clients regarding their animal's health.*

38. *The average number of times that an audience is exposed to a message in a given period.*

39. *Directing a promotional effort toward one or more identifiable groups.*

For Questions 40 through 43, select the correct answer from the 4 choices below.

a. personal selling
b. publicity
c. public relations
d. advertising

40. *Any paid form of mass communication designed primarily to attract new clients to the hospital.*

41. *Any activity initiated by the hospital to create a positive image with current and potential clients.*

42. *Personal communication to inform a client about their animal's health.*

43. *Any unpaid communication conveyed through the media.*

44. *Which of the following is **not** a form of public relations?*

a. practice newsletters
b. Yellow Pages advertising
c. sympathy letters and charitable donations in the name of deceased pets
d. hospital brochures and handouts
e. talks to schools, kennel clubs and scout groups

45. *Which of the following is **not** a piece of computer hardware (machinery or equipment)?*

a. mouse
b. word processing program
c. printer
d. video display terminal
e. modem

46. *In a computer, a hard-disk drive:*

a. is easily damaged by dust and animal hair
b. can be easily removed from the computer in seconds and without tools
c. holds more information than floppy disks
d. locates information more slowly than floppy-disk drives
e. is not a component of laptop or portable computers

47. Computers have become very popular in veterinary hospitals because they:

a. have replaced receptionists
b. are very inexpensive
c. have vast ability to store and access information
d. automatically correct errors in data entered
e. have replaced hospital accountants and attorneys

48. Adding a service charge or interest on an account receivable (unpaid bill) is:

a. illegal
b. legal but must be explained to the client
c. not a good business practice
d. difficult to calculate if your accounts receivable are computerized
e. a way to encourage clients to defer payment of fees

*49. Which of the following is **not** a valid reason for an animal hospital to own a computer?*

a. inventory control
b. generate vaccination reminders
c. generate public relations materials
d. store medical records
e. impress clients

*50. Which federal agency does **not** regulate legal use of veterinary pharmaceuticals and biologics?*

a. Food and Drug Administration
b. Department of Agriculture
c. Environmental Protection Agency
d. National Institute of Health
e. Drug Enforcement Administration

*51. Which of the following is **not** a purpose of routine staff meetings?*

a. confront problems
b. improve communications
c. improve staff training
d. discuss and agree on new practice policies
e. reprimand staff members

52. Most clients patronize a particular veterinary practice because:

a. they trust the veterinarian
b. the practice is conveniently located
c. the practice has the lowest fees
d. the practice offers full service
e. they are not kept waiting during visits to the practice

*53. Which of these is **not** a reason to have new clients complete an information form?*

a. to keep accurate statistics on numbers of new clients
b. to discover how a new client learned about your practice
c. to discover who referred the new client so that you can send a "thank you" note
d. to learn what new clients want from your practice
e. to learn what new clients want to see improved in your practice

*54. Appointment books are critical to the success of a practice. Which of the following is **not** an important aspect of appointment books?*

a. they help control the flow of client visits
b. they provide a quick visual reference of recent and near-future client visits
c. they help to minimize client waiting time
d. they provide data that can be used to schedule staff work shifts
e. they allow for scheduling of emergencies

55. When a telephoning client is put on hold, which of the following is the most important consideration?

a. the length of time they must remain on hold
b. how courteous you are when you return to the line
c. the music played while the client is on hold
d. the recorded messages presented while the client is on hold
e. ensuring that the call does not involve an emergency before the client is put on hold

Correct answers are on pages 139-140.

56. Clients are most likely to stop patronizing a particular veterinary practice because of:

a. moving to another area
b. death of their animal
c. excessively high fees
d. inconvenient office hours
e. perceived lack of concern by the staff

57. Clients patronize a veterinary practice for 2 main reasons: to resolve their animal's health problems and to:

a. purchase over-the-counter drugs
b. obtain advice on preventive care
c. have elective surgery performed
d. have access to emergency care
e. feel that they are providing excellent care for their animal

58. In interacting with a client, a crucial point in the interaction is:

a. being honest with the client
b. saying "thank you"
c. conceding that you cannot resolve every problem
d. any aspect of the interaction that forms the client's opinion about your practice
e. making a profit

59. A written report, given to the client, of the findings on physical examination of a client's animal is helpful because:

a. it is required by law
b. most clients cannot remember findings reported verbally
c. it enhances the client's perceived value of your services and indicates evaluation of many body systems
d. it precludes the need to record findings in the patient's medical record
e. it reduces paperwork and the requirement of record storage in the practice

60. What is the main reason for marking up the dispensed price of all supplies by a fixed percentage?

a. it preserves your profit margin
b. you make a higher percentage of profit on more expensive items
c. you must shop for the best price all of the time
d. it helps to minimize inventory turnover
e. it facilitates calculation of sales taxes

61. When an animal is admitted to a veterinary hospital for treatment, the client should be given a written estimate of treatment costs because:

a. it is required by law
b. it allows the practice to charge higher fees
c. it prevents misunderstandings about the final cost
d. they are useful for tax audits
e. the American Animal Hospital Association requires it for all member hospitals

62. The major reason cited by employees who quit working for a practice is:

a. inadequate pay
b. poor work environment
c. lack of recognition
d. unsafe practices
e. personality conflict

63. Recording of all transactions, including cash transactions,:

a. should be done at the end of the day from memory
b. should be done on a "day sheet"
c. requires a computer
d. is required by law
e. is not necessary

64. Marketing veterinary services by personal interaction with clients:

a. is usually unproductive
b. typically antagonizes clients
c. tends to build trust between the client and the seller

d. necessitates higher fees
e. requires a course in salesmanship

65. Inventory should be stored:

a. where the doctor thinks it should be located
b. in alphabetical order by generic name
c. on open shelves in the center of activity
d. in any special convenient arrangement, as long as storage conditions and security are adequate
e. in the front desk area to improve clients' perception of value

---

Answers

1. **c**
2. **a**
3. **d**
4. **c**
5. **d**
6. **d**
7. **c**
8. **c**
9. **a**
10. **c**
11. **d**
12. **c**
13. **b**
14. **b**
15. **d**
16. **c**
17. **c**
18. **e**
19. **a**
20. **c**
21. **d**
22. **b**
23. **b**
24. **d**
25. **c**
26. **c**
27. **d**
28. **d**
29. **b**
30. **a**
31. **d**
32. **c**
33. **d** According to Helen Kubler Ross, the 4 stages of grief are denial, anger, guilt and depression.
34. **d**
35. **a**
36. **a**
37. **d**
38. **b**
39. **c**
40. **d**
41. **c**
42. **a**
43. **b**
44. **b**
45. **b**
46. **c**
47. **c**
48. **b**
49. **e**
50. **d**
51. **e** Reprimands should be given in private.
52. **a** Convenience is often touted as the most important factor in practice success. However, over the long run, if clients do not have confidence in the veterinarian, they will patronize another practice.
53. **e** A new client cannot suggest improvements if s/he has not yet used your services.
54. **e**
55. **e**

56. **e** Clients' perception of your care and concern is most important.

57. **e**

58. **d** Any interaction that causes a client to form an opinion of your business is important.

59. **c** Clients will perceive the exam as having more value if they receive a written report of your findings.

60. **a** It allows you to pass on any price increases to the client, so your profit margin is maintained.

61. **c**

62. **c**

63. **b**

64. **c**

65. **d**

Notes

Section 14

Dentistry

G.J. Baker, R.B. Wiggs

Recommended Reading

Bojrab MJ and Tholen M: *Small Animal Oral Medicine and Surgery.* Lea & Febiger, Philadelphia, 1990.
Emily P and Penman S: *Handbook of Small Animal Dentistry.* Pergammon Press, Oxford, 1990.
Harvey CE: Feline dentistry. *Vet Clin No Am* (Small Anim Pract) 22:1265-1495, 1992.
Harvey CE: *Veterinary Dentistry.* Saunders, Philadelphia, 1985.
Holmstrom SE *et al: Veterinary Dental Techniques.* Saunders, Philadelphia, 1992.
Marretta-Manfra S: Dentistry. *Problems in Veterinary Medicine* 2:1-278, 1990.
Wiggs RB: Canine oral anatomy and physiology. *Comp Cont Ed Pract Vet* 11:1475-1482, 1989.

Practice answer sheet is on page 371.

Questions

For Questions 1 through 5, select the correct answer from the 5 choices below.

a. posterior crossbite
b. base-narrow mandibular canines
c. wry mouth
d. anterior crossbite
e. open bite

1. *Malocclusion in which one side of the mandible or maxilla is disproportionate to its other side, and the incisor midline of the mandible does not match the incisor midline of the maxilla.*

2. *When the mouth is closed as fully as possible, a gap or space remains between the upper and lower incisors.*

3. *Malocclusion of the permanent incisors resulting from retained deciduous teeth displacing their normal eruption position, with no indications of disproportionate jaw length.*

4. *Malocclusion in which the upper fourth premolars lie medial to the lower first molars.*

5. *Malocclusion of the permanent lower canine teeth resulting from retained deciduous teeth displacing their normal eruption position and causing trauma to the hard palate.*

Correct answers are on pages 147-148.

For Questions 6 through 10, select the correct answer from the 5 choices below.

a. 2 x (I 3/3; C 1/1; P 3/2) = 26
b. 2 x (I 3/3; C 1/1; P 4/4; M 2/3) = 42
c. 2 x (I 3/3; C 1/1; P 3/2; M 1/1) = 30
d. 2 x (I 3/3; C 1/1; P 3/3) = 28
e. 2 x (I 3/3; C 1/1; P 4/4; M 3/3) = 44

6. *Dental formula for deciduous or temporary teeth of dogs.*

7. *Dental formula for permanent teeth of dogs.*

8. *Dental formula for deciduous or temporary teeth of cats.*

9. *Dental formula for permanent teeth of cats.*

10. *Dental formula for permanent teeth of swine.*

For Questions 11 through 15, select the correct answer from the 5 choices below.

a. premolars
b. molars
c. incisors
d. carnassials
e. canines or cuspids

11. *Teeth anatomically suited to grooming, nibbling and cutting.*

12. *Teeth anatomically suited to holding, grasping and tearing.*

13. *Teeth anatomically suited to holding, shearing and cutting.*

14. *Teeth anatomically suited to grinding.*

15. *Largest shearing cheek teeth.*

For Questions 16 through 20, select the correct answer from the 5 choices below.

a. enamel
b. dentin
c. cementoenamel junction
d. enamodentinal junction
e. cementum

16. *The outside coating of the normally exposed portion of a cat's tooth.*

17. *The hard portion of the tooth that constitutes the majority of the tooth's hard structure.*

18. *The modified bone-like structure on the outer surface of the root of a dog's tooth.*

19. *Juncture on the outside of the tooth where crown and root meet.*

20. *Juncture of the enamel and the hard tissue immediately deep to it.*

For Questions 21 through 25, select the correct answer from the 5 choices below.

a. apex
b. crown
c. root
d. neck
e. pulp cavity

21. *Normally exposed portion of the tooth.*

22. *Juncture of the crown and root.*

23. *Portion of the tooth normally embedded in the periodontium.*

24. *Deep tip of the root.*

25. *Open area within the tooth, occupied by soft tissues.*

26. *In regard to periodontal disease, all of the following are considered part of the peridontium* ***except:***

 a. alveolar bone
 b. pulp
 c. cementum
 d. peridontal ligament
 e. gingiva

For Questions 27 through 31, select the correct answer from the 5 choices below.

 a. root canal
 b. pulp
 c. apical foramen
 d. pulp chamber
 e. apical delta

27. *Interior soft tissue of the tooth.*

28. *Normal part of the cavity within the tooth root.*

29. *Normal portion of the cavity within the tooth crown.*

30. *A single opening in the apex of a tooth root that provides passage for vascular, neural and connective tissues.*

31. *A multiple opening at the apex of the tooth.*

For Questions 32 through 36, select the correct answer from the 5 choices below.

 a. dental elevator
 b. probe
 c. curette
 d. explorer
 e. sickle scaler

32. *Used to scale below the gum line (subgingival).*

33. *Used to scale above the gum line (supragingival).*

34. *Aids in removal of a tooth.*

35. *Used to check teeth for decay, canal exposures and cavities.*

36. *Used to check the depth of the gingival sulcus.*

37. *How often should curettes and hand-scaling instruments be sharpened?*

 a. with each use
 b. once daily
 c. once weekly
 d. once monthly
 e. when chipped or broken

For Questions 38 through 42, select the correct answer from the 5 choices below.

 a. rotosonic
 b. sonic
 c. piezoelectric
 d. magnetostrictive
 e. sickle scaler

38. *Claw-like scaler held by a modified "pen grasp."*

39. *Scaler vibrating at 20-40 kHz, producing an elliptic oscillating pattern through a ferromagnetic rod.*

40. *Scaler vibrating at 20-40 kHz, producing a linear oscillating pattern through changes in shape of a crystal by electric charge.*

41. *Scaler with a tip that vibrates at less than 20 kHz.*

42. *Six-sided soft steel bur, used on a high-speed handpiece.*

Correct answers are on pages 147-148.

43. *The factor primarily contributing to periodontal disease is:*

a. tartar
b. plaque
c. calculus
d. salivary polysaccharides
e. salivary minerals

44. *All of the following predispose to periodontal disease* ***except****:*

a. overcrowded and rotated teeth
b. retained deciduous teeth
c. hard, crunchy diet
d. malocclusions
e. some endocrine and systemic diseases

For Questions 45 through 47, select the correct answer from the 5 choices below.

a. polishing
b. sulcal lavage
c. subgingival curettage
d. scaling
e. root planing

45. *Curettage of rough and disease cementum.*

46. *Curettage of the sulcal epithelium.*

47. *Flushing of the sulcus with a solution.*

For Questions 48 through 52, select the correct answer from the 5 choices below.

a. splinting
b. closed curettage
c. gingivoplasty
d. open curettage
e. odontoplasty

48. *Removal of hyperplastic gingival tissue.*

49. *Root planing in association with a releasing flap.*

50. *Root planing without a gingival flap.*

51. *Removal of a portion of the tooth structure.*

52. *Bonding of loose teeth together to stabilize them during a healing process.*

Questions 53 through 58

In extracting teeth, it is important to know how many roots each type of tooth has.

53. *How many roots do the incisor teeth of dogs have?*

a. 1
b. 2
c. 3
d. usually 1, but sometimes 2
e. usually 3, but sometimes 2

54. *How many roots do the cuspid or canine teeth of dogs have?*

a. 1
b. 2
c. 3
d. usually 1, but sometimes 2
e. usually 3, but sometimes 2

55. *How many roots do the upper fourth premolar teeth of dogs have?*

a. 1
b. 2
c. 3
d. usually 1, but sometimes 2
e. usually 3, but sometimes 2

56. *How many roots do the lower fourth premolar teeth of dogs have?*

a. 1
b. 2
c. 3
d. usually 1, but sometimes 2
e. usually 3, but sometimes 2

57. *How many roots do the upper first molar teeth of dogs have?*

a. 1
b. 2
c. 3
d. usually 1, but sometimes 2
e. usually 3, but sometimes 2

58. *How many roots do the lower first molar teeth of dogs have?*

a. 1
b. 2
c. 3
d. usually 1, but sometimes 2
e. usually 3, but sometimes 2

For Questions 59 through 61, select the correct answer from the 5 choices below.

a. composite
b. acrylic
c. porcelain
d. glass ionomer
e. amalgam

59. *Has a silver and mercury base.*

60. *Most commonly used to treat cervical line lesions in cats.*

61. *A tooth-colored material commonly used to treat lesions or close access sites in dogs' teeth.*

62. *Which substance should* **not** *be used for routine brushing of the teeth of a 14-year-old dog with congestive heart failure?*

a. enzymatic tooth paste
b. baking soda
c. 0.12% chlorhexidine gluconate solution
d. 0.4% stannous fluoride gel
e. zinc ascorbate solution

63. *An adult dog is presented to you for treatment of a tooth with a broken crown and exposed pulp. The injury occurred several weeks before presentation. What is the most appropriate type of treatment?*

a. composite filling
b. application of a crown
c. extraction or root canal therapy
d. amalgam filling
e. glass ionomer filling

64. *All of the following are indications for tooth extraction* ***except:***

a. advanced periodontal disease
b. retained deciduous teeth
c. abscessed tooth
d. chipped tooth without pulpal exposure or pulpitis
e. root fractured near the periodontal sulcus

65. *Under normal conditions, the teeth of a horse wear at the rate of:*

a. 1/16 inch per year
b. 1/8 inch per year
c. 3/16 inch per year
d. 1/4 inch per year
e. 5/16 inch per year

66. *In horses, wolf teeth:*

a. are vestigial in mares
b. are more common in the mandible than in the maxilla
c. have 2 roots
d. have roots half the size of the crown
e. do not make occlusal contact

67. *Periodontal disease in equids:*

a. is caused by accumulation of supragingival calculus
b. is initiated by malocclusion
c. is seen more frequently in ponies
d. is easily treated by gingival resection
e. cannot be prevented

Correct answers are on pages 147-148.

68. In horses, dental prophylaxis (floating) is recommended to:

a. maintain normal occlusion
b. improve appearance (cosmetics)
c. use as a "practice builder"
d. prevent dental caries
e. ensure accuracy in determining the horse's age

69. The lower canine and lateral incisor teeth of baby pigs are routinely clipped soon after birth to:

a. improve weaning weights
b. prevent fighting
c. prevent damage to the dam's teats
d. prevent mandibular malalignment
e. prevent periodontal disease

70. Abnormal wear of cheek teeth in pigs is usually the result of:

a. chewing on bars, pens or partitions
b. dental caries
c. periodontal disease
d. atrophic rhinitis
e. dietary calcium/phosphorus imbalance

71. The most important function of the periodontal ligament is to:

a. provide an adequate blood supply to the tooth
b. serve as a shock absorber
c. provide a reservoir of cementoblasts
d. serve as a reservoir of T-cells
e. provide venous drainage for the tooth

*72. Tooth eruption is a complex physiologic process involving all of the following **except**:*

a. root development
b. periodontal ligament traction
c. apexification
d. selective bone resorption and deposition
e. hydrostatic pressure

73. Lateral jaw movement is greatest during mastication in:

a. horses
b. pigs
c. primates
d. camels
e. rhinoceros

74. In horses, mandibular retraction during mastication leads to development of:

a. periodontal disease
b. rostral hooks on the first mandibular cheek teeth
c. rostral hooks on the first maxillary cheek teeth
d. caries of cementum
e. enamel points

*75. Concerning the canine teeth, which statement is **least** accurate?*

a. They are vestigial in mares.
b. They are subject to supragingival calculus in horses.
c. They function as incisors in ruminants.
d. They are void of cementum in ponies.
e. They do not make occlusal contact.

76. In horses, dental calculus:

a. contains more calcium than calculus in ruminants
b. develops when there is malocclusion
c. is related to fiber content of the diet
d. does not involve plaque formation
e. is rare in horses less than 15 years old

For Questions 77 through 80, select the correct answer from the 4 choices below.

a. 2 x (I 3/3; C 1/1; P 3 or 4/3; M 3/3) = 40 or 42
b. 2 x (I 0/4; C 0/0; P 3/3; M 3/3) = 32
c. 2 x (I 3/3; C 0/0; P 3/3) = 24
d. 2 x (I 3/3; C 1/1; P 4/4; M 3/3) = 44

77. Dental formula for deciduous teeth of horses.

78. Dental formula for permanent teeth of pigs.

79. Dental formula for permanent teeth of horses.

80. Dental formula for permanent teeth of sheep.

81. A horse's teeth should be floated:

a. only upon request by the owner or trainer
b. every 2 years
c. every year or more frequently, depending on diet
d. only when clinical signs of dental disease are present
e. more frequently in driven rather than ridden horses

82. Broken incisor teeth in sheep lead to development of:

a. calculus and gingival recession
b. apical cysts
c. draining mandibular sinuses
d. periodontal fibrous epulis
e. esophageal obstruction

*83. Complications of tooth extractions in horses may include all of the following **except**:*

a. palatine artery hemorrhage
b. persistent sinusitis
c. persistent fistula
d. mandibular fracture
e. ameloblastoma formation

Answers

1. **c**
2. **e**
3. **d** Some upper incisors are caudal to the lower incisors.
4. **a**
5. **b**
6. **d**
7. **b**
8. **a**
9. **c**
10. **e** A phenotypically correct dentition consists of a formula of I3, C1, P4, M3 in each of the 4 jaw quadrants. Swine are the most common animals in this classification.
11. **c**
12. **e**
13. **a**
14. **b**
15. **d**
16. **a** Enamel covers the crown of the tooth.
17. **b** Dentin constitutes the bulk of the tooth under the enamel and cementum.
18. **e**
19. **c** This is the neck of the tooth.
20. **e**
21. **b**
22. **d**
23. **c**
24. **a**
25. **e** This inner cavity consists of the root canal (root) and the pulp chamber (crown).
26. **b** The periodontium comprises the supporting structures of the tooth.
27. **b**
28. **a**
29. **d**
30. **c**
31. **e**

32. **c** A curette with a rounded toe is safer to use subgingivally.

33. **e** A sickle scaler with a sharp tip and edges should be used supragingivally.

34. **a** An elevator is used to loosen the periodontal ligament for tooth extraction.

35. **d** An explorer has a sharp, hooked end.

36. **b** A probe is marked in millimeters to measure pockets.

37. **a** Instruments must be sharp to remain effective.

38. **e** This is a hand instrument.

39. **d** This is an ultrasonic scaler.

40. **c**

41. **b**

42. **a**

43. **b** Plaque is associated with bacterial infection.

44. **c** Crowding facilitates retention of plaque and inflammation. Hard, crunchy foods help reduce plaque and calculus accumulation.

45. **e** Root planing involves use of a curette in several different directions to scale the root.

46. **c** Subgingival curettage involves use of a curette to gently remove diseased tissue from the sulcus lining.

47. **b** Sulcular lavage flushes out debris, plaque and prophylaxis paste.

48. **c**

49. **d**

50. **b**

51. **e** Odontoplasty involves restructuring the shape of a tooth.

52. **a**

53. **a**

54. **a**

55. **c**

56. **b**

57. **c**

58. **b**

59. **e**

60. **d** Glass ionomer needs no mechanical undercuts and releases fluoride.

61. **a**

62. **b** Baking soda (sodium bicarbonate) can cause sodium loading.

63. **c** Pulpal tissue exposed for several weeks is infected and necrotic. It should be removed and the cavity filled with inert material or the tooth should be extracted.

64. **d** Without pulpal insult, the tooth should be preserved.

65. **b**

66. **e**

67. **b**

68. **a**

69. **c**

70. **a**

71. **b**

72. **c**

73. **d**

74. **c**

75. **d**

76. **b**

77. **c**

78. **d**

79. **a**

80. **b**

81. **c**

82. **a**

83. **e**

Section 15

Diagnostic Imaging and Recordings

Recommended Reading

Bowen JM, in Oliver JE *et al: Veterinary Neurology.* Saunders, Philadelphia, 1987.

Brearley MJ *et al: Color Atlas of Small Animal Endoscopy.* Mosby, St. Louis, 1991.

Chrisman CL: *Problems in Small Animal Neurology.* 2nd ed. Lea & Febiger, Philadelpia, 1991.

Douglas SW *et al: Principles of Veterinary Radiography.* 4th ed. Bailliere Tindall, Philadelphia, 1987.

Edwards NJ: *Bolton's Handbook of Canine and Feline Electrocardiography.* 2nd ed. Saunders, Philadelphia, 1987.

Fox PR: *Canine and Feline Cardiology.* Churchill Livingston, New York, 1988.

Gompf B *et al: Nomenclature and Criteria in Diseases of the Heart and Vessels (Small Animal Medicine).* American Animal Hosp Assn and Acad Vet Cardiology, Denver, 1986.

Jones BD: Veterinary endoscopy. *Vet Clin No Am* (Small Animal Pract) 20: 1 *et seqq,* 1990.

Klemm WR: *Animal Electroencephalography.* Academic Press, New York, 1969.

Klemm WR: *Applied Electronics for Veterinary Medicine and Animal Physiology.* Charles C Thomas, Springfield, IL, 1976. pp 287-351.

Klemm WR, in Indrieri RJ: Epilepsy. *Problems Vet Med* 1:535-556, 1989.

McIlwraith CW: *Diagnostic and Surgical Arthroscopy in the Horse.* Lea & Febiger, Philadelphia, 1990.

Morgan JP and Silverman S: *Techniques of Veterinary Radiography.* 3rd ed. Veterinary Radiology Assoc, Davis, CA, 1982.

Thrall DE: *Textbook of Veterinary Diagnostic Radiology.* Saunders, Philadelphia, 1986.

Ticer JW: *Radiographic Technique in Veterinary Practice.* 2nd ed. Saunders, Philadelphia, 1984.

Tilley LP: *Essentials of Canine and Feline Electrocardiography: Interpretation and Treatment.* 3rd ed. Lea & Febiger, Philadelphia, 1992.

Tilley LP and Owen J: *Manual of Small Animal Cardiology.* Churchill Livingstone, New York, 1985.

Tilley LP and Miller MS, in Kirk RS: *Current Veterinary Therapy IX.* Saunders, Philadelphia, 1986

Traub-Dargatz JL and Brown CM: *Equine Endoscopy.* Mosby, St. Louis, 1990..

Practice answer sheet is on page 373.

Correct answers are on pages 158-160.

Radiography

C.M. Han, D.E. Thrall

Questions

1. *You make a radiograph of a dog's pelvis that measures 16 cm in diameter. You manually process the film for 5 minutes in the developer and 10 minutes in the fixer. The radiograph is too dark. What is the most likely reason the film turned out too dark?*

   a. a grid was used
   b. slow-speed screens were used
   c. chemicals were 73 F
   d. chemicals were stirred
   e. rinse time was 30 seconds

2. *Which technique produces an image with the greatest radiographic density?*

   a. 100 mA, 1/10 sec
   b. 150 mA, 1/30 sec
   c. 200 mA, 1/20 sec
   d. 200 mA, 1/10 sec
   e. 100 mA, 1/60 sec

3. *What happens when radiographic film is stored past the expiration date listed on the carton?*

   a. the film becomes brittle
   b. the film becomes fogged
   c. the film does not respond to exposure
   d. the emulsion slips when processed
   e. the film develops branching light artifacts resembling lightning

4. *Which grid requires the highest exposure technique?*

   a. 8:1
   b. 12:1
   c. 5:1
   d. 10:1
   e. 15:1

5. *You make a radiograph using 10 mAs and 60 kVp. You decide to double the radiographic density for a second film. Which technique should you use?*

   a. 200 mA, 0.10 sec, 60 kVp
   b. 150 mA, 0.20 sec, 60 kVp
   c. 100 mA, 0.20 sec, 70 kVp
   d. 300 mA, 0.03 sec, 60 kVp
   e. 300 mA, 0.10 sec, 60 kVp

6. *When making vertebral radiographs, it is important to collimate the beam down to the width of the vertebra. Why is this necessary?*

   a. collimation strengthens the beam
   b. collimation makes the x-rays travel in a line, rather than diverging
   c. collimation reduces scatter radiation
   d. collimation allows your attention to focus only on the area of interest
   e. collimation increases the penetrating power of the beam

7. *Why are screens used in veterinary radiography?*

   a. screens produce a more detailed radiograph than direct exposure film
   b. screens are less expensive to use than direct exposure film
   c. screens are easier to care for than direct exposure film
   d. screens do not require as much radiation to produce the same radiographic density as direct exposure film
   e. screens require more exposure than direct exposure film, but they produce a better image

8. mAs controls the:

a. quality of the beam
b. quantity of electrons emitted
c. speed of electrons emitted
d. wavelength of the beam
e. focal spot size

9. Why should a radiation film badge be worn at collar level?

a. so it can be worn outside the lead gown
b. to determine the type of radiation exposure
c. to monitor exposure of the thyroid gland and lenses of the eyes
d. to monitor primary beam exposure
e. to inform everyone you are radiographing an animal

10. What element clears the remaining silver halide crystals from exposed x-ray film?

a. developer
b. fixer
c. wash water
d. infrared light
e. room air

11. When radiographing the thorax, when should the x-ray film be exposed?

a. peak expiration
b. peak inspiration
c. between inspiration and expiration
d. mid-expiration
e. early inspiration

12. Which of the following controls the contrast on the radiograph?

a. mAs
b. kVp
c. focal-film distance
d. focal spot size
e. amount of collimation

13. On skull radiographs of a cat, you observe damage to the upper right canine tooth. The veterinarian would like to see that tooth without superimposition of the other teeth. Which view can best accomplish this?

a. lateral
b. ventrodorsal
c. dorsoventral
d. ventral 45 degrees left – dorsal right oblique
e. ventral 45 degrees right – dorsal left oblique

14. A clear strip at the top of a manually processed film may be caused by:

a. low fixer level
b. low developer level
c. low water level
d. no agitation of developer solution
e. weak acid bath

15. What is the maximum intensity of the safelight in developing rooms?

a. 7.5 watts
b. 15 watts
c. 60 watts
d. 100 watts
e. 2.5 watts

16. If kVp is used to increase radiographic density, by how much must 70 kVp be increased to double the density?

a. 4 kVp
b. 10 kVp
c. 14 kVp
d. 20 kVp
e. 35 kVp

17. If mAs is used to decrease radiographic density, by how much must 40 mAs be decreased to halve the density?

a. 5 mAs
b. 10 mAs
c. 15 mAs
d. 20 mAs
e. 25 mAs

Correct answers are on pages 158-160.

Radiography, continued

18. *If your focal-film distance is increased from 36 inches to 72 inches, how must the mAs be adjusted to maintain the same radiographic density?*

    a. decreased by a factor of 4
    b. decreased by a factor of 2
    c. increased by a factor of 4
    d. increased by a factor of 2
    e. decreased by a factor of 8

For Questions 19 through 25, select the correct answer from the 7 choices below.

a. electrons
b. filament
c. anode
d. cathode
e. target
f. focusing cup
g. x-rays

19. *The area of the anode that is struck by the electrons during an exposure.*

20. *Tungsten coil that emits electrons when heated.*

21. *Negative electrode.*

22. *Travels from the filament to the target when a positive electrical potential is applied to the target.*

23. *Small depression where the filament is placed.*

24. *Positive electrode.*

25. *Produced at the anode.*

26. *Which of the following* **decreases** *the effect of scatter radiation on x-ray film?*

    a. detailed screens
    b. increased kVp and decreased mAs
    c. decreased focal-film distance
    d. increased object-film distance and increased focal-film distance
    e. nonscreen film

27. *An animal is presented to your clinic with clinical signs suggesting kidney disease. The veterinarian wants to do a contrast study. Which of the following is best for evaluating renal function?*

    a. celiogram
    b. myelogram
    c. arthrogram
    d. excretory urogram
    e. pneumocystogram

28. *The veterinarian wants to do an upper gastrointestinal contrast study on a dog with possible bowel perforations. Why is a water-based iodide contrast medium used instead of barium sulfate?*

    a. it is quickly cleared from the stomach and intestines and can be absorbed by the body
    b. it is less expensive than barium
    c. it provides better mucosal detail
    d. it will not dehydrate the dog
    e. it cannot be absorbed by the body and will better delineate the perforation

For Questions 29 through 39, select the correct answer from the 11 choices below.

a. ventral
b. dorsal
c. medial
d. lateral
e. cranial
f. caudal
g. rostral
h. palmar
i. plantar
j. proximal
k. distal

29. *Situated toward the nose.*

30. *Situated closer to a point of attachment or origin.*

31. *Situated farther from the median plane or midline.*

32. *Situated toward the tail.*

33. *Situated on the caudal aspect of the rear limb, distal to the tarsocrural (hock) joint.*

34. *Situated toward the belly or underside of quadrupeds (downward).*

35. *Situated toward the median plane or midline.*

36. *Situated farther from a point of attachment or origin.*

37. *Situated on the caudal aspect of the front limb, distal to the antebrachiocarpal joint (carpus).*

38. *Situated toward the head.*

39. *Situated toward the back or topline area of quadrupeds (upward).*

40. *kVp controls the:*

a. quality of the beam
b. quantity of the beam
c. number of electrons emitted
d. wavelength of the beam
e. focal spot size

41. *For which of the following radiographic examinations would a grid provide the greatest improvement in detail?*

a. lateral view, body, parakeet
b. craniocaudal view, antebrachium, Great Dane
c. lateral view, abdomen, German Shepherd
d. lateral view, thorax, 6-week-old Siamese
e. lateral view, metacarpal bones, adult Thoroughbred

42. *Which of the following would cause a film to be too dark after processing?*

a. 2 films in the same cassette
b. kVp too low
c. film stored in area of high room temperature
d. focal-film distance too long
e. mA too low

43. *Which technique would produce an abdominal radiograph with the greatest contrast?*

a. 1 mAs, 108 kVp
b. 2 mAs, 90 kVp
c. 4 mAs, 72 kVp
d. 8 mAs, 58 kVp
e. 16 mAs, 46 kVp

44. *A radiograph made using 20 mAs and 80 kVp is too dark. Which technique is reasonable to use for the second attempt?*

a. 20 mAs, 160 kVp
b. 20 mAs, 40 kVp
c. 10 mAs, 80 kVp
d. 40 mAs, 80 kVp
e. 40 mAs, 60 kVp

45. *The optimal developer temperature for manual processing of x-ray film is:*

a. 60 F
b. 60 C
c. 68 F
d. 68 C
e. 76 F

Correct answers are on pages 158-160.

Radiography, continued

46. Rare-earth intensifying screens were introduced in the 1970s. Their biggest advantage over calcium-tungstate intensifying screens is:

a. increased detail
b. increased contrast
c. increased cost
d. increased speed
e. decreased cost

47. Ideally, thoracic radiographs of dogs should be made:

a. at the time of full inspiration
b. at the time of full expiration
c. at any time during the respiratory cycle
d. only in left lateral and ventral recumbency
e. only in right lateral and sternal recumbency

48. In comparison with low-mAs, high-kVp techniques, high-mAs, low-kVp techniques are recommended for abdominal radiography in dogs because high-mAs, low-kVp techniques:

a. are safer for technical personnel
b. produce radiographs of higher contrast
c. require shorter exposure times
d. do not necessitate use of a grid
e. do not necessitate use of protective aprons and gloves

49. Protective lead aprons and gloves:

a. should be worn whenever holding a patient or cassette during radiography
b. should be worn only when a part of the body will be in the primary x-ray beam
c. should be worn whenever mAs values greater than 10 are used
d. are designed primarily for protection against the primary x-ray beam
e. have essentially an infinite useful life

50. Pregnant or possibly pregnant women:

a. may safely remain in the x-ray room during an exposure but must not restrain the patient
b. may safely remain in the x-ray room and restrain a patient during an exposure, as long as they wear protective aprons and gloves
c. may safely remain in the x-ray room and restrain a patient during an exposure, as long as they are not in the first trimester of gestation
d. should not remain in the x-ray room during an exposure at any time
e. should not be in a building where radiographs are made

51. A 14 x 17-inch sheet of x-ray film is developed manually following exposure to x-rays. When the film is dry, you notice a green stripe at the edge of one of the 14-inch ends. The most likely cause is:

a. the fixer solution level is too low
b. the green region was not exposed to x-rays
c. the developer solution level is too low
d. both the developer and fixer solution levels are too low
e. the wash water level is too low

52. Following processing of a radiograph, you note an intensely black artifact with the appearance of arborized (branching) black lines. The most likely cause is:

a. underdevelopment
b. overdevelopment
c. light fog
d. developer was splashed on the film in the darkroom
e. static electricity

53. Detail is the degree of sharpness of an object on a radiograph. Which of the following does ***not*** *affect detail?*

a. focal spot size
b. object-film distance
c. film-screen contact
d. focal spot-object distance
e. milliamperage

54. In myelography, contrast medium should be injected into the:

a. subarachnoid space
b. epidural space
c. vertebral canal
d. spinal canal
e. central canal

55. *Masses within the lung parenchyma are frequently not apparent on radiographs made with the affected lung in a dependent position. The reason for this is:*

a. increased air volume in the dependent lung
b. decreased air volume in the dependent lung
c. increased fluid volume in the dependent lung
d. decreased fluid volume in the dependent lung
e. compression of the mass in the dependent lung

56. *Skeletal mineralization in canine fetuses is usually detectable radiographically at about what stage of gestation?*

a. 20-25 days
b. 30-35 days
c. 40-45 days
d. 50-55 days
e. 56-60 days

57. *Which radiographic sign is **least** suggestive of fetal death?*

a. gas within the fetus
b. peritoneal effusion in the dam
c. gas within the dam's uterus
d. overlapping of fetal cranial bones at the skull sutures
e. a shrunken, distorted fetal skeleton

58. *What is the most appropriate contrast medium for positive-contrast cystography in dogs?*

a. barium sulfate paste
b. barium sulfate solution
c. air
d. nonionic, iodinated, water-soluble contrast medium
e. ionic, iodinated, water-soluble contrast medium

59. *The best radiographic contrast procedure to assess the urinary bladder mucosa is:*

a. excretory urography
b. positive-contrast cystography
c. negative-contrast cystography
d. double-contrast cystography
e. retrograde urography

60. *The contrast medium of choice for a negative-contrast cystogram is:*

a. room air
b. carbon dioxide
c. helium
d. argon
e. 100% oxygen

Ultrasonography

C.M. Han

For Questions 61 through 65, select the correct answer from the 5 choices below.

a. near-field gain
b. far-field gain
c. power
d. depth
e. delay

61. *Controls the brightness in the far field.*

62. *Controls the point at which gain is applied.*

63. *Controls overall brightness.*

64. *Controls the brightness in the near field.*

65. *Controls the amount of tissue being displayed.*

Correct answers are on pages 158-160.

Ultrasonography, continued

66. *As compared with a 3.5-mHz transducer, a 7.5-mHz transducer has:*

a. better resolution
b. worse resolution
c. equal resolution
d. equal axial resolution
e. equal lateral resolution

For Questions 67 through 69, select the correct answer from the 3 choices below.

a. anechoic tissue
b. hypoechoic tissue
c. hyperechoic tissue

67. *Tissue that reflects a low proportion of sound waves back to the transducer, producing a relatively dark image.*

68. *Tissue that does not reflect sound waves back to the transducer, producing a black image.*

69. *Tissue that reflects a high proportion of sound waves back to the transducer, producing a relatively bright image.*

Endoscopy

P.W. Pratt

70. *In a fiberoptic endoscope,:*

a. a coherent fiber bundle transmits light from the light source to the distal tip
b. a noncoherent fiber bundle transmits images from the distal tip to the eyepiece
c. about 80% of the light from the light source has been dissipated when it reaches the distal tip
d. each glass fiber is clad with a substance of low refractive index
e. water is circulated around the fiber bundles to reduce heat

71. *The major reason for unproductive or unsuccessful colonoscopic examination is:*

a. bowel perforation
b. iatrogenic intussusception
c. inadequate bowel cleansing
d. underinsufflation of the bowel
e. atresia ani

72. *In preparing small animals for colonoscopy,:*

a. magnesium citrate should not be given to cats for colonic cleansing
b. polyethylene glycol should not be given to dogs for colonic cleansing
c. several warm-water enemas are superior to oral electrolyte lavage solutions
d. metoclopramide is given to stimulate vomiting and delay gastric emptying
e. enema solution should be repeatedly infused at 75 ml/kg

73. *In endoscopic examination of the guttural pouches,:*

a. the endoscope is introduced into the dorsal nasal meatus
b. general anesthesia is necessary
c. the slit-like openings are located rostroventral to the pharyngeal recess
d. the stylohyoid bone can be identified by its mediolateral course, dividing the guttural pouch into dorsal and ventral compartments
e. the internal carotid artery can be identified by its rostroventral location in the dorsal compartment

74. *In determining the gender of a bird by laparoscopy,:*

a. the laparoscope is inserted into the cloaca
b. the abdominal air sac must be avoided
c. the bird should be kept anesthetized for at least 30 minutes after laparoscopy so as to prevent air sac eventration
d. the gonad can be found caudal to the caudal lobe of the kidney
e. the bird should be placed in right lateral recumbency

Electrocardiography

L.P. Tilley

75. *A 10-mm upward deflection of the ECG stylus in response to 1 mV of electrical current is known as:*

a. depolarization
b. polarity
c. standardization
d. conductivity
e. automaticity

76. *Left-axis deviation occurs when:*

a. Lead I is positive and aV_F is positive
b. Lead I is positive and aV_F is negative
c. aV_F is positive and Lead I is negative
d. aV_F is negative and Lead I is negative
e. Lead I is negative, aV_F is negative and Lead II is negative

77. *A rhythm characterized by slowing and speeding of the heart rate related to respiration is known as:*

a. sinus arrhythmia
b. normal sinus rhythm
c. sinus bradycardia
d. sinoatrial block
e. sinus tachycardia

78. *The QRS complex on the ECG represents:*

a. atrial depolarization
b. ventricular repolarization
c. ventricular depolarization
d. atrioventricular conduction
e. atrial repolarization

79. *The P wave on the ECG represents:*

a. firing of the sinus node
b. ventricular repolarization
c. atrial repolarization
d. atrial depolarization
e. ventricular depolarization

80. *The QT interval on the ECG represents:*

a. ventricular depolarization
b. atrial depolarization
c. ventricular repolarization
d. conduction through the atrioventricular node
e. ventricular depolarization and repolarization

81. *An arrhythmia that can progress to ventricular fibrillation and for which one must continually monitor is:*

a. first-degree atrioventricular block
b. sinus tachycardia
c. atrial premature complexes
d. sinoatrial arrest
e. ventricular tachycardia

Correct answers are on pages 158-160.

Electrocardiography, continued

82. *The normal PR interval in dogs is:*

a. 0.06-0.13 second
b. 0.10-0.16 second
c. 0.12-0.20 second
d. 0.16-0.24 second
e. 0.04-0.10 second

Electroencephalography

W.R. Klemm

83. *The electroencephalogram (EEG) can most accurately be described as:*

a. the best way to measure intelligence
b. the only way to monitor consciousness
c. a plot of microvolts vs time
d. a reflection of the amount of brain activity
e. the best way to detect epilepsy

Electromyography

J.M. Bowen

84. *The major use of electromyography is in:*

a. suppressing excessive electrical activity in muscle
b. neurologic diagnosis
c. acupuncture
d. diagnosing electrical diseases of muscle
e. promoting reinnervation of skeletal muscles

Answers

1. **c** In manual film processing, the film must be immersed for 5 minutes in chemicals held at 68 F. The higher the temperature, the more fogged the image becomes, making it nondiagnostic.
2. **d** 200 mA x 1/10 sec = 20 mAs.
3. **b** Film kept past its expiration date becomes fogged.
4. **e** The higher the grid ratio, the more efficient it is at improving the image. This requires an increased technique to compensate.
5. **a** Doubling the mAs doubles the radiographic density.
6. **c** Collimation reduces the amount of scatter radiation and increases detail.

7. **d** Intensifying screens do not require as much exposure as direct exposure film. With unanesthetized animals, the fastest exposure time possible is necessary to prevent motion on the radiograph.
8. **b** mAs controls the number of electrons produced.
9. **c** Film badges are worn at collar level so as to monitor the amount of exposure to the lenses of the eyes and the thyroid gland.
10. **b** Developer solution changes the sensitized silver halide crystals into black metallic silver. Fixer solution clears all remaining silver halide crystals from the film.
11. **b** When radiographing the thorax, the film should be exposed at peak inspiration.
12. **b** kVp controls contrast on the radiograph. The higher the kVp, the longer the scale of contrast (more grays).
13. **d** A ventral 45 degree left – dorsal right oblique projection places the tooth in question close to the film, without other teeth superimposed.
14. **b** If the level of developer solution is low, the portion of the film not in the developer retains silver halide crystals. Once it is placed in the fixer, the silver halide crystals on the undeveloped part are cleared, leaving the clear film base.
15. **a**
16. **c** When kVp is used to double the radiographic density, it must increase by 20%. 70 kVp x 20% = 14 kVp.
17. **d** Halving the mAs halves the radiographic density. 40 mAs x 1/2 = 20 mAs.
18. **c** The inverse square law states that if the focal-film distance is doubled, you must increase the mAs 4 times to produce a radiograph with the same density.
19. **e** The target is the area of the anode struck by the electrons during an exposure.
20. **b** The filament is a tungsten coil that emits electrons when heated.
21. **d** The cathode is the negative electrode.
22. **a** Electrons travel from the filament to the target when a positive electrical potential is applied to the target.
23. **f** The focusing cup is a small depression where the filament is placed.
24. **c** The anode is the positive electrode.
25. **g** X-rays are produced at the anode.
26. **d** By increasing the object-film distance and the focal-film distance, the effects of scatter radiation can be decreased. This is helpful when making radiographs of large animals, and grids are not available.
27. **d** An excretory urogram best demonstrates renal function.
28. **a** Water-based iodide solution is used because it is rapidly cleared from the stomach and can be absorbed by the body.
29. **g**
30. **j**
31. **d**
32. **f**
33. **i**
34. **a**
35. **c**
36. **k**
37. **h**
38. **e**
39. **b**
40. **a** kVp controls the quality of the x-ray beam.
41. **c** Grids are indicated for parts thicker than 10 cm.
42. **c** Film should not be stored in areas of high temperature.
43. **e** High-mAs, low-kVp techniques produce the highest contrast. All listed techniques are equivalent in terms of film blackness.
44. **c** Halving the mAs is a reasonable adjustment to correct an exposure that is too dark.
45. **c**
46. **d** Rare-earth screens have increased speed as their main advantage.
47. **a** This provides contrast in the lung to identify regions of increased opacity.
48. **b**
49. **a** Protective attire should be worn at all times when assisting with patient radiography.
50. **d**
51. **d** Unprocessed x-ray film is naturally green to gray.
52. **e** Static often causes this type of artifact.
53. **e** Milliamperage does not affect detail.

54. **a**

55. **b** The dependent lung is partially collapsed and of increased opacity, and may silhouette a mass.

56. **c**

57. **b** There are many causes of peritoneal effusion other than fetal death.

58. **e** This offers the optimal combination of safety and low cost.

59. **d** Other choices will not allow the mucosa to be visualized in comparable detail.

60. **b** The high solubility decreases the chance of fatal air embolism.

61. **b** Far-field gain controls the brightness in the far field.

62. **e** The delay controls the point at which the gain is applied to the image.

63. **c** The power controls the overall brightness of the field.

64. **a** Near-field gain controls the brightness in the near field.

65. **d** The depth controls the amount of tissue displayed on the screen.

66. **a** Transducers with higher frequencies cannot penetrate as deeply into tissues but have better resolution than lower-frequency transducers.

67. **b** Hypoechoic images result when fewer echoes are reflected back to the transducer, appearing darker than other tissues on the screen. The liver is hypoechoic as compared with the spleen.

68. **a** Anechoic images result when no echoes are reflected back to the transducer, appearing black on the screen. Some types of fluid may be anechoic.

69. **c** Hyperechoic images result when many echoes are reflected back to the transducer, appearing brighter than other tissues on the screen. Fat is hyperechoic as compared with the spleen.

70. **d** Unless the fibers are clad, light tends to leak as it traverses the fibers toward the distal tip of the endoscope.

71. **c** Fasting and administration of oral electrolyte solutions help cleanse the colonic mucosa in preparation for colonoscopy.

72. **a** Some treated cats may develop hypermagnesemia.

73. **c**

74. **e**

75. **c** The other possible choices describe electrical activity within the myocardial cell.

76. **b** Using at least 2 limb leads (I, aVF) and the different angles at which they record the heart's electrical activity, one can estimate the mean electrical axis in the frontal plane.

77. **a** Sinus arrhythmia is represented by alternating periods of slower and more rapid heart rates, usually related to respiration. The heart rate increases with inspiration and decreases with expiration.

78. **c** Atrial depolarization and repolarization represent the P wave and subsequent T wave, while ventricular repolarization represents the T wave following a QRS complex.

79. **d** The depolarization waves spread from the sinoatrial node through the right atrium, toward the left atrium and the atrioventricular node, resulting in a P wave. This indicates depolarization.

80. **e** The QT interval is the summation of ventricular depolarization and repolarization.

81. **e** The other possible choices are not primary ventricular arrhythmias and are also arrhythmias that usually do not lead to ventricular fibrillation.

82. **a** The normal PR interval range is 0.06-0.13 seconds.

83. **c** All of the other choices are incomplete or ambiguous. Some of the other choices, such as b and e, are only half-truths, because there are other ways to evaluate consciousness and epilepsy.

84. **b** Electromyography is an important adjunct to neurologic examination. By itself, electromyography does not provide a definitive diagnosis of a nerve or muscle disease.

Section 16

Epidemiology and Public Health

J.S. Reif and G.T. Woods

Recommended Reading

Martin SW *et al: Veterinary Epidemiology.* Iowa State University Press, Ames, 1987.

Reif JS, in Ettinger SJ: *Textbook of Veterinary Internal Medicine.* 2nd ed. Saunders, Philadelphia, 1982.

Smith RD: *Veterinary Clinical Epidemiology: A Problem-Oriented Approach.* Butterworth-Heinemann, Boston, 1991.

Practice answer sheet is on page 375.

Questions

1. *The study of the frequency, distributions and determinants of disease in populations is known as:*

   a. biostatistics
   b. public heath
   c. preventive medicine
   d. epidemiology
   e. herd health

2. *The major component of epidemiology that differentiates it from other medical specialties is its focus on:*

   a. animals
   b. diseased animals
   c. healthy animals
   d. populations
   e. the environment

3. *The continuous, longitudinal collection of data on the occurrence and spread of disease in a specified population and geographic area is known as:*

   a. a disease survey
   b. sampling
   c. surveillance
   d. epidemiology
   e. preventive medicine

Correct answers are on page 167.

4. *The term endemic (enzootic) refers to:*

   a. the occurrence in a community or region of a group of illnesses of similar nature clearly in excess of normal expectancy
   b. a world-wide epidemic/epizootic
   c. the usual prevalence of a disease or an infectious agent in a given geographic area
   d. a disease cluster
   e. a low level of ongoing disease in a community or region, with periodic outbreaks or epidemics/epizootics

5. *The occurrence in a community or region of a group of illnesses of similar nature clearly in excess of normal expectancy is known as:*

   a. an enzootic (endemic)
   b. a parazootic
   c. its endemicity
   d. the attack rate
   e. an epidemic (epizootic)

6. *"Test and slaughter" is a control procedure employed most beneficially in a disease:*

   a. that is spreading rapidly through a population
   b. in which 50% of the cattle population may be infected
   c. with a low prevalence and for which a sensitive and specific diagnostic test exists
   d. with serious economic implications and that does not currently exist in the United States
   e. with a wildlife reservoir

7. *The length of a quarantine period in disease control is based on the:*

   a. duration of communicability of the disease
   b. duration of agent shedding (patent period)
   c. latent period
   d. incubation period
   e. exposure period

8. *Complete elimination of a disease and its etiologic agent from a large portion of the world (eg, the Western Hemisphere) is called:*

   a. control
   b. eradication
   c. primary prevention
   d. disinfection
   e. secondary prevention

9. *Depopulation in a disease-control program involves:*

   a. elimination of all susceptible species populations (hosts), regardless of their disease or exposure status
   b. elimination of all susceptible species populations (hosts) that have been exposed or may have been exposed to the disease agent
   c. elimination of the disease agent from the population using vaccination
   d. elimination of all food-producing animals in the region, regardless of their disease status
   e. elimination of all vectors from the area

10. *With a disease for which a sensitive and specific diagnostic test is available, elimination of carriers of an infectious agent from a population to protect uninfected animals is best accomplished by:*

    a. selective removal or slaughter
    b. depopulation
    c. quarantine
    d. environmental sanitation
    e. reservoir elimination

11. *Which disease-control measure is **least** likely to be applied during an outbreak of viral respiratory disease in horses?*

    a. isolation
    b. segregation
    c. quarantine
    d. immunization
    e. depopulation

12. *Efforts directed toward reducing the frequency of existing disease to biologically or economically "acceptable" levels is known as:*

    a. disease prevention
    b. disease control
    c. disease eradication

d. disease minimization
e. selective slaughter

13. *Screening for heartworm microfilariae in dogs and treatment to remove adult heartworms and microfilariae from infected dogs before signs of cardiopulmonary disease develop are an example of:*

a. primary prevention
b. secondary prevention
c. eradication
d. disease control
e. vector control

14. *Presumptive identification of unrecognized disease by the application of tests, examinations or other procedures that can be applied rapidly is known as:*

a. surveillance
b. test and slaughter
c. screening
d. prevention
e. survey

15. *The ability of a screening test to correctly identify individuals in a population that are truly diseased is a measure of the test's:*

a. sensitivity
b. specificity
c. reliability
d. positive predictive value
e. negative predictive value

16. *The ability of a screening test to correctly identify individuals in a population that are truly free of disease (nondiseased) is a measure of the test's:*

a. sensitivity
b. specificity
c. reliability
d. positive predictive value
e. negative predictive value

17. *The probability that an individual with a positive test result actually has the disease is referred to as the:*

a. sensitivity
b. specificity
c. reliability
d. predictive value of a positive test
e. predictive value of a negative test

18. *The capacity of an agent to cause disease in a susceptible host defines its:*

a. virulence
b. pathogenicity
c. infectivity
d. invasiveness
e. aggressiveness

19. *The species or environment in which a pathogenic organism is maintained and upon which the organism depends for survival is called a:*

a. carrier
b. vector
c. source
d. reservoir
e. fomite

20. *An infection that results in* ***no*** *perceptible clinical signs is called:*

a. a clinical infection
b. a convalescent infection
c. an inapparent infection
d. a "dead end" infection
e. an atypical infection

21. *In a herd of 120 llamas, 75 have had diarrhea and vomiting within the last 24 hours. All of the animals were normal 48 hours ago. Only adult animals are affected. The most likely source for the outbreak is:*

a. exposure to a common source
b. an infection propagated in the herd and spread from animal to animal
c. a change in the diet of younger animals
d. an organism transmitted through water
e. an enteric virus

Correct answers are on page 167.

22. *During an outbreak of strangles, a feedbucket contaminated with* Streptococcus equi *is part of the chain of transmission from one horse to another. The feedbucket is an example of a:*

a. vector
b. vehicle
c. fomite
d. carrier
e. portal of entry

23. *In arthropod-borne infections, the time the agent spends in the arthropod host is known as the:*

a. prepatent period
b. latent period
c. extrinsic incubation period
d. patent period
e. maturation period

24. *Arthropods that transmit microorganisms from one animal to another without multiplication or maturation of the microorganisms in the arthropod are known as:*

a. biological vectors
b. mechanical vectors
c. incidental hosts
d. alternate reservoirs
e. biovars

25. *Animals that begin shedding an infectious agent before showing clinical signs are known as:*

a. incubationary carriers
b. convalescent carriers
c. intermittent shedders
d. chronic carriers
e. healthy carriers

26. *The place from which an etiologic agent passes directly to a susceptible host is known as the:*

a. source
b. reservoir
c. vehicle
d. vector
e. portal of entry

27. *An agent transmissible from animals to people under natural conditions is described as:*

a. endemic
b. pandemic
c. epizootic
d. enzootic
e. zoonotic

28. *An inapparent carrier is an animal that is:*

a. showing atypical clinical signs of disease
b. hyperimmunized
c. immunodeficient
d. infected but manifesting no clinical signs
e. infected but mounting an IgM antibody response

29. *The interval between effective exposure to an infectious agent and the onset of clinical signs of that disease describes the:*

a. patent period
b. period of communicability
c. latent period
d. prepatent period
e. incubation period

30. *Which of the following is **not** an example of direct transmission of an infectious agent?*

a. aerosol transmission
b. venereal transmission
c. bite wound
d. skin contact
e. food-borne transmission

31. *Which of the following is **not** approved for humane slaughter of livestock at federal- and state-inspected meat-packing plants:*

a. rifle shot and kosher slaughter
b. carbon dioxide
c. penetrating or nonpenetrating captive bolt

d. electrical stunning
e. knocking hammer

32. At federally inspected meat-packing plants, meat is preserved with:

a. heating, freezing, application of a wax coating, smoking
b. smoking, irradiation, pickling, freezing
c. dehydration, heating, smoking, application of a wax coating
d. cold, irradiation, dehydration, heat, addition of chemicals
e. application of a wax coating

33. Nitrites are added to some cured meat products to:

a. increase the protein content
b. reduce the meat's odor
c. inhibit fungal action
d. act as filler
e. improve flavor, fix the meat's colorand inhibit bacterial action

34. Phosphates are added to certain meat products to:

a. neutralize salt
b. neutralize bacterial action
c. improve water-holding capacity
d. increase pH
e. decrease pH

35. Ascorbates are added to some meat products to:

a. help fix the meat's color
b. prevent bone souring
c. inhibit bacterial action
d. control molds
e. help fix the meat's color and prevent fading

36. After pasteurization, Grade A milk must be free of:

a. butterfat
b. casein
c. bacteria
d. active phosphatase
e. solids not fat

37. The 3 major causes of confirmed food-borne disease outbreaks in American people are:

a. salmon poisoning, shigellosis and *Streptococcus* Group A contamination
b. ptomaine poisoning, trichinosis and undulant fever
c. mercury poisoning, typhoid fever and cholera
d. trichinosis, typhoid fever and typhus
e. salmonellosis, *Clostridium perfringens* contamination and *Staphylococcus aureus* contamination

38. Prepared foods are most commonly contaminated with Staphylococcus aureus *by:*

a. ingredients containing contaminated milk
b. ingredients containing contaminated eggs
c. air-borne fomites
d. handling by food-preparation workers
e. ingredients containing contaminated condiments

39. Concerning botulism in human infants, which statement is most accurate?

a. The botulinus toxin must be pre-formed if a clinical effect is to be observed.
b. Infant formula containing honey is considered a risk factor.
c. Affected infants are typically 7-10 months old.
d. Botulism in infants usually is asymptomatic.
e. Botulism in infants is characterized by peracute onset of fulminant clinical signs.

40. Food-borne Clostridium perfringens *infection in people is usually associated with:*

a. food from dispensing machines
b. fish prepared in a home kitchen or in fast-food establishments where employee turnover is high
c. cultured dairy products
d. bacon bits packaged for use in salads
e. institutions or commerical food sites where many people handle a food before it is served and where larger quantities are prepared

Correct answers are on page 167.

41. *Foods canned improperly in a home kitchen have often been the source of:*

a. botulism
b. brucellosis
c. tuberculosis
d. pseudotuberculosis
e. tularemia

42. *Outbreaks of salmonellosis in people are best controlled and prevented by:*

a. health education and preventing contamination of food products
b. avoidance of poultry products
c. irradiation of all fish-based food products
d. using only eggs that have been hard-boiled
e. using only cake mixes that have been irradiated or pasteurized

43. *Brucellosis (undulant fever) in people results most commonly from:*

a. occupational exposure and drinking unpasteurized milk
b. eating meat from infected animals
c. exposure to infected dogs
d. accidents during vaccination of cattle
e. exposure to infected ticks

44. *Food-borne disease caused by* Vibrio parahemolyticus *has been associated with all of the following* ***except:***

a. shellfish
b. raw, improperly cooked or improperly handled seafood
c. fish-based canned cat food
d. boiled shrimp
e. boiled crabs

45. *A method used to prevent and control* Taenia saginata *infection in people is:*

a. irradiation of all pork products
b. thoroughly cooking any beef product
c. administration of pyrantel pamoate to feedlot cattle
d. chilling poultry carcasses immediately after slaughter
e. avoiding contact with infected pets

46. *Concerning tuberculosis in cattle in the United States, which statement is most accurate?*

a. It cannot be transmitted to household pets.
b. Reduction of human tuberculosis in the US has proceeded at a faster pace than reduction of tuberculosis infection in cattle.
c. Cattle may be asymptomatically infected and not react to intradermal tuberculin tests.
d. The disease has been eradicated in cattle.
e. Only 5 infected herds remain in the US.

47. *Concerning plague, which statement is* ***least*** *accurate?*

a. It is primarily a disease of rodents.
b. Control of fleas and rats is sufficient to control the disease in the US.
c. It has been reported in the US, including Indian reservations in New Mexico and Arizona.
d. Dogs and cats may be affected.
e. It occurs in bubonic and pneumonic forms.

48. Toxoplasma *infection in people can be prevented by any of the following methods* ***except:***

a. emptying the cat's litterbox daily
b. covering the children's sandbox
c. saturating the cat's litterbox with 1% available chlorine solution before handling it
d. cooking all meats thoroughly before eating
e. washing hands thoroughly after petting cats

49. *You have accidentally injected yourself with strain 19* Brucella abortus *vaccine. The most appropriate action is to:*

a. cleanse the wound thoroughly with soap and water to prevent bacterial infection; no other treatment is indicated because strain 19 does not produce clinical disease in people

b. cleanse the wound and seek prophylactic treatment with broad-spectrum antibiotics
c. take no special precautions
d. cleanse the wound and seek prophylactic treatment with large doses of penicillin
e. wait until clinical disease is verified before seeking medical treatment

50. *Concerning rabies, which statement is* ***least*** *accurate?*

a. If exposed to rabies, people vaccinated before exposure but never developing a demonstrable antibody response should proceed as though they had never been vaccinated against rabies.
b. Because the efficacy of postexposure prophylaxis in animals is so uncertain, any exposed animal should be destroyed.
c. It is doubtful that aerosol transmission of rabies virus occurs under any but extremely limited circumstances.
d. If sufficiently sensitive tests are used, rabies virus can be detected in nearly every portion of the body of an infected animal.
e. In the US, insectivorous bats have been found to harbor rabies virus, but they cannot transmit the infection to people.

Answers

1. **d**
2. **d**
3. **c**
4. **c**
5. **e**
6. **c**
7. **d**
8. **b**
9. **b**
10. **a**
11. **e**
12. **b**
13. **b**
14. **c**
15. **a**
16. **b**
17. **d**
18. **b**
19. **d**
20. **c**
21. **a**
22. **c**
23. **c**
24. **b**
25. **a**
26. **a**
27. **e**
28. **d**
29. **e**
30. **e**
31. **e**
32. **d**
33. **e**
34. **c**
35. **e**
36. **d**
37. **e**
38. **d**
39. **b**
40. **e**
41. **a**
42. **a**
43. **a**
44. **c**
45. **b**
46. **c**
47. **b**
48. **c**
49. **b**
50. **e**

Notes

Section 17

Ethics, Law and Animal Welfare

R.W. Lewis, P.W. Pratt, M.D. Steele

Recommended Reading

Lewis RW: Amputation of the tail of a horse as the basis for a malpractice suit. *JAVMA* 198:2056-2058, 1991.
Tannenbaum J: *Veterinary Ethics.* Williams & Wilkins, Baltimore, 1989.
Wilson JF: *Law and Ethics of the Veterinary Profession.* Priority Press, Yardley, PA, 1990.

Practice answer sheet is on page 377.

Questions

Questions 1 through 3

Two dogs are brought to Dr. X's clinic on Monday afternoon. One is brought in for teeth cleaning and the other for castration. The receptionist gives 2 cage cards to the licensed veterinary technician, who puts the dogs in cages and puts the cards on the cages. One of the cards indicates teeth cleaning, while the other indicates castration. Dr X has 2 partners, Dr. Y and Dr. Z. Dr. Y is a small animal practitioner, while Dr. Z does large animal work. Dr. X, Dr. Z and Dr. Y had no prior contact with the 2 dogs or their owners. Dr. X arrives early Tuesday morning after being off work the prior day. Dr. X does not recognize the dogs or the owners' names on the dogs' cages, and castrates one dog and cleans the teeth of the other, according to the cage card information. When the owner of the castrated dog comes to pick it up Tuesday evening, Dr. X learns he has castrated the wrong dog, a very valuable breeding animal. After cursing Dr. X and his clinic, the castrated dog's owner stomps out. Her last words are, "You'll be hearing from my attorney."

Correct answers are on page 175.

1. *Who is **least** likely to be sued for the damages resulting from castration of the wrong dog?*

   a. Dr. X
   b. Dr. X's veterinary technician
   c. Dr. X's receptionist
   d. Dr. Y
   e. Dr. Z

2. *What money damages are **least** likely to be awarded to the castrated dog's owner for the negligent castration?*

   a. money for the value of the dog before castration
   b. money for lost potential breeding fees
   c. the price of the teeth cleaning for which the dog's owner had already paid
   d. money for the dog owner's mental anguish
   e. money paid by the dog's owner to another veterinarian to treat an abscess that developed at the castration site

3. *Assuming that the receptionist incorrectly indicated the dogs on their respective cage cards and that the master patient record cards in fact correctly identified which dog was to receive a teeth cleaning and which was to be castrated, which person is **least** likely to be sued for the negligent castration?*

   a. Dr. X
   b. Dr. Y
   c. the receptionist
   d. the technician
   e. Dr. Z

4. *Dr. X's part-time kennel attendant assaults a client in the cage room. He has never previously assaulted anyone and Dr. X had no reason to believe he ever would commit such an act. Concerning the potential liability of Dr. X, which statement is most accurate?*

   a. Dr. X probably would be liable for the client's injuries because he is the employer of the kennel attendant.
   b. Dr. X probably would not be liable for the client's injuries because the assault was beyond the scope of the employee's duties and Dr. X had no reason to know the employee presented a risk of assault.
   c. Dr. X could not be liable, even if he knew the employee had a history of assaulting people, because Dr. X did not commit the assault.
   d. Dr. X could not be liable because he did not witness the assault.
   e. Dr. X could not be liable if his insurance did not cover that type of risk.

5. *Dr. X's part-time groomer has a history of losing her temper with fractious grooming subjects, and Dr. X knows that she has struck an animal more than once with her hand and various objects. To date, the groomer has not seriously injured an animal, but this time she loses control and strikes a poodle on the head with her clippers, killing it. Dr. X was not present. Concerning the potential liability of Dr. X, which statement is most accurate?*

   a. Dr. X could not be liable because he was not present.
   b. Dr. X could not be liable because he did not kill the dog.
   c. Dr. X could be liable because he knew the groomer presented a risk and he failed to take adequate precautions.
   d. Dr. X could be liable only if the groomer had previously killed someone's pet.
   e. Dr. X could not be liable because the groomer obviously had a psychological condition entitling her to a defense of insanity.

Questions 6 and 7

Dr. X castrates a dog for a new client. The new client does not show up to reclaim the dog until 7 days later. He refuses to pay the bill and demands his dog back.

6. *Concerning the rights of Dr. X in this situation, which statement is most accurate?*

   a. Under the laws and ethical rules of all states, Dr. X has a right to keep the dog until the bill is paid.
   b. Depending on the law and ethical rules in his state, Dr. X may have a right to keep the dog until the bill is paid.

c. Under the laws and ethical rules of all states, Dr. X may consider the dog abandoned and immediately euthanize the dog.
d. Under the laws of any state, Dr. X would not have a right to keep the dog.
e. Under the laws of all states, Dr. X can immediately sell the dog.

7. *If the dog's owner never shows up at all to reclaim the dog and it has been 4 weeks since the surgery, which statement is most accurate?*

a. Under the laws and ethical rules of all states, Dr. X may consider the animal abandoned and immediately euthanize it.
b. Under the laws of most states, Dr. X may be entitled to euthanize the dog after first attempting to notify the owner by mail.
c. Under the laws of some states, Dr. X must keep the animal until the owner claims it, regardless of how long that is.
d. Under the laws and ethical rules of all states, if Dr. X has been told by the owner over the telephone to "keep the dog," he may immediately euthanize the dog.
e. Under the laws and ethical rules of some states, Dr. X must keep the dog but need not feed it.

8. *Animals are legally classified as:*

a. real property
b. fixtures
c. personal property
d. "persons" with legal rights
e. nonentities with no legal rights

9. *If a client's dog bites the client while a veterinarian is examining the animal,:*

a. the veterinarian cannot be held liable for the client's injuries because it is the client's dog
b. the veterinarian could not be held liable if the attack was unprovoked
c. the veterinarian could be held liable for the client's injuries if the veterinarian knew the dog was dangerous and asked the client to restrain it anyway
d. the veterinarian could not be held liable if the owner voluntarily offered to restrain the dog
e. the veterinarian could not be held liable if she immediately washed and treated the owner's wound

10. *A veterinarian dehorns an 8-month-old pygmy goat without using any anesthetic. Concerning the ethics of such a practice, which statement is most accurate?*

a. The veterinarian could be held liable for violation of the animal cruelty laws of some states.
b. There is no risk that the veterinarian would be guilty of violation of any state law or ethical rule.
c. The owner who watched the procedure and heard the screams of the goat will likely be very pleased that he will not be charged for any anesthetic.
d. Because the goat is just an animal, there are no restrictions on what an owner or veterinarian can do to it.
e. It is not appropriate to use anesthetics to dehorn a goat, so the veterinarian has committed no ethical violation.

11. *Under the Federal Controlled Substances Act,:*

a. Schedule-II drugs have a low human abuse potential and are currently accepted for use in treatment in the United States
b. Schedule-V drugs have a high human abuse potential and are currently not accepted for use in treatment in the United States
c. Schedule-III drugs have a low human abuse potential and are currently accepted for use in treatment in the United States
d. Schedule-IV drugs have a high human abuse potential and are currently not accepted for use in treatment in the United States
e. Schedule-I drugs have a high human abuse potential and are currently not accepted for use in treatment in the United States

Correct answers are on page 175.

12. *The Food and Drug Administration has promulgated regulations for veterinary prescription drugs. Among other requirements, a manufacturer must indicate on the label of such a drug:*

a. "Keep out of reach of children."
b. "Sold only to graduate veterinarians."
c. "Caution: Federal law restricts this drug to use by or on the order of a licensed veterinarian."
d. "Caution: Use only as directed by a licensed veterinarian."
e. "For veterinary use only."

13. *Records of controlled substance inventories and their subsequent dispensing:*

a. must be maintained separately from all other records of the registrant veterinarian, or in such form that the information required is readily retrievable from the registrant veterinarian's other business and patient records
b. may be included in patient records, provided that such records are maintained for 2 years after the patient's record becomes inactive
c. must be maintained in locked storage areas off the premises for 3 years
d. require no special precautions, other than accurate recording of patient, client and inventory data
e. must be stored separately from patient medical records and other files in the case of Schedule-II substances

14. *Prescribing of drugs by a veterinarian for direct use by another person:*

a. is permissible if the prescription involved is not a Schedule-II drug
b. is permissible if there is a valid veterinarian-client relationship
c. is not permissible, except in bona fide emergencies in which that person's life is in imminent danger
d. is not permissible under any circumstances
e. is not permissible, except where specifically approved by the Drug Enforcement Administration

15. *A particularly common source of malpractice suits against practitioners involves:*

a. accidents involving practice vehicles driven after business hours
b. falls caused by puddles or urine on the floor of the reception area
c. injury of clients while they are physically restraining their animal
d. chronic misscheduling of appointments
e. charging excessively high fees for routine elective surgery

Animal Welfare and Ethics

P.W. Pratt

16. *According to the general and most widely held views of Western society, which of the following is considered an* ***illegitimate*** *and* ***unnecessary*** *reason to subject animals to pain or discomfort?*

a. dog fighting
b. slaughter of food animals
c. medical research
d. confinement of certain food animals, such as chickens
e. use of horses or oxen for work

17. *An animal's biologically determined nature ("telos") sometimes conflicts with the interests of people. This conflict is exemplified by all of the following* ***except:***

a. cats sharpening their claws on rugs and furniture
b. dogs barking in residential areas
c. roosters crowing in residential areas
d. coyotes preying on domestic sheep
e. owls preying on mice and rats

Questions 18 and 19

18. *The American Veterinary Medical Association (AVMA) has taken a position against merchandising of certain products by veterinarians. As defined in the AVMA's Principles of Veterinary Medical Ethics, "professional products" include all of the following* ***except:***

a. prescription diets
b. pharmaceuticals
c. prescription drugs
d. food dishes
e. anthelmintics

19. *As defined in the AVMA's Principles of Veterinary Medical Ethics, "nonprofessional products" include all of the following* ***except:***

a. nonprescription commercial diets
b. biologicals
c. grooming equipment
d. collars
e. identification tags

20. *Ethical guidelines concerning exterior signs identifying a veterinary hospital or clinic include all of the following* ***except:***

a. of reasonable size
b. no garish colors or flashing lights used
c. made of wood and affixed to the building rather than to a pole
d. no claims made of superior service
e. no commercial slogans used

21. *Concerning euthanasia of a beloved companion animal, which statement is* ***least*** *accurate?*

a. Euthanasia is best performed without the client present, regardless of the client's wishes.
b. The client should be allowed ample time alone with the animal for a final goodbye.
c. The veterinarian should explain to the client the technical aspects of the procedure of euthanasia.
d. The client should be allowed a quiet period with the animal's body after euthanasia, if desired.
e. The animal's body should be treated with respect and dignity after euthanasia.

22. *Moral considerations regarding the propriety of euthanasia of a companion animal include all of the following* ***except:***

a. client's expense for continuing the animal's treatment
b. probability that the animal will achieve a certain quality of life with dedicated treatment
c. pain or discomfort the animal will likely suffer without euthanasia
d. client's inconvenience or emotional upset with continued treatment of the animal
e. veterinarian's inconvenience or emotional upset with continued treatment of the animal

23. *What is the position of the American Veterinary Medical Association on the ethics of declawing domestic cats?*

a. it is acceptable if the owner signs a written statement promising not to allow the cat outdoors
b. it is justified if the cat cannot be deterred from using its claws destructively
c. it is unacceptable under any circumstances
d. it is justified if the owner has been physically injured (scratched) by the cat
e. it is generally unacceptable unless the veterinarian performs the procedure at the same time as castration or ovariohysterectomy

Correct answers are on page 175.

Question 24

Certain husbandry practices used with food animals have stirred controversy regarding the welfare of food animals kept under certain conditions.

24. *Welfare concerns regarding husbandry practices used in raising veal calves include all of the following* ***except:***

    a. isolation in single-animal crates or stalls
    b. poor ventilation and insufficient light
    c. stressful transition to the feedlot
    d. feeding of low-iron, low-fiber diets
    e. poor sanitation of stalls or crates

25. *Valid issues concerning the welfare of animals used in medical research include all of the following* ***except:***

    a. size and construction of animal enclosures
    b. ventilation and ambient temperature
    c. nature and quantity of bedding for nesting animals
    d. natural, nonmanufactured feeds
    e. group housing of social species

Answers

1. **c**
2. **d**
3. **c**
4. **b**
5. **c**
6. **b**
7. **b**
8. **c**
9. **c**
10. **a**
11. **e** See section 812(b) *et seqq* of the Controlled Substances Act of 1970. Schedule-I drugs have no current acceptable use in treatments in the United States.
12. **c** This is specified in the Code of Federal Regulations section 201.105.
13. **a** The record-keeping requirements for controlled substances are complex and not easily understood. They are, however, important for the protection of the registrant veterinarian. They can be found in several sections of the Code of Federal Regulations.
14. **d** Many state laws provide for such a blanket prohibition. Veterinarians are not physicians, and as such should never undertake treatment of a person.
15. **c** Malpractice is different from ordinary business negligence. The AVMA Professional Malpractice Insurance Trust warns veterinarians not to allow clients to hold or restrain their own animals at any time.
16. **a** Despite the opposing views of certain individuals or groups, all of the other choices listed are generally approved by Western society as legitimate reasons to subject animals to pain or discomfort.
17. **e** If society had an economic, religious or other interest in mice or rats, predation by owls would likely be considered undesirable. However, society generally views this type of predation as desirable because it keeps rodent populations in check.
18. **d** According to the AVMA, all of the other items listed require a veterinarian's knowledge to use safely and appropriately, and so are classified as professional products.
19. **b** Biologicals are classified as the AVMA as professional products requiring a veterinarian's knowledge for safe and proper use.
20. **c** While such signs are desirable, other types of signs, such as a discreet metal sign on a well-maintained, unobtrusive pole, are acceptable.

21. **a** The veterinarian should ask if the client wishes to be present during the procedure.

22. **e** This should have no bearing on a client's decision to euthanize a companion animal.

23. **b**

24. **c** Veal calves typically are not shipped to feedlots, but rather go directly to slaughter from the crate.

25. **d** Commercial, nutritionally balanced "chows" have been formulated for various species used in research. Natural feeds are not always available.

Notes

Notes

Section 18

Hematology and Cytology

R.L. Cowell, W.J. Dodds, B.L. Hines

Recommended Reading

Cowell RL and Tyler RD: *Cytology and Hematology of the Horse.* American Veterinary Publications, Goleta, CA, 1992.

Cowell RL and Tyler RD: *Diagnostic Cytology of the Dog and Cat.* American Veterinary Publications, Goleta, CA, 1989.

Jain NC *et al: Schalm's Veterinary Hematology.* 4th ed. Lea & Febiger, Philadelphia, 1986.

Kaneko JJ: *Clinical Biochemistry of Domestic Animals.* 4th ed. Academic Press, New York, 1989.

Meyers JR *et al: Veterinary Laboratory Medicine.* Saunders, Philadelphia, 1992.

Thrall MA and Weiser MG, in Pratt PW: *Laboratory Procedures for Veterinary Technicians.* 2nd ed. American Veterinary Publications, Goleta, CA, 1992.

Young KM *et al*, in Morgan RV: *Handbook of Small Animal Practice.* 2nd ed. Churchill Livingstone, New York, 1992.

Practice answer sheet is on page 379.

Questions

1. *Viral infection is classically associated with:*

    a. lymphocytosis
    b. lymphopenia
    c. eosinophilia
    d. neutrophilia
    e. target cells

2. *Smears of blood from dogs with autoimmune hemolytic anemia often show:*

    a. rouleaux formation
    b. spherocytosis
    c. Heinz bodies
    d. elliptocytosis
    e. hypochromasia

3. *The immune-mediated form of thrombocytopenia is characterized by:*

    a. leukocytosis
    b. giant platelets
    c. small platelets
    d. autoagglutination
    e. platelet clumping

Correct answers are on pages 187-189.

4. *Autoagglutinated red blood cells usually indicate:*

   a. hypoproteinemia
   b. hyperosmolarity
   c. collection artefact
   d. erythrocyte fragility
   e. autoimmune hemolytic disease

5. *Disseminated intravascular coagulation produces red blood cell fragmentation. These fragments of red blood cells are called:*

   a. schistocytes
   b. microcytes
   c. target cells
   d. leptocytes
   e. Howell-Jolly bodies

6. *The red blood cells of animals with iron-deficiency anemia are classically:*

   a. hyperchromic and normocytic
   b. polychromatophilic
   c. hypochromic and macrocytic
   d. hypochromic and microcytic
   e. hypochromic and normocytic

7. *The nonregenerative anemia that accompanies chronic renal failure is caused by:*

   a. chronic blood loss
   b. erythropoietin deficiency
   c. erythrophagocytosis
   d. elevated blood urea nitrogen
   e. hypoparathyroidism

8. *A marked regenerative response to anemia is characterized by:*

   a. microcytosis and reticulocytosis
   b. normochromia and reticulocytosis
   c. hyperchromia and reticulocytosis
   d. normocytosis and reticulocytosis
   e. macrocytosis and reticulocytosis

9. *A common cause of chronic blood loss anemia in young animals is:*

   a. parasitism (fleas, hookworms)
   b. rodenticide toxicosis (warfarin)
   c. primary bleeding disorder
   d. immune-mediated hemolytic disease
   e. copper deficiency

10. *Basophilic stippling of erythrocytes is characteristic of:*

    a. magnesium poisoning
    b. copper toxicosis
    c. lead poisoning
    d. hemobartonellosis
    e. babesiosis

11. *The cause of feline infectious anemia is:*

    a. feline leukemia virus
    b. coronavirus
    c. parvovirus
    d. *Hemobartonella felis*
    e. feline immunodeficiency virus

12. *Dehydration is characterized by:*

    a. increased packed cell volume and decreased plasma protein level
    b. decreased packed cell volume and decreased plasma protein level
    c. decreased packed cell volume and increased plasma protein level
    d. increased packed cell volume and normal plasma protein level
    e. increased packed cell volume and increased plasma protein level

13. *Polychromatophilic red blood cells are called:*

    a. reticulocytes
    b. poikilocytes
    c. leptocytes
    d. target cells
    e. acanthocytes

14. Variation in erythrocyte size on a blood smear is called:

a. spherocytosis
b. poikilocytosis
c. anisocytosis
d. elliptocytosis
e. acanthocytosis

15. Variation in erythrocyte shape on a blood smear is called:

a. spherocytosis
b. poikilocytosis
c. anisocytosis
d. elliptocytosis
e. acanthocytosis

16. The "LE cell" is characteristic of:

a. acute leukemia
b. chronic leukemia
c. Hodgkin's disease
d. systemic lupus erythematosus
e. lymphosarcoma

17. A leukocyte with a nucleus in the shape of a "spoked wheel" is called a:

a. plasma cell
b. leukemoid cell
c. chromatid body
d. polychromatophilic cell
e. monocyte

18. The test for erythrocyte antiglobulin is called the:

a. Schmidt's test
b. Shirmer test
c. Cooley's anemia test
d. Howell-Jolly test
e. Coombs' test

19. Monocytosis is a characteristic sign of:

a. systemic toxicity
b. severe viral disease
c. severe parasitic infection
d. acute lymphoblastic leukemia
e. systemic inflamatory response

20. Which blood cells have the longest life span?

a. leukocytes
b. erythrocytes
c. thrombocytes
d. megakaryocytes
e. macrophages

21. Cyclic hematopoiesis of gray Collie dogs is characterized by:

a. cyclic thrombocytosis
b. cyclic leukocytosis
c. cyclic neutropenia
d. intermittent polycythemia
e. erythrophagocytosis

22. The congenital, hereditary anemia of Basenji dogs is called:

a. glucose-6-phosphate dehydrogenase deficiency
b. phosphofructokinase deficiency
c. porphyria
d. pyruvate kinase deficiency
e. methemoglobinemia

23. Toxic anemia caused by oxidant drugs or toxins is characterized by deposits of denatured hemoglobin called:

a. Howell-Jolly bodies
b. Heinz bodies
c. LE bodies
d. refractile bodies
e. *Ehrlichia* bodies

24. Tropical pancytopenia is a tick-borne rickettsial infection known as:

a. babesiosis
b. ehrlichiosis
c. trypanosomiasis
d. piroplasmosis
e. anaplasmosis

Correct answers are on pages 187-189.

25. The most common severe inherited coagulation defect of companion animals is:

a. hemophilia A
b. von Willebrand's disease
c. factor X deficiency
d. Christmas disease
e. factor XII deficiency

26. Platelet adhesion, an important initial event in the control of bleeding, is primarily mediated by:

a. fibrin
b. platelet factor 3
c. von Willebrand factor
d. thromboxanes
e. subendothelial elastin

27. The most common inherited bleeding disorder of people and dogs is:

a. thrombocytopenic purpura
b. von Willebrand's disease
c. hemophilia
d. factor VII deficiency
e. factor X deficiency

28. The inheritance pattern of hemophilia is:

a. sex-linked recessive
b. autosomal recessive
c. sex-linked dominant
d. autosomal incompletely dominant
e. sex-linked codominant

29. A common cause of bleeding tendency in aged patients is:

a. rodenticide toxicosis (warfarin)
b. capillary fragility
c. platelet dysfunction secondary to uremia (end-stage kidney disease)
d. hepatosplenomegaly secondary to production of defective red blood cells
e. cardiopulmonary failure

30. Adverse effects of trimethoprim-sulfa antibacterials include bleeding tendency because they:

a. inhibit vitamin K-dependent clotting factors
b. enhance fibrinolysis
c. cause thrombocytopenia and platelet dysfunction
d. sterilize the bowel
e. impair production of von Willebrand factor

31. The results of which hemostatic tests are usually normal in animals with von Willebrand's disease?

a. bleeding time, erythrocyte sedimentation rate
b. platelet retention (adhesion), von Willebrand factor activity
c. activated partial thromboplastin time, prothrombin time
d. ristocetin cofactor activity, bleeding time
e. factor VIII activity, von Willebrand factor activity

32. Hemophilia A is characterized by:

a. low factor VIII activity
b. low von Willebrand factor activity
c. low factor IX activity
d. prolonged primary bleeding time
e. normal factor VIII activity

33. Hemophilia B is characterized by:

a. low factor VIII activity
b. low von Willebrand factor activity
c. prolonged primary bleeding time
d. normal factor IX activity
e. low factor IX activity

34. The recently developed second-generation rodenticides are more toxic because they:

a. affect platelet function as well as coagulation
b. affect coagulation and fibrinolysis
c. are more potent and slowly metabolized
d. are more potent and rapidly metabolized
e. are hepatotoxic

35. Patients with hypothyroidism have a bleeding tendency primarily related to:

a. altered hepatic protein synthesis
b. reduced platelet function and von Willebrand factor activity
c. capillary fragility
d. chronic intravascular coagulation
e. hyperactive fibrinolysis

36. Parvovirus infection in people and animals can produce:

a. septic arthritis
b. urticaria
c. abruptio placentae
d. muscle atrophy
e. transient bone marrow failure

37. Coagulation profiles performed in animals with liver disease typically show:

a. low von Willebrand factor activity
b. reduced fibrinolysis
c. elevated prothrombin time
d. thrombocytosis
e. hypercoagulability

38. Fibrin clot formation is the result of:

a. thrombin interaction with fibrinogen
b. plasmin interaction with fibrinogen
c. thrombin interaction with plasminogen
d. plasmin interaction wtih plasminogen
e. prothrombin interaction with thrombin

39. The 3 major events in hemostasis involve:

a. platelets, thrombosis and fibrinolysis
b. the blood vessel, coagulation and fibrinolysis
c. the blood vessel, thrombosis and platelets
d. the blood vessel, platelets and coagulation
e. platelets, coagulation and fibrinolysis

40. Vitamin K-dependent clotting factors are synthesized in the:

a. spleen
b. liver
c. lung
d. kidney
e. heart

41. Inherited platelet function defects have been recognized in:

a. German Shepherds and Doberman Pinschers
b. Beagles and Basenjis
c. Otterhounds and Basset Hounds
d. Poodles and Cocker Spaniels
e. Lhasa Apsos and Keeshonds

42. The dog breed most commonly affected with von Willebrand's disease is the:

a. Scottish Terrier
b. Shetland Sheepdog
c. Standard Poodle
d. Doberman Pinscher
e. Akita

43. A typical sign of thrombocytopenic bleeding is:

a. hematoma formation and joint pain
b. epistaxis and exercise intolerance
c. petechiae and ecchymoses
d. melena and retinal hemorrhage
e. hematuria and splenomegaly

44. The classic sign of bleeding in animals with hemophilia is:

a. hematoma formation
b. epistaxis
c. petechiae and ecchymoses
d. melena
e. hematuria

45. The characteristic type of bleeding in animals with von Willebrand's disease involves the:

a. skin and subcutaneous tissue
b. muscles
c. mucosal surfaces
d. joints
e. medullary cavity of long bones

Correct answers are on pages 187-189.

46. Aspirin is used to prevent and treat thrombosis because it:

a. impairs coagulation
b. impairs platelet function
c. enhances fibrinolysis
d. stimulates thrombopoiesis
e. produces thrombocytopenia

47. Rodenticide poisoning causes bleeding by:

a. inhibiting platelet function and fibrin deposition
b. inhibiting platelet function and fibrinolysis
c. preventing formation of fibrin in the liver
d. blocking synthesis of vitamin K-dependent clotting factors
e. inhibiting prothrombin activation of blood vessels

48. The most common cause of chronic recurrent thrombocytopenia is:

a. onion poisoning
b. parvoviral infection
c. adverse reaction to modified-live-virus vaccine
d. bone marrow failure
e. immune-mediated disease

49. The most common inheritance pattern in von Willebrand's disease is:

a. sex-linked recessive
b. autosomal recessive
c. autosomal incompletely dominant
d. sex-linked dominant
e. sex-linked codominant

50. The bone marrow precursor cell of the blood platelet is the:

a. megakaryocyte
b. macrokaryoblast
c. mononuclear giant cell
d. Reed-Sternberg cell
e. pluripotent stem cell

51. A 5-yr-old St. Bernard is presented to your small animal practice because of lethargy and anorexia of 2 weeks' duration. Physical examination reveals generalized lymphadenopathy. Microscopic examination of a fine-needle aspirate shows a monotonous population (>90%) of round cells with a high nucleus to cytoplasm ratio and prominent nucleoli. These cells are larger than the rare neutrophils you find. Based on this description, what is the most likely diagnosis?

a. inflammation
b. osteosarcoma
c. lymphosarcoma
d. benign hyperplasia
e. immune stimulation

52. What is the predominant cell type seen in most chylous effusions?

a. mast cell
b. eosinophil
c. neutrophil
d. lymphocyte
e. macrophage

53. Which of the following is typical of fluid removed from the peritoneal cavity of a cat with effusive feline infectious peritonitis?

a. clear, high-protein fluid containing primarily lymphocytes
b. straw-colored, low-protein fluid containing primarily neutrophils
c. straw-colored, high-protein fluid containing primarily eosinophils
d. straw-colored, high-protein fluid containing primarily neutrophils
e. straw-colored, high-protein fluid containing primarily lymphocytes

54. A Kurloff body is an eosinophilic-staining inclusion seen normally within the lymphocytes of:

a. rats
b. rabbits
c. reptiles
d. hamsters
e. guinea pigs

*55. Which of the following is **not** classified as a round-cell tumor?*

a. histiocytoma
b. mastocytoma
c. osteosarcoma
d. lymphosarcoma
e. transmissible venereal tumor

56. On an impression smear made from an ulcerated area on the forelimb of a cat, you find multiple, small (2-4 μ), basophilic-staining organisms whose shape varies from round to oval to fusiform (cigar-shaped), with a thin, clear halo. The most likely cause of the lesion in this cat is:

a. leishmaniasis
b. toxoplasmosis
c. sporotrichosis
d. histoplasmosis
e. cytauxzoonosis

57. Which organism commonly affects the central nervous system and might be found on cytologic evaluation of cerebrospinal fluid?

a. *Sporothrix schenckii*
b. *Coccidioides immitis*
c. *Histoplasma capsulatum*
d. *Blastomyces dermatitidis*
e. *Cryptococcus neoformans*

For Questions 58 through 62, select the correct answer from the 5 choices below.

a. metaplasia
b. dysplasia
c. crenation
d. carcinoma
e. sarcoma

58. Morphologic change of red blood cells typically caused by dehydration and characterized by multiple indentations in the cell membrane.

59. Malignant neoplasm of epithelial-cell origin.

60. Tissue change caused by chronic irritation and characterized by replacement of one mature cell type with another mature cell type.

61. Malignant neoplasm of mesenchymal-cell origin.

62. Non-neoplastic tissue change associated with various factors, such as inflammation, and characterized by irregular, atypical and proliferative changes in cell populations.

63. Steatitis defines:

a. inflammation of the mammary glands
b. excessive lipid globules in feces, associated with enteritis
c. inflammation of adipose tissue
d. excessive conjugated bilirubin in the serum, associated with hepatitis
e. inflammation of lymph vessels

64. You find rare, small, round, pale blue- to gray-staining, mulberry-like morulae in the cytoplasm of neutrophils of a 3-year-old English Pointer with polyarthritis. The most likely cause of this finding is:

a. distemper
b. babesiosis
c. ehrlichiosis
d. leptospirosis
e. histoplasmosis

65. From which cell type does multiple myeloma arise?

a. astrocytes
b. plasma cells
c. endothelial cells
d. precursor cells of granulocytes
e. myelin-producing cells of the central nervous system

Correct answers are on pages 187-189.

66. *In a vaginal swab from a 2-year-old intact Miniature Schnauzer, you find 96% superficial cells, with small pyknotic nuclei. This finding indicates that this bitch is most likely:*

a. in estrus
b. in diestrus
c. in anestrus
d. in proestrus
e. infected with a fungus

67. *Which cell type may occasionally be observed in synovial fluid and is diagnostic of systemic lupus erythematosus?*

a. lupus erythematosus (LE) cells
b. Mott cells
c. giant cell
d. leptocyte
e. siderocyte

68. *A Coombs' test is used to help diagnose:*

a. neonatal isoerythrolysis
b. feline infectious anemia
c. equine infectious anemia
d. autoimmune hemolytic anemia
e. microangiopathic hemolytic anemia

69. *Which organisms are referred to as "marginal bodies"?*

a. *Babesia*
b. *Anaplasma*
c. *Eperythrozoon*
d. *Hemobartonella*
e. *Ehrlichia*

70. *In a transtracheal wash from a horse, you find ciliated and nonciliated columnar and cuboidal cells, alveolar macrophages, an occasional neutrophil, and approximately 20% of cells as eosinophils. You observe no superficial squamous epithelial cells or* Simonsiella *organisms. Which of the following is the most appropriate cytologic interpretation?*

a. This is a normal cell population.
b. There is evidence of malignant neoplasia.
c. There is evidence of a hypersensitivity reaction.
d. There is evidence of bacterial or fungal inflammation.
e. There is evidence of oropharyngeal contamination.

71. *Concerning the procedure of percutaneous transtracheal/ bronchial wash, which statement is most accurate?*

a. It cannot be done without general anesthesia.
b. It is preferred in fractious animals.
c. It requires use of a sterilized endotracheal tube.
d. It reduces the risk of oropharyngeal contamination.
e. It involves passage of a needle and catheter through the thyroid cartilage.

72. *Which of the following best characterizes a septic exudate?*

a. low protein content (<3.0 g/dl), predominantly lymphocytes present, no bacteria seen or cultured
b. low protein content (<3.0 g/dl), predominantly nondegenerate neutrophils present, no bacteria seen or cultured
c. high protein content (>3.0 g/dl), predominantly degenerate neutrophils present, intracellular and/or extracellular bacteria present
d. low protein content (<3.0 g/dl), predominantly nondegenerate neutrophils present, intracellular and/or extracellular bacterial present
e. high protein content (>3.0 g/dl), predominantly foamy macrophages and nondegenerate neutrophils present, intracellular and/or extracellular bacteria present

73. *Which cell type comprises the lining of the pleural, peritoneal and visceral surfaces?*

a. Kupffer cell
b. epithelial cell
c. endothelial cell
d. mesothelial cell
e. reticuloendothelial cell

74. *Concerning normal cerebrospinal fluid in dogs, which statement is most accurate?*

a. It should contain fewer than 8 nucleated cells/μl.
b. Nucleated cells should consist primarily of nondegenerate neutrophils.
c. Cell counts should be performed 2-24 hours after collection of the sample.
d. Normal cerebrospinal fluid is clear and pink, with a total protein concentration of 50-100 mg/dl.
e. Normal cerebrospinal fluid is clear and yellow, with a total protein concentration of 50-100 mg/dl.

75. *Which of the following best describes an osteoblast?*

a. arises from the granulocytic cell line
b. a giant cell containing 6-10 randomly arranged nuclei
c. a cell that produces calcitonin within the parathyroid gland
d. the precursor cell to other skeletal system cells, such as chondrocytes and fibrocytes
e. an ovoid, plump cell resembling a large plasma cell, with a round, eccentric nucleus and dark blue cytoplasm

76. *Concerning cytologic evaluation of synovial fluid of dogs, which statement is* ***least*** *accurate?*

a. The presence of lupus erythematosus (LE) cells in synovial fluid is diagnostic of lupus erythematosus.
b. Normal synovial fluid is of low cellularity (less than 3,000 cells/μl).
c. Osteoclasts are not unusual in synovial fluid because these cells are present in articular cartilage.
d. Organisms are often difficult to identify in inflammatory arthropathies of bacterial origin.
e. An increased nucleated cell count with more than 90% mononuclear cells suggests degenerative joint disease.

77. *Concerning cytologic evaluation of lymph nodes, which statement is* ***least*** *accurate?*

a. Ruptured cells are a common artifact due to the fragility of lymphoid tissue.
b. There is no true cytologic difference between normal and hyperplastic lymph nodes.
c. Small lymphocytes typically comprise at least 75% of a normal lymph node cell population.
d. Lymphadenitis can be reliably diagnosed when neutrophils make up greater than 10% of the nucleated cell population.
e. Aspiration of foamy epithelial cells in the area of the mandibular lymph node usually indicates neoplasia.

78. *The linear distribution of cells seen on pull smears of fluids of high viscosity is termed:*

a. rouleaux
b. windrowing
c. pyriformation
d. castellation
e. coronification

79. *Which of the following is* ***not*** *a cytologic criterion of malignancy for epithelial-cell tumors?*

a. angular nucleoli
b. uniform nuclear size
c. large, prominent nucleoli
d. high nucleus:cytoplasm ratio
e. large numbers of abnormal mitotic figures

Correct answers are on pages 187-189.

80. *Concerning cytologic examination of the external ear canal, which statement is* ***least*** *accurate?*

a. Cerumen, an oily, yellow secretion, stains poorly or not at all.
b. A sweet-smelling, pale yellow exudate is most likely attributed to *Pseudomonas* infection.
c. *Malassezia* is a broad-based, budding yeast that is the most common cause of mycotic otitis externa.
d. The ear mite that produces a dry, black, granular discharge associated with parasitic otitis externa in companion animals is *Otobius megnini.*
e. Some of the most common causes of otitis externa (*Malassezia* and bacteria) are often normal inhabitants of the external ear canal.

81. *Concerning cytologic examination of the eye, which statement is* ***least*** *accurate?*

a. Keratoconjunctivitis sicca produces a lymphocytic exudate.
b. The anterior uvea is a site for metastasis of systemic carcinomas.
c. Neutrophilic infiltration of aqueous humor is characteristic of most causes of anterior uveitis.
d. In cats, corneal scrapings containing primarily eosinophils indicate eosinophilic keratitis.
e. Most intraocular tumors, either primary or secondary, do not exfoliate into aqueous humor; the exception is lymphosarcoma.

82. *Concerning cytologic examination of nasal masses and exudates, which statement is* ***least*** *accurate?*

a. Most nasal tumors are of mesenchymal origin.
b. *Rhinosporidium* infection in dogs causes a polypoid growth.
c. Transmissible venereal tumor can occur in the nasal areas, particularly in males.
d. Ciliated pseudostratified columnar epithelial cells originate from the nasal turbinates.
e. *Cryptococcus neoformans* infections produce a mucoid exudate and are most common in cats.

83. *Concerning cytologic examination of squamous-cell carcinomas, which statement is* ***least*** *accurate?*

a. They are often secondarily infected.
b. The tumor masses tend to yield groups of cells.
c. Perinuclear vacuolation is a common cytologic finding.
d. They are found only in poorly pigmented areas of the skin exposed to ultraviolet radiation.
e. They are tumors of epithelial origin.

84. *Which of the following best describes lipemic plasma from a normal, nonfasted dog?*

a. clear and yellow
b. opaque and white
c. clear and colorless
d. opaque and yellow
e. clear and pink to red

85. *Which of the following is associated with an exudate?*

a. hypoproteinemia
b. right heart failure
c. lymphatic obstruction
d. mycobacterial pneumonia
e. congestive heart failure with ascites

86. *Concerning transudates and exudates, which statement is most accurate?*

a. Both have similar cell counts, but exudates have higher protein concentrations.
b. Both have similar cell counts, but transudates have higher protein concentrations.
c. Exudates have lower protein concentrations but higher cell counts than transudates.
d. Transudates have lower protein concentrations but higher cell counts than exudates.

e. Exudates have higher protein concentrations and higher cell counts than transudates.

87. *Which of the following is **not** a typical finding in a long-standing or resolving hemorrhagic effusion?*

a. thrombocytosis
b. erythrophagocytosis
c. hypersegmented neutrophils
d. pink or xanthochromic supernatant
e. macrophages containing black pigment (hemosiderin)

88. *Which plasma protein of large animals is used to detect internal inflammatory lesions?*

a. kallikrein
b. thrombin
c. serotonin
d. fibrinogen
e. plasminogen

89. *Which term describes an intravascular deposit comprised of fibrin and formed elements of blood?*

a. embolus
b. thrombin
c. thrombus
d. infarct
e. plaque

90. *In a centrifuged microhematocrit tube containing whole blood, the area containing platelets and leukocytes is called the:*

a. band layer
b. white band
c. buffy coat
d. white line
e. myelochrome band

Answers

1. **b**
2. **b**
3. **c**
4. **e**
5. **a**
6. **d**
7. **b**
8. **e**
9. **a**
10. **c**
11. **d**
12. **e**
13. **a**
14. **c**
15. **b**
16. **d**
17. **a**
18. **e**
19. **e**
20. **b**
21. **c**
22. **d**
23. **b**
24. **b**
25. **a**
26. **c**
27. **b**
28. **a**
29. **c**
30. **c**
31. **c**
32. **b**
33. **e**
34. **a**

35. **b**

36. **e**

37. **c**

38. **a**

39. **d**

40. **b**

41. **c**

42. **d**

43. **c**

44. **a**

45. **c**

46. **b**

47. **d**

48. **e**

49. **c**

50. **a**

51. **c** St Bernards are predisposed to lymphosarcoma. Finding over 50% lymphoblasts in a cytologic preparation of an enlarged lymph node is considered diagnostic of lymphosarcoma.

52. **d** Neutrophils can predominate, but this is much less common.

53. **d**

54. **e**

55. **c** Osteosarcoma is a spindle-cell tumor of mesenchymal origin. All the others listed are round-cell tumors.

56. **c** Many *Sporothrix* organisms are found in infected cats but the organisms are difficult to find in infected dogs and horses. Fusiform (cigar) shapes are characteristic of *Sporothrix schenckii*.

57. **e**

58. **c**

59. **d**

60. **a**

61. **e**

62. **b**

63. **c**

64. **c** Pale blue inclusions in neutrophils are seen with some *Ehrlichia ewingii* infections. Parvoviral infection does not cause inclusion bodies in circulating cells. Distemper inclusions are homogeneous, basophilic or eosinophilic staining structures in neutrophils and erythrocytes or mononuclear cells.

65. **b** Multiple myeloma is a tumor of plasma cells, which generally produce excessive amounts of a single type of immunoglobulin. Another characteristic of this tumor in dogs is bone lysis.

66. **a**

67. **a** Mott cells are vacuolated plasma cells. Giant cells are seen with chronic granulomatous disease. Siderocytes are red blood cells containing iron particles. Leptocytes are thin, folded red blood cells.

68. **d** Neonatal isoerythrolysis is diagnosed by clinical behavior and serologic tests. Equine infectious anemia is confirmed using the Coggins test. Feline infectious anemia can be confirmed by examination of the blood smear, as can microangiopathies.

69. **b**

70. **c** If greater than 10% of the cells are eosinophils and no criteria of malignancy or oropharyngeal contamination exist (superficial squamous cells), then an allergic or parasitic infection is most likely.

71. **d** It reduces the risk of oropharyngeal contamination. The landmark used for this technique is the cricothyroid ligament. Because general anesthesia is usually not needed, this would not be a good choice for a fractious or aggressive animal.

72. **c**

73. **d**

74. **a** Normal CSF is also clear and colorless and has a total protein concentration of less than 50 mg/dl.

75. **e** Osteoblasts are ovoid, plump cells with a rounded eccentric nucleus and dark blue cytoplasm. They resemble large plasma cells. Osteoclasts are large multinucleated cells that arise from the macrophage/monocyte cell line. There is not a single precursor cell to all other skeletal system cells.

76. **c** Finding an osteoclast is not unusual because these cells are present in articular cartilage. Osteoclasts are present in subchondral bone. Their presence in synovial fluid suggests erosion of articular cartilage to subchondral bone.

77. **e** Aspiration of foamy epithelial cells in the area of the mandibular lymph node usually indicates neoplasia. The submandibular salivary gland is often aspirated in this area, revealing a uniform population of foamy cells in a pink background when stained with Wright's stain.

78. **b**

79. **b** Uniform nuclear size. Typically, malignant neoplasia shows a large variation in nuclear size. An exception is lymphosarcoma. Lymphosarcoma is a round-cell tumor, not an epithelial-cell tumor.

80. **d** The ear mite that produces a dry, black, granular discharge is *Otodectes cynotis. Otobius megnini* is the spinose ear tick of food animals.

81. **a** Keratoconjunctivitis sicca produces a neutrophilic exudate, usually containing bacteria.

82. **a** Most nasal tumors are of epithelial origin.

83. **d** Tumors are only found in poorly pigmented areas of the skin exposed to ultraviolet radiation. Squamous-cell carcinoma may be found in any area of the skin in dogs and cats.

84. **b** Clear and colorless plasma is seen normally in most dogs and cats. Horses and cattle have slightly yellow plasma. Icteric samples are yellow, while hemolyzed samples are pink to red.

85. **d** Mycobacterial pneumonia. The other disorders listed would produce a transudate or modified transudate.

86. **e** Exudates have higher protein concentrations and cell counts than transudates. An exudate generally has a protein concentration of >3.0 g/dl and a high cell count.

87. **a** Platelets are generally absent.

88. **d**

89. **c** Thrombin is a coagulation protein. An infarct is an area of tissue necrosis, often caused by a thrombus or embolus. An embolus is a freely circulating thrombus. A plaque is a flat area or patch.

90. **c**

Notes

Notes

Section 19

Immunology

I. Tizard

Recommended Reading

Abbas AK *et al: Cellular and Molecular Immunology.* Saunders, Philadelphia, 1991.

Colloqium on Clinical Immunology. *JAVMA* 181:962-1182, 1982.

Halliwell REW and Gorman NT: *Veterinary Clinical Immunology.* Saunders, Philadelphia, 1989.

Tizard I: *Veterinary Immunology: An Introduction.* 4th ed. Saunders, Philadelphia, 1992.

Practice answer sheet is on page 381.

Questions

1. *Cellular immunity involves activities of which cells?*

   a. B-cells, mast cells and plasma cells
   b. neutrophils, mast cells and histiocytes
   c. macrophages, NK cells and T-cells
   d. mast cells, macrophages and histiocytes
   e. B-cells and histiocytes

2. *Mature antibody-producing cells are called:*

   a. immunoblasts
   b. histiocytes
   c. T-cells
   d. neutrophils
   e. plasma cells

3. *The major function of eosinophils is probably to:*

   a. phagocytose bacteria
   b. neutralize mast cell-derived factors
   c. neutralize viruses
   d. promote inflammation
   e. caused delayed hypersensitivity

4. *The Coombs' (antiglobulin) test was designed to:*

   a. detect red blood cell antigens
   b. diagnose brucellosis
   c. detect reaginic antibody
   d. detect immune reactants on cells
   e. measure the ability of complement to cause hemolysis

Correct answers are on page 193.

5. *A 3-week-old foal with recurrent infections has normal blood lymphocyte numbers and low serum immunoglobulin levels. The most likely cause of these findings is:*

   a. neonatal isoerythrolysis
   b. failure to absorb colostrum
   c. severe combined immunodeficiency
   d. selective IgM deficiency
   e. viral rhinopneumonitis

6. *"Blue eye" is a complication encountered in dogs vaccinated with:*

   a. live canine distemper virus vaccine
   b. inactivated canine adenovirus vaccine
   c. inactivated canine parainfluenza vaccine
   d. *Leptospira* bacterin
   e. live canine adenovirus vaccine

7. *The reaction to intradermal injection of tuberculin is an example of:*

   a. graft versus host reaction
   b. delayed hypersensitivity
   c. immediate hypersensitivity
   d. autoimmunity
   e. lymphocytotoxicity

8. *In animals that are allergic to penicillin, the drug molecule acts as:*

   a. an antibody
   b. a carrier
   c. a hapten
   d. an antigen
   e. an adjuvant

9. *In dogs, the organ most profoundly affected by systemic anaphylaxis is the:*

   a. lungs
   b. gastrointestinal tract
   c. liver
   d. spleen
   e. skin

10. *False-negative tuberculin tests may occur in:*

   a. very young cattle
   b. heavily parasitized cattle
   c. heavily pregnant cows
   d. very old cattle
   e. Jersey cattle

11. *The reaction to intradermal injection of tuberculin is of maximal intensity within:*

   a. 30-40 minutes
   b. 6-10 hours
   c. 20-24 hours
   d. 48-72 hours
   e. 7-10 days

12. *Puppies should be initially vaccinated against canine distemper at an approximate age of:*

   a. 1 week
   b. 4 weeks
   c. 8 weeks
   d. 12 weeks
   e. 16 weeks

13. *The most likely cause of vaccine failure in a 14-week-old puppy given canine distemper vaccine is:*

   a. distemper infection before vaccination
   b. persistent maternal immunity
   c. immunodeficiency
   d. ineffective vaccine
   e. heavy parasite burden

14. *Bacteria are cleared from the circulation mainly by:*

   a. filtration in the pulmonary capillary bed
   b. phagocytosis by macrophages in the liver and spleen
   c. phagocytosis by circulating neutrophils
   d. phagocytosis by marginated neutrophils
   e. excretion through the renal glomeruli

15. The intestine of newborn domestic animals becomes impermeable to colostral immunoglobulins by approximately:

a. 10 hours of age
b. 24 hours of age
c. 20 hours of age
d. 36 hours of age
e. 7 days of age

Answers

1. **c**
2. **e**
3. **d**
4. **d**
5. **b**
6. **e**
7. **b**
8. **c**
9. **c**
10. **c**
11. **d**
12. **c**
13. **a**
14. **b**
15. **b**

Notes

Notes

Section **20**

Laboratory Procedures

B.T. Mitzner, R.E. Raskin

Recommended Reading

Cowell RL and Tyler RD: *Cytology and Hematology of the Horse.* American Veterinary Publications, Goleta, CA, 1992.

Cowell RL and Tyler RD: *Diagnostic Cytology of the Dog and Cat.* American Veterinary Publications, Goleta, CA, 1989.

Duncan JR and Prasse KW: *Veterinary Laboratory Medicine.* 2nd ed. Iowa State University Press, Ames, 1986.

Goldston RT *et al: Practitioner's Laboratory.* Veterinary Medicine Publishing, Lenexa, KS, 1983.

Henry JB *et al: Clinical Diagnosis and Management by Laboratory Methods.* 17th ed. Saunders, Philadelphia, 1984.

Meyer DJ *et al: Veterinary Laboratory Medicine: Interpretation and Diagnosis.* Saunders, Philadelphia, 1992.

Mitzner BT: In-house Laboratory. Column published regularly in *DVM Newsmagazine.*

Osborne CA and Stevens JB: *Handbook of Canine and Feline Urinalysis.* Ralston Purina, St. Louis, 1981.

Pratt PW: *Laboratory Procedures for Veterinary Technicians.* 2nd ed. American Veterinary Publications, Goleta, CA, 1992.

Schalm OW: *Manual of Feline and Canine Hematology.* Veterinary Practice Publishing, Santa Barbara, CA, 1980.

Willard MD *et al: Small Animal Clinical Diagnosis by Laboratory Methods.* Saunders, Philadelphia, 1989.

Practice answer sheet is on page 383

Questions

1. *Specimens for hematologic analysis should be collected in vacuum tubes with a stopper of what color?*

   a. lavender
   b. blue
   c. red
   d. green
   e. gray

2. *Before staining, blood smears should be fixed in:*

   a. acetone
   b. xylene
   c. isopropyl alcohol
   d. ethanol
   e. methanol

Correct answers are on pages 208-210.

3. *When scanning a blood smear, a finding of 4-6 white blood cells per high-power field indicates an estimated white blood cell count of:*

   a. 7000-10,000/μl
   b. 2000-4000/μl
   c. 13,000-15,000/μl
   d. 16,000-18,000/μl
   e. >20,000/μl

4. *The blood smear of a normal patient should have how many platelets per oil-immersion field?*

   a. <3
   b. 3-5
   c. 6-10
   d. 11-15
   e. >16

5. *Methods for obtaining the total white blood cell count include all of the following* ***except:***

   a. estimation from blood smear
   b. dilution pipet
   c. volumetric impedence analyzer
   d. filtration
   e. Unopette method

6. *Why are blood cell counts done with automated hematology analyzers likely to be more accurate than those done manually?*

   a. automated counts are free from human influence
   b. automated analyzers count a greater number of cells
   c. automated analyzers use light to count cells
   d. cells become distorted during preparation for microscopic viewing
   e. specimens for manual counts require further dilution to be as accurate as specimens counted with an automated system

7. *Automated blood cell counts require manual or electronic coincidence correction. Concerning automated blood cell counts, which statement is most accurate?*

   a. As the count gets higher, accuracy increases.
   b. The procedure corrects for any clots that might have formed in the sample.
   c. Coincidence correction is only necessary for specimens that have been held overnight.
   d. As the count gets higher, the probability of 2 or more cells simultaneously passing through the aperture becomes greater.
   e. As the count gets higher, certain cells in the diluent tend to sediment out of solution.

8. *The most important periodic maintenance procedure required by impedence-type hematology analyzers is:*

   a. oiling the vacuum pump
   b. changing the vacuum tubing
   c. deproteinizing the counting aperture
   d. cleaning the dilutor probe
   e. adjusting the vacuum pressure

9. *When using an impedence-type hematology analyzer, the background count is performed on:*

   a. a normal blood sample
   b. a diluted control sample
   c. deionized water
   d. an aliquot of isotonic diluent
   e. an aliquot of cleaning solution

10. *Hematology quality-control tests are used to assess the:*

    a. performance of the operator
    b. accuracy of the counting method
    c. accuracy of the sample dilutions
    d. integrity of the reagents
    e. performance of the entire system

11. *Most errors that occur with automated hematology analyzers can be traced back to:*

    a. improper specimen collection
    b. inadequate premixing of the specimen
    c. improper dilution of the specimen
    d. lack of familiarity with the analyzer
    e. improper transposition of results

12. *Most practices use a refractometer to perform a quick "total solids" measurement. When the specimen is taken from a spun hematocrit tube, the measurement includes **only**:*

a. total protein
b. total protein and fibrinogen
c. plasma protein
d. albumin
e. albumin and globulin

13. *When using a refractometer to measure total solids, a lipemic sample:*

a. decreases the result
b. increases the result
c. has no effect on the result
d. makes the result impossible to read
e. gives accurate results in fasted patients only

14. *In which species are reticulocytes **least** likely to be found?*

a. dogs
b. cats
c. horses
d. cattle
e. pigs

15. *Which cell type is **not** found in an avian blood smear?*

a. erythrocyte
b. thrombocyte
c. heterophil
d. neutrophil
e. eosinophil

16. *Which cell type is **not** in the red cell series?*

a. prorubricyte
b. metamyelocyte
c. rubricyte
d. reticulocyte
e. erythrocyte

17. *Which of the following is a platelet precursor?*

a. megakaryocyte
b. metamyelocyte
c. metarubricyte
d. thrombocyte
e. myeloblast

18. *What artificial change in the complete blood count is most likely to occur if the blood sample is collected from an excited or agitated patient?*

a. leukocytosis
b. decreased hematocrit
c. platelet aggregation
d. left shift
e. leukopenia

19. *A Barr body is a small, spherical extension of the nucleus of some peripheral granulocytes. Barr bodies indicate that the patient:*

a. is anemic
b. is stressed
c. is female
d. is in critical condition
e. has vitamin B_{12} deficiency

20. *Rouleaux formation (stacking or linear clumping of erythrocytes) is a common finding in:*

a. dogs
b. cats
c. cattle
d. horses
e. pigs

21. *In which species are nucleated erythrocytes a normal finding?*

a. cats
b. pigs
c. rabbits
d. chickens
e. horses

Correct answers are on pages 208-210.

22. *Which cell type is **least** likely to be found on a peripheral blood smear from a dog with autoimmune hemolytic anemia?*

a. reticulocyte
b. spherocyte
c. target cell
d. erythrocyte
e. metamyelocyte

23. *The formula* $\frac{PCV(\%) \times 10}{RBC\ count}$ *is used to calculate:*

a. the maturation index
b. the reticulocyte count
c. the mean corpuscular volume
d. corrected nucleated red blood cell count
e. the mean corpuscular hemoglobin

24. *Microcytic anemia is characterized by:*

a. nucleated red blood cells
b. abnormally small red blood cells
c. abnormally large red blood cells
d. pale red blood cells
e. schistocytes

25. *Variation in the size of erythrocytes is known as:*

a. macrocytosis
b. poikilocytosis
c. polychromasia
d. erythrocytosis
e. anisocytosis

26. *Abnormally shaped erythrocytes are collectively referred to as:*

a. stomatocytes
b. poikilocytes
c. macrocytes
d. heterocytes
e. polychromatocytes

27. *In a complete blood count, a left shift refers to:*

a. movement of the microscope slide to the left
b. decreased numbers of platelets
c. an abundance of immature white blood cell forms
d. increased numbers of nucleated red blood cells
e. a trend toward macrocytosis

28. *An abundance of eosinophils on a peripheral blood smear is most commonly associated with:*

a. neoplastic disease
b. infection
c. trauma
d. allergic conditions
e. stress

29. *How long should microhematocrit tubes be centrifuged?*

a. 1 minute
b. 5 minutes
c. 10 minutes
d. 3 minutes
e. depends on centrifuge calibraton

30. *If the sealant clay fails to stay in the microhematocrit tube during centrifugation, the most likely cause is:*

a. worn tube cushions or gasket
b. old clay sealant
c. tube of incorrect diameter
d. centrifuge not properly balanced
e. not enough clay sealant used

31. *Punctate reticulocytes are most frequently found in:*

a. dogs
b. cats
c. horses
d. pigs
e. cattle

32. *Which stain is **not** appropriate for routine staining of blood smears?*

a. Wright's
b. Wright's-Giemsa
c. Diff-Quik
d. trichrome
e. Giemsa

33. *As a minimum standard, blood collection tubes containing EDTA should be filled:*

a. to the top
b. one-fourth of the way to the top
c. half way to the top
d. three-quarters of the way to the top
e. to any desired level, as the amount is not critical

34. *The most common bleeding disorders seen in companion animals are related to:*

a. decreased clotting factor activity
b. thrombocytopenia
c. platelet dysfunction
d. hemophilia A and B
e. hypocalcemia

35. *The activated clotting time (ACT) is prolonged in animals with:*

a. platelet dysfunction
b. anemia
c. platelet deficiency
d. clotting factor deficiency
e. reticulocytosis

36. *Bleeding time is the best test to detect:*

a. platelet dysfunction
b. anemia
c. platelet deficiency
d. clotting factor deficiency
e. reticulocytosis

37. *Specimens for coagulation testing should be collected in tubes containing:*

a. EDTA
b. ammonium heparin
c. sodium citrate
d. potassium oxalate
e. no anticoagulant

38. *Which of the following is **not** a test of hemostasis?*

a. activated clotting time
b. prothrombin time
c. partial thromboplastin time
d. bleeding time
e. erythrocyte sedimentation rate

39. *While a serum specimen is preferred for chemistry analysis, a plasma specimen may be used for most chemistry assays, provided that the specimen is:*

a. collected from a fasted patient
b. collected in a tube containing lithium heparin
c. collected in a tube containing EDTA
d. collected only from the jugular vein
e. analyzed within 15 minutes after collection

40. *Which abnormality is **least** likely to be found in a non-separated blood sample collected for serum chemistry analysis?*

a. increased potassium level
b. increased aspartate aminotransferase activity
c. increased phosphorus level
d. decreased glucose level
e. decreased cholesterol level

41. *Which method **cannot** be used to avoid or clear most lipemic blood specimens?*

a. allow the specimen to stand upright in the refrigerator for several hours or overnight
b. treat the specimen with chemical "clearing agents"
c. use an ultracentrifuge to separate the specimen
d. obtain the specimen from a fasted patient
e. collect the specimen in a heparinized tube

Correct answers are on pages 208-210.

42. *Which technique is most likely to prevent hemolysis during blood collection?*

a. use a large-gauge (<19-ga) needle
b. use a small-gauge (>21-ga) needle
c. soak the skin well with alcohol before venipuncture
d. shake the specimen vigorously after collection
e. use a large (>10 ml) collection tube

43. *Which clinicopathologic abnormality is* ***least*** *likely to be found in a patient with advanced renal disease?*

a. increased blood urea nitrogen level
b. increased serum creatinine level
c. decreased serum calcium level
d. decreased hematocrit
e. increased serum phosphorus level

44. *Which of the following does* ***not*** *reflect liver function?*

a. serum albumin level
b. serum alanine aminotransferase activity
c. serum alkaline phosphatase activity
d. serum creatinine level
e. serum aspartate aminotransferase activity

45. *Serum amylase activity generally is* ***not*** *increased in animals with:*

a. pancreatitis
b. renal disease
c. dehydration
d. pancreatic abscess
e. colitis

46. *Icteric patients usually exhibit an increased:*

a. serum bilirubin level
b. serum albumin level
c. serum creatinine level
d. serum lipase activity
e. serum creatine phosphokinase activity

47. *Total serum bilirubin reflects serum levels of:*

a. direct bilirubin
b. direct bilirubin and conjugated bilirubin
c. conjugated bilirubin and unconjugated bilirubin
d. indirect bilirubin and unconjugated bilirubin
e. indirect bilirubin

48. *Total plasma protein values in excess of 10 g/dl are usually associated with:*

a. increased serum albumin levels
b. increased serum creatinine levels
c. increased red blood cell hemoglobin content
d. increased serum globulin levels
e. dehydration

49. *Increased serum amylase and lipase activities usually suggest:*

a. liver disease
b. kidney disease
c. intestinal disease
d. pancreatic disease
e. pulmonary disease

50. *Elevated serum creatine phosphokinase activity is usually associated with:*

a. renal disease
b. liver disease
c. intestinal disease
d. muscular disease
e. pancreatic disease

51. ***Decreased*** *serum cholinesterase activity often accompanies:*

a. renal disease
b. trauma
c. organophosphate insecticide toxicity
d. diabetes mellitus
e. pancreatitis

52. The d-xylose test is used as a screening test to detect:

a. malabsorption syndrome
b. diabetes mellitus
c. adrenal disease
d. liver tumors
e. renal disease

53. In an endpoint analysis,:

a. several light-absorbence readings are taken at intervals
b. a standard is not necessary
c. a conversion coefficient is required
d. a stable, colored product is formed at the conclusion
e. light absorbence is not proportional to solute concentration

*54. Which of the following is **not** used to calculate anion gap?*

a. serum sodium level
b. serum calcium level
c. serum CO_2 level
d. serum potassium level
e. serum chloride level

55. The constituents in most serum chemistry control samples are stable for approximately 7 days after reconstitution. Which control sample is stable for the shortest time after reconstitution?

a. glucose
b. albumin
c. creatinine
d. carbon dioxide
e. urea nitrogen

56. A microscope should be professionally cleaned:

a. yearly or more often, as needed
b. every 5 years
c. when more than 30 samples a week are examined for 6 consecutive months
d. when the focal field is obscured
e. when the focusing mechanism breaks

57. The proper immersion oil for normal light microscopy is:

a. type A
b. type B
c. mineral oil
d. linseed oil
e. SAE 30 automotive oil

*58. Which of the following is **not** an acceptable fecal flotation solution?*

a. sodium nitrate
b. Sheather's (sugar)
c. zinc sulfate
d. potassium chromate
e. glycerin

*59. In an infected animal, life cycle stages of which parasite are **least** likely to be found on a fecal flotation preparation?*

a. *Giardia cati*
b. *Toxocara canis*
c. *Trichuris vulpis*
d. *Ancylostoma caninum*
e. *Isospora*

60. Ova of Capillaria plica *are most likely to be found in:*

a. feces
b. urine
c. saliva
d. blood
e. nasal discharge

61. Ova of which parasite are usually seen in the larvated form?

a. *Ancylostoma* (hookworm)
b. *Isospora* (coccidia)
c. *Dipylidium* (tapeworm)
d. *Strongyloides* (threadworm)
e. *Toxocara* (roundworm)

Correct answers are on pages 208-210.

62. *The parasite that appears as a punctate small rod-like or ring-like structure on the periphery of red blood cells in peripheral blood smears is:*

   a. *Ehrlichia canis*
   b. *Babesia bigemina*
   c. *Anaplasma marginale*
   d. *Hemobartonella felis*
   e. *Tritrichomonas fetus*

63. *Which method is most reliable for detection of* Ehrlichia canis *infection?*

   a. blood smear examination
   b. buffy coat examination
   c. indirect fluorescent antibody test on serum
   d. wet preparation of peripheral blood stained with new methylene blue
   e. serum titer

64. *The parasite* Hemoproteus *is most likely to infect the erythrocytes of:*

   a. horses
   b. cattle
   c. dogs
   d. birds
   e. cats

65. *Microfilariae of* Dirofilaria immitis *(canine heartworm) are most often confused with those of:*

   a. *Dipetalonema*
   b. *Trypanosoma*
   c. *Babesia*
   d. *Hemobartonella*
   e. *Ehrlichia*

66. *Which method is **not** used for detection of heartworm microfilariae?*

   a. direct blood smear
   b. buffy coat examination
   c. modified Knott's technique
   d. filtration/concentration method
   e. enzyme-linked immunosorbent assay

67. *The test of choice for routine surveillance of dogs treated monthly with heartworm preventives is:*

   a. Knott's technique
   b. filtration/concentration
   c. enzyme-linked immunosorbent assay of high sensitivity
   d. enzyme-linked immunosorbent assay of high specificity
   e. filtration/concentration plus enzyme-linked immunosorbent assay

68. *Cigar-shaped mites in a skin scraping from a dog are most likely of the genus:*

   a. *Sarcoptes*
   b. *Notoedres*
   c. *Otodectes*
   d. *Demodex*
   e. *Psoroptes*

69. *Which method is **least** appropriate for urine collection?*

   a. mid-stream free catch
   b. manual expression of the bladder
   c. aspiration of urine from a cage floor or litterbox
   d. bladder catheterization
   e. cystocentesis

70. *In which type of patient should cystocentesis **not** be performed?*

   a. 3-month-old puppy
   b. obese Beagle
   c. female dog in heat
   d. adult male cat with disease of the bladder wall
   e. old dog with a fever

71. *A normal-colored but slightly opaque urine sample is most likely to contain:*

   a. many white blood cells and/or phosphates crystals
   b. much fat
   c. many uric acid crystals

d. much bilirubin
e. many yeast organisms

72. *A urine specimen with a "fruity" odor is most likely to contain:*

a. metabolized fruit juice
b. bacteria
c. hemolyzed blood
d. acetone
e. myoglobin

73. *A specific gravity reading consistent with isosthenuria is:*

a. <1.001
b. 1.001-1.008
c. 1.008-1.012
d. 1.012-1.025
e. >1.025

74. *What is the most common cause of erroneous results from urine testing with dipsticks?*

a. light damage to the strip
b. moisture damage to the strip
c. failure to time the reaction correctly
d. insufficient quantity of urine applied
e. cross reactions of various urine constituents

75. *What is the normal pH of canine and feline urine?*

a. 7 or greater
b. 7 or less
c. 8-10
d. 10 or greater
e. highly variable pH, from 4 to 9

76. *Highly alkaline urine samples may result in false-positive results when testing for:*

a. protein
b. blood
c. glucose
d. ketones
e. urobilinogen

77. *Myoglobin, a breakdown product of muscle, is eliminated in the urine and produces a positive reaction on which pad of a urine dipstick?*

a. blood
b. bilirubin
c. ketone
d. glucose
e. urobilinogen

78. *When present in the urine, bilirubin can be broken down by:*

a. heating of the specimen
b. exposure of the specimen to light
c. blood in the specimen
d. drugs in the specimen
e. chemicals used to preserve the specimen

79. *When present in urine, which substance can* ***mask*** *a positive glucose reaction on urine dipsticks?*

a. ketones
b. blood
c. penicillin
d. ascorbic acid
e. creatinine

80. *The urine nitrite test is based on the ability of bacteria to convert nitrate to nitrite and is a crude indicator of urinary tract infection in people. Why is it of limited use in dogs and cats?*

a. Dogs and cats are rarely affected by bacterial infections of the urinary tract.
b. The acidic pH of dog and cat urine prevents this reaction.
c. The bacteria tend to react with other proteins in the urine of dogs and cats.
d. The diets of most dogs and cats do not contain sufficient nitrate to cause a positive reaction.
e. Enzymes in the urine of dogs and cats break down nitrate.

Correct answers are on pages 208-210.

81. *For best results, urine specimens for microscopic analysis should be centrifuged for:*

a. 5 minutes at 10,000 RPM
b. 5 minutes at 6000 RPM
c. 1 minute at 3000 RPM
d. 400 RCF for 5 minutes
e. time and speed are of no significance

82. *Squamous epithelial cells found in a urine sample usually originate from the:*

a. kidney
b. renal pelvis
c. ureter
d. bladder
e. genital tract

83. *Transitional epithelial cells found in urine may originate from all of the following sites* ***except*** *the:*

a. renal pelvis
b. ureter
c. renal tubules
d. bladder
e. proximal urethra

84. *White blood cell casts in a urine sample suggest:*

a. lymphoid neoplasia of the bladder
b. disease of the ureter
c. disease of the kidney
d. calculi
e. bacterial cystitis

85. *Cystine crystals are most likely to be found in the urine of:*

a. female Collies
b. female Doberman Pinschers
c. female Cocker Spaniels
d. male Dachshunds
e. male Labrador Retrievers

86. *Calcium oxalate crystals in urine sediment are most often associated with:*

a. ethylene glycol (antifreeze) toxicity
b. gout
c. bacterial cystitis
d. end-stage renal disease
e. organophosphate insecticide poisoning

87. *The sensitivity of enzyme-linked immunosorbent assay is related to the:*

a. stability of the reagents
b. ease with which an assay can be performed
c. number of components in the assay
d. overall accuracy of the assay in detecting true-positive samples
e. ability of the assay to detect minimal concentrations of the antigen in question

88. *The higher the specificity of a test kit, the* ***less*** *likely that:*

a. false-negative results will occur
b. it will be easy to use
c. it will be accurate
d. false-positive results will occur
e. results will be reliable

89. *All commercially available feline leukemia virus (FeLV) test kits are designed to detect:*

a. FeLV antibodies
b. FeLV-infected red blood cells
c. FeLV antigens
d. FOCMA antibodies
e. FeLV-infected lymphoid cells

90. *A positive enzyme-linked immunosorbent assay for feline leukemia virus (FeLV) may indicate any of the following* ***except****:*

a. the cat may be transiently infected
b. the cat may be chronically infected
c. the cat will definitely die from FeLV infection
d. the cat may become a latent carrier
e. the cat may be contagious for other cats

91. *You test a cat's serum for feline leukemia virus using a microwell-type enzyme-linked*

immunosorbent assay kit. Color develops in the negative control and patient sample wells, as well as in the positive well. What is the most likely cause of these results?

a. failure to properly time the test
b. inadequate washing of wells after addition of the enzyme conjugate
c. prolonged storage of the kit at room temperature
d. nonspecific cross-reactive antibodies in the cat's serum
e. failure to add the enzyme conjugate

92. *The commercially available enzyme-linked immunosorbent assay kits for heartworm infection in dogs are designed to detect:*

a. antibodies to microfilariae
b. antibodies to adult heartworms
c. antibodies to migrating microfilariae
d. microfilarial antigens
e. adult heartworm antigens

93. *A 7-year-old outdoor male cat has a history and clinical signs strongly suggestive of heartworm infection. However, filter tests for heartworm microfilariae and enzyme-linked immunosorbent assay are both negative. What is the most likely explanation?*

a. the cat likely does not have heartworm infection
b. the cat may have small numbers of adult heartworms
c. the test procedures were performed incorrectly
d. the tests are designed for use only in dogs
e. the cat is probably infected with feline leukemia virus

94. *You test a 2-year-old clinically normal cat from a single-cat household for feline leukemia virus infection with an enzyme-linked immunosorbent assay kit designed for in-office use. The test is positive. What is the most appropriate advice for the cat's owner?*

a. isolate the cat and repeat the test in 1-2 months
b. euthanize the cat before it develops full-blown infection
c. the result was probably inaccurate
d. isolate the cat but do not bother to retest, as the second test will likely be positive
e. do not breed this cat

95. *Concerning cats whose saliva tests are positive for feline leukemia virus, which statement is most accurate?*

a. They will soon die.
b. They are only transiently infected.
c. They have a latent infection.
d. They can transmit the virus to other cats.
e. They are probably not contagious.

96. *A commonly used antimicrobial susceptibility testing method is:*

a. chromatographic separation
b. agar dilution
c. Kirby-Bauer
d. McFarland's standard technique
e. anaerobic subculture

97. *The medium of choice for antimicrobial susceptibility testing is:*

a. triple sugar-iron agar with 5% sheep blood
b. Mueller-Hinton agar
c. MacConkey agar
d. Sabouraud's dextrose agar
e. Hektoen agar

98. *When interpreting the results of an antimicrobial susceptibility test, a drug that is appropriate for treatment is indicated by a disk:*

a. with a large zone of inhibition
b. with a small zone of inhibition
c. with a zone diameter designated as inhibitory, according to standard charts for antimicrobial susceptibility
d. with a zone of inhibition indicating poor ability to diffuse through the agar
e. that inhibits growth of the greatest number of organisms

Correct answers are on pages 208-210.

99. Precise antimicrobial susceptibility testing requires that the agar plate containing the antimicrobial disks be inoculated:

a. and incubated immediately after the differential media plates have been inoculated
b. with a standard suspension of a single organism selected from the preincubated blood agar plate
c. with a mixed culture of all the organisms present on the preincubated blood agar plate
d. after preincubation of triple sugar-iron agar slants and broth subcultures
e. after preincubation of Sabouraud's dextrose slants and Hektoen broth subcultures

100. For long-term storage, antimicrobial sensitivity disks should be held at:

a. room temperature
b. 2-25 C
c. <2 C
d. >25 C
e. any convenient temperature

101. The urine of horses is normally thick and cloudy. This is due to the presence of:

a. epithelial cells and mucus
b. epithelial cells and crystals
c. mucus and crystals
d. leukocytes and normal bacterial flora
e. leukocytes and hyaline casts

*102. When urine is collected by cystocentesis, any of the following may be normally found **except**:*

a. sperm
b. leukocytes (3/high-power field)
c. bacteria
d. hyaline casts (2/low-power field)
e. epithelial cells (2/low-power field)

103. A practical way to evaluate a patient's platelet function in the clinic, without sending blood samples to the laboratory, is by:

a. clot retraction
b. bleeding time
c. von Willebrand's factor assay
d. platelet count
e. activated clotting time

104. Which flotation solution is best to use for qualitative examination of feces?

a. distilled water (specific gravity 1.000)
b. sodium chloride solution (specific gravity 1.050
c. acetic acid solution (specific gravity 1.100)
d. sugar solution (specific gravity 1.300)
e. copper sulfate solution (specific gravity 1.500)

105. In which area of a blood smear on a glass slide are heartworm microfilariae best observed?

a. area of the droplet
b. immediately adjacent to the droplet
c. thick area of the smear
d. thin area (monolayer) of the smear
e. feathered edge

106. Horses can be screened for neonatal isoerythrolysis by testing:

a. the mare's serum against the sire's red blood cells early in gestation
b. the foal's serum against the mare's red blood cells
c. the mare's colostrum against the foal's red blood cells 1 week after foaling
d. the foal's serum against the sire's red blood cells
e. the mare's serum against the sire's red blood cells just before foaling

107. Reticulocytes are best stained by:

a. direct application of Romanowsky stains
b. Wright's stain, followed by direct application of new methylene blue
c. incubating new methylene blue stain with the blood before making smears

d. direct application of new methylene blue stain to unstained smears
e. dipping the slides in methanol fixative before applying new methylene blue stain

108. Formalin fumes in the vicinity of freshly made blood films:

a. have no adverse effects of staining
b. alter the staining features of erythrocytes
c. enhance the staining features of leukocyte nuclei
d. have no adverse effects on cellular detail
e. give cell outlines a crisper image

109. During evening office hours you collect a blood sample from a patient. You plan to send the sample to a reference laboratory for a complete blood count, and realize that there will be an overnight delay before the sample is processed. So as to preserve blood cell morphology, the appropriate procedure is to immediately make a blood smear and:

a. refrigerate the unfixed blood smear and the tube of blood
b. leave the unfixed blood smear at room temperature and refrigerate the tube of blood
c. freeze the unfixed blood smear and refrigerate the tube of blood
d. fix the blood smear in methanol before freezing it and the tube of blood
e. leave the unfixed blood smear and the tube of blood at room temperature

110. The white blood cell count must be corrected when a blood smear is found to contain:

a. pyknotic leukocytes
b. large clumps of platelets
c. mast cells
d. nucleated red blood cells
e. neoplastic cells

111. In cattle responding to anemia, evidence of red cell regeneration is indicated by all of the following ***except:***

a. anisocytosis
b. basophilic stippling
c. polychromasia
d. Howell-Jolly bodies
e. acanthocytosis

112. If a dog's packed cell volume is 15% and the reticulocyte count is 12%, the corrected reticulocyte count is:

a. 10%
b. 8%
c. 6%
d. 4%
e. 2%

113. Which of the following does ***not*** *affect the reading for protein concentration in a dipstick test?*

a. urine pH
b. urine specific gravity
c. inflammatory cells in urine
d. ketones in urine
e. albumin in urine

114. Which of the following is ***not*** *considered a test of liver function?*

a. serum albumin concentration
b. citrated plasma clotting tests
c. serum alkaline phosphatase activity
d. serum bile acid concentration
e. bromsulphalein retention test

115. A direct smear preparation is generally ***not*** *advisable for cytologic examination of:*

a. pleural fluid
b. pericardial fluid
c. peritoneal fluid
d. cerebrospinal fluid
e. synovial fluid

Correct answers are on pages 208-210.

Answers

1. **a** Lavender-top tubes contain EDTA anticoagulant.
2. **e**
3. **a**
4. **b**
5. **d**
6. **b**
7. **d**
8. **c** Protein accumulation in the aperture can result in erroneous hematocrit readings and an increased frequency of obstructions.
9. **d** Contamination of the diluent with bacteria or other particles results in counting errors. As the count increases, errors increase exponentially.
10. **e** The entire system includes the reagent, instrument and operator.
11. **b** While all of the other choices can cause errors, inadequate mixing is the most common error. An automatic specimen rotator improves mixing.
12. **b**
13. **b**
14. **c**
15. **d** The avian heterophil is analogous to the mammalian neutrophil.
16. **b** The metamyelocyte is a granulocyte precursor. The others are erythrocyte precursors.
17. **a**
18. **a** Physiologic leukocytosis occurs when marginated granulocytes enter the general circulation as a result of excitement or stress.
19. **c**
20. **d**
21. **d** All avian erythrocytes are nucleated.
22. **e** The metamyelocyte is a granulocyte precursor. The other cells are all of the erythrocyte series.
23. **c**
24. **b**
25. **e**
26. **b**
27. **c** Immature forms include band and stab cells.
28. **d** Eosinophilia occurs commonly in response to antigen antibody reactions, as well as with inflammation of certain organs, such as the lungs, which tend to be allergy "targets."
29. **e** Calibration should be performed every 1-3 months to account for changes in the centrifuge that occur as a result of "wear and tear."
30. **a**
31. **b**
32. **d** Trichrome stain is typically used for visualization of parasites in feces.
33. **c** Filling a tube less than half way results in a dilution error that could, among other things, artificially lower the hematocrit value.
34. **b** Thrombocytopenia refers to a reduction in platelet numbers.
35. **d**
36. **a** Bleeding time is also prolonged with platelet deficiency, but a direct count of platelets is a better method to assess thrombocytopenia.
37. **c**
38. **e** Erythrocyte sedimentation rate is not a test of hemostasis.
39. **b**
40. **e** Serum values of potassium, aspartate aminotransferase and phosphorus increase as a result of red blood cell leakage and hemolysis. Glucose levels decrease up to 5% per hour as a result of anaerobic glycolysis by red blood cells.
41. **e**
42. **b** Large-bore needles result in "spiraling" of the cells as they enter the needle. Alcohol and rough handling can result in cell lysis. A 10-ml tube would likely create too much negative

pressure when collecting blood from a small animal.

43. **c** Some renal diseases are related to increased serum calcium levels.

44. **d** The serum creatinine level is a better assessment of renal function.

45. **e** Because amylase is eliminated through the kidneys, any disorder that reduces renal blood flow or impairs kidney function can result in elevated serum amylase activity.

46. **a**

47. **c**

48. **d**

49. **d**

50. **d**

51. **c** Organophosphate insecticides can be cholinesterase inhibitors.

52. **a**

53. **d**

54. **b** Anion gap = (Na + K) – (Cl + total CO_2).

55. **d** Ammonia (NH_3) is also unstable. Such enzymes as alanine aminotransferase and aspartate aminotransferase usually show some loss of activity after a few days unless the reconstituted control is frozen.

56. **a**

57. **b** Type B is a high-viscosity oil and is the best choice for light microscopy.

58. **d**

59. **a** *Giardia* is more likely to be found in direct saline smears.

60. **b**

61. **d**

62. **d**

63. **c** *Ehrlichia* morulae can occasionally be found in peripheral blood smears, but they are rare.

64. **d**

65. **a**

66. **e** Enzyme-linked immunosorbent assays detect adult heartworm antigens.

67. **d** In a low-incidence population, a test with a high positive predictive value is the best choice. Tests of high specificity have a high positive predictive value.

68. **d**

69. **c** Urine specimens collected from the floor or litterbox are likely to be contaminated.

70. **d** Needle puncture of the wall of a diseased bladder may predispose to bladder rupture.

71. **a**

72. **d** The urine of diabetic patients with ketoacidosis may have a fruity odor.

73. **c**

74. **b**

75. **b** The diet of carnivores usually produces acidic urine.

76. **a**

77. **a**

78. **b**

79. **d** Dogs and cats can synthesize ascorbic acid; therefore, an ascorbic acid-resistant urine dipstick is best for veterinary use.

80. **d** Nitrate occurs naturally in plants. Dogs and cats are primarily carnivores.

81. **d** RCF refers to relative centrifugal force. An RCF of 400 can be attained with a 6-inch-radius arm rotated at 1500 RPM.

82. **e**

83. **c**

84. **c**

85. **d** Cystinuria occurs almost exclusively in male dogs. Dachshunds, Basset Hounds, Chihuahuas, Yorkshire Terriers and Irish Terriers have been affected.

86. **a** Calcium oxalate crystals may also be found in small numbers in normal urine.

87. **e**

88. **d**

89. **c** All of these kits test for the p27 FeLV antigen.

90. **c** Some infected cats will die from FeLV infection; however, many more will recover and become immune.

91. **b** Unbound enzyme conjugate was probably left behind in all 3 wells. The unbound conjugate reacted with the added substrate to produce color.

92. **e**

93. **b** The test kits currently on the market lack the sensitivity to repeatedly detect only 1-2 adult worms.

94. **a** Many of these animals are transiently infected and seroconvert in time.

95. **d** FeLV is transmitted primarily through the saliva of infected cats.

96. **c**

97. **b**

98. **c** The extent to which an antimicrobial diffuses through agar is a property of the individual drug. Drugs that diffuse more slowly yield smaller zones of inhibition; however, they may still be effective choices for treatment.

99. **b** Direct sensitivity tests (those performed with mixed cultures) may only yield equivocal results.

100. **c** Unopened disk cartridges are best stored in the freezer. Once opened, however, it may be more convenient to store them with the dispenser in the refrigerator.

101. **c**

102. **c**

103. **b** Using the buccal mucosa and a cutting device, bleeding time is highly sensitive in detecting platelet function abnormalities and severe thrombocytopenia. Clot retraction also may be used but is more crude and less quantitative than bleeding time.

104. **d** The preferred specific gravity is between 1.100 and 1.350.

105. **e**

106. **e**

107. **c**

108. **b** In smears stained with Romanowsky stains, formalin fumes cause red blood cells to stain greenish-blue. Cellular detail appears indistinct.

109. **b**

110. **d**

111. **e**

112. **d** Corrected % reticulocytes = % reticulocytes x patient's PCV/normal PCV. In this dog, corrected reticulocytes = 12% x 15%/45% = 4%.

113. **d**

114. **c**

115. **d** Cell counts in uncentrifuged cerebrospinal fluid are usually too low to count accurately, and preparations must be concentrated before examination.

Section 21

Microbiology

G.R. Carter, M. Ikram

Recommended Reading

Biberstein EL and Zee YC: *Review of Veterinary Microbiology.* Blackwell Scientific, Boston, 1990.

Carter GR and Chengappa MM: *Microbial Diseases: A Veterinarian's Guide to Laboratory Diagnosis.* 2nd ed. Iowa State University Press, Ames, IA, 1993.

Carter GR and Chengappa MM: *Essentials of Veterinary Bacteriology and Mycology.* 4th ed. Lea & Febiger, Malvern, PA, 1991.

Carter GR and Cole, Jr JR: *Diagnostic Procedures in Veterinary Bacteriology and Mycology.* 5th ed. Academic Press, San Diego, 1990.

Fraser CM: *The Merck Veterinary Manual.* 7th ed. Merck, Rahway, NJ, 1991.

Ikram M and Hill E: *Microbiology for Veterinary Technicians.* American Veterinary Publications, Goleta, CA, 1991.

Ikram M, in Pratt PW: *Laboratory Procedures for Veterinary Technicians.* 2nd ed. American Veterinary Publications, Goleta, CA, 1992.

Timoney JF *et al: Hagan and Bruner's Microbiology and Infectious Diseases of Domestic Animals.* 8th ed. Comstock Publishing, Ithaca, NY, 1988.

Practice answer sheet is on page 385.

Questions

Questions 1 and 2

A 9-week-old pup has a fever, mild vomiting, diarrhea and conjunctivitis with a slight serous ocular discharge. There is no history of vaccination.

1. *The most likely cause of these signs is:*

   a. kennel cough
   b. infectious canine hepatitis
   c. parvoviral enteritis
   d. canine distemper
   e. dietary change

Correct answers are on pages 222-224.

2. *To confirm the diagnosis in this pup, one should:*

   a. submit a conjunctival smear for fluorescent antibody testing
   b. perform a fecal examination
   c. culture the ocular discharge
   d. submit paired serum samples for antibody titer
   e. submit serum samples for protein electrophoresis

Questions 3 through 6

A yearling bull suddenly dies at pasture. The hindquarters are extensively swollen and, on palpation, you note a crackling sound.

3. *Culture of tissue samples is most likely to reveal:*

   a. Gram-positive, nonmotile, anaerobic rods
   b. Gram-negative, nonmotile rods with square ends
   c. Gram-positive, motile, spore-forming rods with rounded ends
   d. Gram-positive, motile, spore-forming rods with square ends
   e. Gram-positive rods with terminal spores giving the appearance of a tennis racquet

4. *The most likely cause of this bull's death is:*

   a. salmonellosis
   b. malignant edema
   c. tetanus
   d. black head
   e. blackleg

5. *The causative agent of this disease is:*

   a. *Clostridium chauvoei*
   b. *Clostridium septicum*
   c. *Clostridium novyi*
   d. *Clostridium tetani*
   e. *Clostridium hemolyticum*

6. *A rapid and reliable test that is commonly used to diagnose this disease is:*

   a. direct smear of affected muscle tissue
   b. fluorescent antibody test
   c. mouse inoculation
   d. complement fixation
   e. hemagglutination inhibition

Questions 7 and 8

A farmer has asked the veterinarian to examine a cow that has died. The cow is lying on its side, and a bloody discharge can be seen around the nose, mouth, vulva and anus.

7. *To determine the microbial cause of the cow's death, the technician should:*

   a. collect a fecal sample
   b. open the carcass and collect liver and kidney samples
   c. aseptically cut into the jugular area and collect a blood sample
   d. aseptically puncture an ear vein and collect a blood sample
   e. collect a sample from the cow's nose using a finger

8. *Aerobic culture of bacteria isolated from this cow shows Gram-positive, nonmotile, aerobic, encapsulated rods in a box car arrangement. The most likely organism isolated is:*

   a. *Clostridium tetani*
   b. *Clostridium botulinum*
   c. *Bacillus anthracis*
   d. *Bacillus cerous*
   e. *Clostridium hemolyticum*

Questions 9 through 11

A portion of the intestinal tract from a horse with suspected salmonellosis is submitted for microbiologic examination.

9. *How should the specimen be handled to confirm the diagnosis?*

a. suspend the intestinal contents in tetrathionate-selenite broth and culture on blood agar and MacConkey agar plates
b. suspend the intestinal contents in trypticase-nutrient broth and culture on blood agar and MacConkey agar plates
c. directly swab the intestinal contents onto blood agar and MacConkey agar plates
d. directly swab the intestinal contents onto Sabouraud agar plates
e. directly swab the intestinal contents onto blood agar, MacConkey agar and brilliant green agar

10. *After proper incubation, samples from* Salmonella *cultures should be streaked on:*

a. Hektoen agar and brilliant green
b. Mueller-Hinton and MacConkey agar
c. MacConkey agar and blood agar
d. trypticase agar containing blood serum
e. chocolate agar

11. *Suspected* Salmonella *colonies can be reliably identified by:*

a. carbohydrate fermentation
b. mouse inoculation
c. guinea pig inoculation
d. bacterial cell morphology
e. serologic tests

12. *Which microorganism does **not** form individual colonies on blood agar?*

a. *Pseudomonas*
b. *E coli*
c. *Proteus*
d. *Salmonella*
e. *Klebsiella*

13. E coli *and* Salmonella *differ by:*

a. size and shape
b. production of hemolysis on blood agar
c. fermentation of lactose with gas production
d. motility
e. utilization of urea as a source of nitrogen

14. *A 24-hour culture of a specimen from a dog shows a Gram-negative, motile, oxidase-positive organism with bluish-green colonies on blood agar. On the basis of general and cultural characteristics, this organism most likely is:*

a. *E coli*
b. *Pseudomonas aeruginosa*
c. *Brucella canis*
d. *Actinomyces (Corynebacterium) pyogenes*
e. *Pasteurella hemolytica*

15. *The organism that produces a characteristic fruity odor when grown on blood agar is:*

a. *Pseudomonas*
b. *Pasteurella*
c. *Proteus*
d. *Salmonella*
e. *Corynebacterium*

16. *The indole test is used for biochemical identification of bacteria. In the indole test,:*

a. a protein digest containing an ample quantitiy of tryptophan is used
b. a carbohydrate solution containing an ample quantity of glucose is used
c. carbohydrate in the protein digest promotes indole production
d. a protein digest containing an ample quantity of cystine is used
e. methyl red is used to produce a red layer at the top of the broth

17. *Concerning the cytoplasmic membrane of bacteria, which statement is most accurate?*

a. It is an impermeable layer.
b. It is responsible for maintaining the shape of bacteria.
c. It is structurally different from mammalian cell membranes.
d. It consists of phospholipopeptides.
e. It is the innermost membrane next to the cell wall.

Correct answers are on pages 222-224.

18. *Which of the following is **not** a characteristic of a bacterial endospore?*

a. highly refractile
b. very sensitive to heat
c. means of continuity of bacterial life
d. very low metabolic rate
e. resistant to staining

19. *Which of the following is **not** a characteristic of bacterial flagella?*

a. found in all bacteria
b. long whip-like appendages
c. can be seen with special staining techniques
d. protein in nature
e. a means of locomotion of bacteria

20. *After the iodine step of Gram staining, Gram-positive organisms are:*

a. colorless
b. pink
c. purple
d. red
e. black

21. *After the acetone-alcohol step of Gram staining,:*

a. Gram-positive and Gram-negative bacteria are pink
b. Gram-positive and Gram-negative bacteria are colorless
c. Gram-positive bacteria are black
d. Gram-negative bacteria are red
e. Gram-negative bacteria are colorless

22. *Coagulase production is characteristic of:*

a. *Staphylococcus aureus*
b. *Staphylococcus epidermidis*
c. *Streptococcus uberis*
d. *Actinomyces pyogenes*
e. *Streptococcus agalactiae*

23. *Anaerobic, endospore-forming, nonencapsulated bacteria are found in the genus:*

a. *Bacillus*
b. *Hemophilus*
c. *Actinomyces*
d. *Clostridium*
e. *Corynebacterium*

24. *Bacteria that grow best between 20 and 40 C are referred to as:*

a. psychophiles
b. mesophiles
c. thermodurics
d. capnophiles
e. anaerobes

25. *A candle jar is used to produce an:*

a. anaerobic environment
b. environment with an increased level of carbon dioxide
c. aerobic environment
d. environment with an increased level of nitrogen
e. environment with no water

26. *The technique of isolating bacteria in pure culture form was perfected by:*

a. Louis Pasteur
b. Robert Koch
c. Edward Jenner
d. Alex Fleming
e. Francesco Redi

27. *What component of a MacConkey agar makes this medium selective for Gram-negative organisms?*

a. lactose
b. sodium chloride
c. neutral red
d. glucose
e. bile salts

28. *Beta hemolysis on blood agar cultures refers to:*

a. partial hemolysis of red blood cells in the medium

b. complete hemolysis of red blood cells in the medium
c. a double zone of hemolysis of red blood cells in the medium
d. no hemolysis of red blood cells in the medium
e. selective hemolysis of undersized red blood cells in the medium

29. *Which of the following is* **not** *a characteristic of an exotoxin?*

a. soluble in water
b. protein in nature
c. heat stable
d. antigenic
e. excreted from the bacteria into the surrounding medium

30. *Bacteria with a tuft of flagella at both poles are described as:*

a. amphitrichous
b. peritrichous
c. lophotrichous
d. monotrichous
e. ditrichous

31. *Organisms sharing a set of biological characteristics are called:*

a. a phylum
b. an order
c. a genus
d. a species
e. a family

32. *Concerning mycoplasmas, which statement is* **least** *accurate?*

a. Their colonies have a "fried egg" appearance.
b. They are small, free-living cells with no cell wall.
c. They are very sensitive to antibiotics, particularly penicillins.
d. They affect epithelial or serosal membranes.
e. They require X and V factors for growth.

33. *All of the following subspecies of* Campylobacter fetus *are catalase positive* ***except:***

a. *venerealis*
b. *intestinalis*
c. *fecalis*
d. *sputorum*
e. *coli*

34. *All of the following are characteristics of mycobacteria* ***except:***

a. thin, straight rods
b. aerobic
c. acid fast
d. Gram negative
e. nonmotile

35. *The optichin test is used to identify which species of* Streptococcus*?*

a. *Streptococcus uberis*
b. *Streptococcus agalactiae*
c. *Streptococcus pneumoniae*
d. *Streptococcus equisimilis*
e. *Streptococcus suis*

36. *The test used to differentiate* Staphylococcus *from* Micrococcus *is the:*

a. coagulase test
b. indole test
c. oxidation-fermentation test
d. mouse inoculation test
e. CAMP-esculin test

37. *Microscopic examination of Gram-stained cultures of* Nocardia *reveals:*

a. Gram-positive rods with delicate branching hyphae
b. Gram-positive cocci with peritrichous flagella
c. Gram-negative short rods with a perimeter fringe
d. Gram-negative cigar-shaped rods with terminal spores
e. Gram-positive small rods in Chinese letter arrangements

Correct answers are on pages 222-224.

38. *Concerning* Listeria *and* Erysipelothrix, *which statement is most accurate?*

a. Both organisms are catalase positive and nonmotile.
b. *Listeria* is catalase positive and *Erysipelothrix* is catalase negative, and both organisms are motile.
c. Both organisms are catalase positive and motile.
d. Both organisms are catalase negative and nonmotile.
e. *Listeria* is catalase positive and motile, while *Erysipelothrix* is catalase negative and nonmotile.

39. *Which of the following is* **not** *a characteristic of* Bacillus anthracis?

a. Gram-positive rod
b. nonmotile
c. anaerobic
d. catalase positive
e. has a central spore

40. *Which organism forms colonies with a typical inverted pine tree appearance in motility media?*

a. *Erysipelothrix*
b. *Listeria*
c. *Moraxella*
d. *Pasteurella*
e. *Salmonella*

41. *Which of the following is an anaerobe?*

a. *Bacillus*
b. *Clostridium*
c. *Listeria*
d. *Pseudomonas*
e. *Erysipelothrix*

42. *The term ectothrix refers to:*

a. dermatophyte spores located on the outside of infected hair shafts
b. bacterial spores located on the inside of infected hair shafts
c. bacterial spores located on the outside and inside of infected hair shafts
d. dermatophyte spores located in the dermis
e. dermatophyte spores located in the germinal bed of claws

43. *In the germ tube test,* Candida albicans *is inoculated into human or bovine serum and incubated at 37 C for:*

a. 30 minutes
b. 2-4 hours
c. 10-12 hours
d. 24 hours
e. 48 hours

44. *Which genus has characteristics resembling those of* E coli, *except that it is nonmotile and usually has a capsule?*

a. *Bacillus*
b. *Clostridium*
c. *Salmonella*
d. *Klebsiella*
e. *Arizona*

45. *Which of the following is* **not** *a general characteristic of bacteria in the family Enterobacteriaceae?*

a. Gram-negative rods
b. catalase positive
c. oxidase positive
d. motile and nonmotile species
e. fermentation of sugars by several genera

46. *To differentiate between bacteria of the family Staphylococcaceae and those of Streptococcaceae, which test is most appropriate?*

a. bacitracin test
b. optichin test
c. catalase test
d. coagulase test
e. oxidation-fermentation test

47. *How do molds differ from bacteria and yeasts?*

a. growth curve
b. plant-like
c. saprophytes
d. Gram reaction
e. multinucleated

Questions 48 through 50

A 1-year-old calf has circumscribed raised skin lesions, and hair loss around the head, neck and flank.

48. *The most likely cause of these lesions is:*

a. ringworm
b. roundworm infection
c. mange
d. pinworm infection
e. tapeworm infection

49. *To confirm the diagnosis, which type of specimen should you collect from the calf and submit to the diagnostic laboratory?*

a. fecal specimen
b. skin scrapings
c. blood sample
d. urine sample
e. skin biopsy

50. *Upon culturing the specimen on medium enriched with thiamin and inositol, you are most likely to isolate:*

a. *Trichophyton verrucosum*
b. *Trichophyton mentagrophytes*
c. *Microsporum nanum*
d. *Microsporum gypseum*
e. *Trichophyton equinum*

51. *You isolate several small, round, budding, encapsulated organisms from the cerebrospinal fluid of a cat. This organism most likely is:*

a. *Candida albicans*
b. *Cryptococcus neoformans*
c. *Coccidioides immitis*
d. *Sporothrix schenckii*
e. *Histoplasma capsulatum*

52. *In dogs, a Wood's lamp can sometimes be used to diagnose infection with:*

a. *Microsporum canis*
b. *Trichophyton mentagrophytes*
c. *Sarcoptes scabiei*
d. *Cryptococcus neoformans*
e. *Trichophyton verrucosum*

53. *Which of the following are produced by streptococci?*

a. neurotoxin and coagulase
b. coagulase and enterotoxin
c. hemolysin and hyaluronidase
d. leukocidin and hemolysin
e. enterotoxin and streptolysin

54. *A strain of* E coli *isolated from a 2-week-old calf that died from complications of diarrhea is most likely to be:*

a. hemolytic
b. of the K99 strain
c. oxidase negative
d. resistant to tetracycline
e. catalase positive

55. *Which organism grows best at room temperature?*

a. *Pseudomonas*
b. *Corynebacterium equi*
c. *Staphylococcus aureus*
d. *Aspergillus niger*
e. *E coli*

56. *Viruses are commonly classified by their:*

a. mode of infection
b. cultural characteristics
c. tissue affinities
d. staining characteristics
e. physical and chemical properties

Correct answers are on pages 222-224.

57. Structural components of all viruses include:

a. a capsule, a cell wall and a cell membrane
b. a cell wall, a cytoplasmic membrane and nucleic acid
c. a capsid and nucleic acid
d. an envelope, DNA, RNA and a cell wall
e. an envelope, a cell wall, a cytoplasmic membrane and nucleic acid

*58. Which of the following is **not** a property of interferon?*

a. virus specific
b. stable under acidic conditions
c. heat stable
d. nontoxic to cells
e. weakly antigenic

59. The correct sequence of virus replications in animals is:

a. attachment, uncoating, penetration, latent period, replication, assembly and release
b. attachment, penetration, latent period, uncoating, replication, assembly and release
c. attachment, penetration, uncoating, assembly, replication and release
d. attachment, penetration, uncoating, latent period, replication, assembly and release
e. attachment, penetration, uncoating, replication, latent period, assembly and release

60. On a culture plate inoculated with material from an abscess in a dog, you grow a large number of Staphylococcus aureus *colonies and several colonies of large Gram-positive rods with Chinese letter arrangement. The colonies of Gram-positive rods are most likely those of:*

a. *Actinomyces (Corynebacterium) pyogenes*
b. *Bacillus pisiformis*
c. *Pasteurella multocida*
d. *Clostridium novyi*
e. *Pseudomonas aeruginosa*

61. Skin and nail scrapings are best examined microscopically for fungal elements after:

a. Gram staining
b. suspension in physiologic saline
c. soaking in pancreatic enzyme solution
d. crushing beneath a coverslip
e. clearing with 10% potassium hydroxide solution

62. The microscopic structures most useful in identification of dermatophytes are:

a. septate, branching hyphae
b. microconidia and nonseptate, nonbranching hyphae
c. chlamydospores and microconidia
d. macroconidia and microconidia
e. macroconidia and colony morphology

63. Brucellosis is diagnosed by:

a. demonstration of small Gram-negative rods on direct smears
b. typical clinical signs
c. a history of ingesting contaminated feed
d. a history of abortion
e. determining the serum titer

64. In cultures of Candida albicans, *production of germ tubes can be stimulated by:*

a. using blood agar
b. adding human serum to the culture medium
c. using corn meal medium
d. using brain-heart infusion broth
e. doubling the dextrose concentration in Sabouraud's dextrose agar

65. The CAMP-esculin test is used to differentiate:

a. staphylococci from streptococci
b. *Streptococus agalactiae* from other streptococci causing mastitis
c. *Staphylococcus aureus* from *Staphylococcus epidermidis*
d. *Micrococcus* from staphylococci causing pyoderma
e. *Streptococcus equi* from *Streptococcus zooepidemicus*

66. A microorganism that is unique for its bipolar staining is:

a. *Pasteurella*
b. *Listeria*
c. *Clostridium*
d. *Bacillus*
e. *Klebsiella*

67. In order of occurrence, the growth curve of bacteria consists of:

a. lag phase, stationary phase, logarithmic phase, death phase, dormant phase
b. lag phase, logarithmic phase, stationary phase, death phase, dormant phase
c. stationary phase, lag phase, log phase, death phase, dormant phase
d. dormant phase, lag phase, stationary phase, death phase, logarithmic phase
e. lag phase, logarithmic phase, stationary phase, dormant phase, death phase

68. The typical biochemical and physiologic characteristics of bacteria are most obvious during the:

a. lag phase
b. logarithmic phase
c. death phase
d. dormant phase
e. stationary phase

69. Bacteria are most resistant to destruction during the:

a. lag phase
b. logarithmic phase
c. stationary phase
d. dormant phase
e. death phase

70. Electron microscopy can be used to identify viruses:

a. to the family level
b. to the genus level
c. to the species level
d. without staining
e. in living infected cells

71. The steps involved in bacteriophage replication are similar to those of virus replication. Concerning bacteriophages, which statement is most accurate?

a. The entire bacteriophage enters the bacterium.
b. Bacteriophage uncoating occurs soon after it enters a bacterium.
c. Only the head of the bacteriophage enters the bacterium.
d. Bacteriophages enter bacteria with the tail part inserted first.
e. There is a latent period or eclipse in bacteriophage replication.

72. Dark-field microscopy is used in studies of Leptospira *because:*

a. it is easier on the microscopist's eyes
b. *Leptospira* is more evident when viewed this way
c. it provides greater magnification
d. it is easier to perform
e. it is less expensive than bright-light illumination

73. A horse has lesions involving the superficial layer of the skin. The hair is matted as if painted with a brush, and scabs have formed. A Gram stain of a sample collected from the undersurface of the scab is most likely to reveal:

a. Gram-negative rods
b. Gram-positive rods
c. Gram-positive branching hyphae
d. Gram-positive cocci
e. Gram-positive rods in pairs

74. Concerning rhabdoviruses, which statement is ***least*** *accurate?*

a. They are single-stranded RNA viruses.
b. They are helical, bullet-shaped viruses.
c. They cause rabies.
d. They replicate in the nucleus of host cells.
e. They have an envelope.

Correct answers are on pages 222-224.

75. *Transmissible gastroenteritis is an important disease of unweaned piglets. It is caused by:*

a. coronaviruses, which are single-stranded RNA viruses with pleomorphic morphology
b. rotaviruses, which are double-stranded RNA viruses with icosahedral morphology
c. togaviruses, which are single stranded with icosahedral morphology
d. herpesviruses, which are single-stranded DNA viruses with icosahedral morphology
e. parvoviruses, which are single-stranded DNA viruses with icosahedral morphology

76. *Concerning viruses, which statement is* ***least*** *accurate?*

a. Viruses do not grow on artificial media and require living cells to grow.
b. Viruses do not have cellular organelles for metabolism.
c. Viruses contain both DNA and RNA.
d. Viruses do not contain ribosomes.
e. Viruses are not destroyed by antibiotics.

77. *The potassium hydroxide test is used to differentiate:*

a. staphylococci from streptococci
b. *Streptococcus agalactiae* from other streptococci
c. *Staphylococcus aureus* from *Staphylococcus epidermidis*
d. Gram-positive bacteria from Gram-negative bacteria
e. *Brucella* from *Nocardia*

78. *In the California mastitis test, gel forms when the test reagent reacts with:*

a. proteins in the milk sample
b. cellular DNA in the milk sample
c. fat and protein in the milk sample
d. organic salts in the milk sample
e. trace elements in the milk sample

79. *The California mastitis test is used to determine the:*

a. protein content of mastitic milk
b. degree of mastitis as reflected by somatic cell numbers
c. fat content in mastitic milk, as reflected by increases associated with inflammation
d. number of bacteria in mastitic milk
e. type of bacteria causing mastitis, as reflected by the character of gel formation

80. *Distemper virus can be cultured in:*

a. trypticase soy broth with 10% glucose
b. the yolk sac of embryonated duck eggs
c. the chorioallantoic membranes of embryonated chicken eggs
d. the amnionic sac of embryonated duck eggs
e. the allantoic cavity of embryonated chicken eggs

81. *Various types of cells have been used for tissue culture of viruses. The term "continuous cell line" refers to cells that:*

a. divide to form a large sheet-like cell or syncytium
b. divide indefinitely
c. divide for up to 5 generations
d. divide for up to 10 generations
e. divide slowly

82. *In identification of members of the family Enterobacteriaceae, triple sugar-iron agar is used as a culture medium. Concerning use of this medium in identifying enterobacteria, which statement is most accurate?*

a. Glucose, sucrose and lactose fermentation can be detected independently.
b. Glucose fermentation can be detected if sucrose and lactose are not fermented.
c. Glucose fermentation can be detected if sucrose is fermented but not if lactose is fermented.
d. Lactose fermentation can be detected if glucose and sucrose are fermented.
e. Sucrose and lactose fermentation can be detected if glucose is not fermented.

83. A pathogen of animals that stains with fluorescent acid-fast stain is:

a. *Corynebacterium pyogenes*
b. *Mycobacterium avium*
c. *Actinomyces bovis*
d. *Escherichia coli*
e. *Mycoplasma mycoides*

84. Diagnosis of rabies has been greatly facilitated in recent years by use of the:

a. complement fixation test
b. gel diffusion precipitation test
c. guinea pig inoculation test
d. fluorescent antibody test
e. hemagglutination inhibition test

85. The factors required for growth of certain strains of Hemophilus *bacteria are:*

a. porphyrin and nicotinic acid
b. coenzyme A and nicotinic acid
c. hemin and nicotinamide adenine dinucleotide (NAD)
d. hemin, sodium tellurite and beta hydroxy butyric acid
e. myoglobin and nicotinic acid

86. Which agent causing human infections is associated with pigeon feces?

a. *Candida albicans*
b. *Histoplasma capsulatum*
c. *Cryptococcus neoformans*
d. *Aspergillus fumigatus*
e. *Blastomyces dermatitidis*

87. A fungus associated with ear infections in dogs is:

a. *Aspergillus fumigatus*
b. *Cryptococcus neoformans*
c. *Malassezia pachydermatis (Pityrosporum canis)*
d. *Rhinosporidium seeberi*
e. *Sporothrix schenckii*

88. Which fungus is most frequently transmitted from animals to children?

a. *Blastomyces dermatitidis*
b. *Coccidioides immitis*
c. *Histoplasma capsulatum*
d. *Microsporum canis*
e. *Trichophyton mentagrophytes*

89. A Wood's lamp is most effective in demonstrating fluorescence in hair infected with:

a. *Trichophyton verrucosum*
b. *Microsporum gypseum*
c. *Microsporum canis*
d. *Trichophyton mentagrophytes*
e. *Microsporum nanum*

90. The best stain to use for wet mounts of mycelial fungal cultures is:

a. Gram's stain
b. India ink
c. lactophenol cotton blue
d. modified Ziehl-Neelsen
e. silver nitrate

91. An acidic reaction in the slant and butt portions of a triple sugar-iron agar medium indicates:

a. carbohydrate utilization
b. deamination
c. desulfurylation
d. fermentation
e. anaerobic growth

92. Which is the preferred clinical specimen to submit for laboratory diagnosis of rhodococcal pneumonia in foals?

a. tracheal wash
b. cotton swab from the nasal passages, without immersion in transport medium
c. cotton swab from the nasal passages, immersed in transport medium
d. cotton swab from the nasopharynx
e. unclotted blood sample

Correct answers are on pages 222-224.

93. *Sporulation of* Bacillus anthracis *is most likely to occur in:*

a. an anaerobic atmosphere
b. healthy tissue
c. necrotic tissue
d. an aerobic atmosphere
e. the bloodstream

94. *How long can the causal agent of contagious footrot in sheep survive on pasture?*

a. 1 week
b. 2 weeks
c. 4 weeks
d. 6 weeks
e. 2 months

95. *Which Gram-negative organism has been frequently associated with mastitis in cows bedded on sawdust or wood shavings?*

a. *Proteus mirabilis*
b. *Serratia*
c. *Klebsiella*
d. *Providencia*
e. *Yersinia enterocolitica*

96. *The diarrhea and dehydration seen in calves with colibacillosis are mainly attributable to the effects of:*

a. enterotoxin
b. endotoxin
c. capsular antigen
d. lipopolysaccharide
e. verotoxin

97. Anaplasma marginale *infects:*

a. monocytes
b. neutrophils (polymorphonuclear leukocytes)
c. eosinophils
d. red blood cells
e. hepatocytes

98. *Concerning cat scratch disease or cat scratch fever, which statement is* **least** *accurate?*

a. It affects mainly kittens.
b. It affects mainly children.
c. It is noncontagious.
d. A skin test is used in diagnosis.
e. A small bacterium is considered to be the cause.

99. *Rabies and vesicular stomatitis viruses are classified in the family:*

a. Reoviridae
b. Rhabdoviridae
c. Coronaviridae
d. Caliciviridae
e. Paramyxoviridae

100. *The principal reservoir for pseudorabies virus is thought to be:*

a. pigs
b. sheep
c. rats
d. raccoons
e. insects

Answers

1. **d** Most unvaccinated pups are susceptible to distemper at 8-12 weeks of age. The history and clinical signs are suggestive of distemper.
2. **a** Laboratory tests, such as fluorescence of antigens in conjunctival smears, are important to exclude diseases causing similar signs, such as canine parvoviral enteritis and rabies.
3. **c**
4. **e** Swelling over the hindquarters and gas in the tissues causing crackling sounds on palpation suggest blackleg (malignant edema, gas gangrene).
5. **a**

6. **b**

7. **d** *Bacillus anthracis* is aerobic. Therefore, samples of blood should be collected from a site that releases the minimum number of bacteria into the environment.

8. **c** *Bacillus anthracis* is an aerobic, nonmotile, encapsulated rod with typical morphologic arrangement.

9. **a** Tetrathionate and selenite broths are selective and enrichment broths for *Salmonella*. The intestinal contents should be inoculated into either of these broths, in addition to routine plating on blood agar or MacConkey agar.

10. **a** Hektoen agar and brilliant green agar are selective media for *Salmonella*.

11. **e** Serologic tests can identify salmonellae on the basis of antigenic structure.

12. **c** *Proteus* produces swarming growth on blood agar.

13. **c** *Salmonella* does not ferment lactose, whereas *E coli* is a lactose fermenter and produces gas.

14. **b**

15. **b** This is a characteristic of *Pasteurella*.

16. **a** Indole is a nitrogenous compound formed when the amino acid tryptophan is broken down.

17. **e** The cytoplasmic membrane is the innermost layer separating the cytoplasm from the cell wall.

18. **b** Bacterial spores are very resistant to heat and can withstand boiling temperatures for several hours.

19. **a** Not all bacteria have flagella.

20. **c** The iodine fixes the crystal violet in the bacterial cell wall, producing a purple color. Iodine does not impart its own color to the cell.

21. **e** Acetone alcohol removes crystal violet from the cell wall of Gram-negative bacteria. Gram-negative bacteria are colorless.

22. **a** *Staphylococcus aureus* produces coagulase, an enzyme that coagulates rabbit plasma.

23. **d** *Clostridium* is a large, anaerobic, nonencapsulated, endospore-forming rod.

24. **b** Mesophilic bacteria grow at 20-40 C, which is the temperature range preferred by most pathogenic bacteria.

25. **b** After a candle burns until extinguished, the atmosphere in the jar contains approximately 5-10% carbon dioxide.

26. **b** Robert Koch perfected the technique by the use of solidifying materials, such as agar.

27. **e** Bile salts inhibit the growth of Gram-positive organisms.

28. **b** Beta hemolysis refers to complete hemolysis of red blood cells in the medium, producing a clear zone around the bacterial colonies.

29. **c** Exotoxins are very heat sensitive.

30. **a**

31. **d**

32. **c** Penicillin stops bacterial proliferation by inhibiting cell wall synthesis. Because *Mycoplasma* has no cell wall, penicillin is not effective against mycoplasmal infections.

33. **d**

34. **d** *Mycobacterium* is Gram positive.

35. **c** Growth of *Streptococcus pneumoniae* is inhibited by optichin.

36. **c** *Micrococcus* is oxidative and *Staphylococcus* is fermentative.

37. **a**

38. **e** *Listeria* is catalase positive with tumbling motility, whereas *Erysipelothrix* is catalase negative and nonmotile.

39. **c** *Bacillus anthracis* is aerobic.

40. **b**

41. **b** *Clostridium* is strictly anaerobic.

42. **a**

43. **b**

44. **d**

45. **c** All Enterobacteriaceae are oxidase negative.

46. **c** Staphylococcaceae are catalase positive, whereas Streptococcaceae are catalase negative.

47. **e**

48. **a** In cattle, ringworm produces raised, crusted lesions resembling a patch of asbestos.

49. **b** Skin scrapings are the preferred sample.

50. **a** *Trichophyton verrucosum* requires thiamin or inositol for growth.

51. **b** None of the other organisms has a capsule.

52. **a** Some strains of *Microsporum canis* fluoresce on exposure to ultraviolet rays from a Wood's lamp.

53. **c**

54. **b** *E coli* strain K99 is very pathogenic.

55. **d** Most molds grow best near room temperature.

56. **e**

57. **c**

58. **a** Interferon is not virus specific and can be used against a variety of viral infections.

59. **d**

60. **a** This species was named *pyogenes* (pus producer) because it is commonly associated with pus production. This Gram-positive bacillus is often "clubbed" at one end and occurs in palisades or "Chinese letter" arrangement.

61. **e** 10% potassium hydroxide solution allows partial digestion of proteinaceous skin debris before microscopic examination.

62. **e**

63. **e**

64. **b** Human or bovine serum helps stimulate germ tube formation.

65. **b** *Streptococcus agalactiae* produces an arrow-shaped zone, while *Streptococcus uberis* produces brown colonies. *Streptococcus dysgalactiae* produces no special effects.

66. **a**

67. **b**

68. **b**

69. **c**

70. **c**

71. **e** The cycle of virus replication, including replication of bacteriophages, is characterized by a latent period or eclipse.

72. **b** *Leptospira* is difficult to stain and is more easily observed by dark-field microscopy.

73. **c** These lesions are most likely caused by *Dermatophilus congolensis,* a Gram-positive mycelial fungus.

74. **d** Rhabdoviruses replicate in the cytoplasm of host cells.

75. **a**

76. **c** Viruses may contain DNA or RNA, but never both.

77. **d** This chemical test is performed when there is a doubtful Gram reaction.

78. **b**

79. **b** When the reagent reacts with cellular DNA, gel formation is proportional to the degree of mastitis or number of somatic cells.

80. **c**

81. **b**

82. **b**

83. **b** Fluorescent acid-fast stain is used to detect mammalian *Mycobacterium*. The fluorescent staining procedure does not require heat or carbol fuchsin.

84. **d**

85. **c**

86. **c**

87. **c**

88. **d**

89. **c**

90. **c**

91. **d**

92. **a** *Rhodococcus equi* is not apt to be isolated from blood. Cultures from sources other than tracheal wash are likely to be overgrown with other bacteria.

93. **d** For this reason, it is not advisable to open the carcasses of animals that have died from anthrax.

94. **b**

95. **c**

96. **a**

97. **d**

98. **a**

99. **b**

100. **a**

Section 22

Necropsy

P.W. Pratt

Recommended Reading

Andrews JJ: Necropsy techniques. *Vet Clin No Am* (Food Animal Pract) 2: 1 *et seqq*, 1986.

Buck WB *et al: Clinical and Diagnostic Veterinary Toxicology*. 2nd ed. Kendall/Hunt Publishing, Dubuque, IA, 1976.

Rooney JR: *Autopsy of the Horse: Technique and Interpretation*. Williams & Wilkins, Baltimore, 1970.

Strafuss AC: *Necropsy Procedures and Basic Diagnostic Methods for Practicing Veterinarians*. Charles C Thomas, Springfield, IL, 1988.

Strafuss AC, in Pratt PW: *Laboratory Procedures for Veterinary Technicians*. 2nd ed. American Veterinary Publications, Goleta, CA, 1992.

Practice answer sheet is on page 387.

Questions

1. *The species traditionally placed in right lateral recumbency for necropsy is the:*

   a. dog
   b. cat
   c. horse
   d. pig
   e. sheep

2. *When submitting a recently dead bird to the diagnostic laboratory for necropsy, the bird should be:*

   a. quick-frozen in liquid nitrogen
   b. immediately soaked in a water plus detergent solution, then refrigerated
   c. submitted unrefrigerated and unfrozen
   d. allowed to cool slowly to room temperature before freezing
   e. plucked of feathers and then immediately refrigerated

3. *Samples collected from animals found dead are of limited diagnostic value because:*

   a. postmortem autolysis causes enzymatic digestion and bacterial contamination of organs and tissues
   b. rigor mortis causes organ contamination by enzymes released from muscle cells
   c. any microorganisms present in tissues die immediately
   d. reticuloendothelial cells engulf bacteria soon after an animal dies
   e. natural cooling of the cadaver eliminates any microorganisms present and halts all enzymatic action

Correct answers are on pages 228-229.

4. *The increased postmortem temperature of ruminant cadavers, leading to accelerated tissue liquefaction and gas production, is caused by:*

   a. release of enzymes from muscle cells
   b. proliferation of bacteria in the rumen
   c. escape of intestinal protozoa into the peritoneal cavity
   d. rapid hemolysis and subsequent release of hemoglobin
   e. the relatively small body surface area in proportion to alimentary system capacity

5. *To increase the likelihood of a definitive diagnosis by necropsy and subsequent histologic examination of tissue specimens, you should:*

   a. submit only 2 or 3 tissue specimens so as to avoid confusing the pathologist
   b. immediately freeze all collected tissues
   c. sample only tissues suggested by antemortem clinical signs
   d. submit the animal's history to the laboratory
   e. submit tissue samples in sterile saline

6. *Concerning shipment by mail, U.S. Postal Service regulations stipulate that veterinary specimens:*

   a. can be shipped in a single leak-proof container, rigid or flexible
   b. must be shipped in an inner container surrounded by absorbent material, with an outer shipping container with more absorbent material
   c. can be shipped in any type of inner container but must be surrounded by a rigid outer shipping container
   d. must be vacuum packed, regardless of contents
   e. cannot be shipped by mail

7. *After euthanasia, a procedure that should be done immediately so as to prevent obscuring of lesions in tissues or body cavities is to:*

   a. immerse the cadaver in hot water containing a detergent and a germicide
   b. remove all organs in the thoracic and abdominal cavities, and refrigerate them for later examination
   c. exsanguinate the cadaver by severing the jugular vein, axillary vessels or femoral vessels
   d. freeze the cadaver
   e. remove and refrigerate the cadaver's skin and major organs for later examination, and commence the necropsy by grossly examining the cadaver

8. *Before commencing a necropsy, you should:*

   a. disinfect all instruments and the immediate area around the cadaver
   b. assess the animal's body condition, haircoat, mucous membranes and body orifices
   c. infuse the cadaver with formalin solution to retard postmortem autolysis and bloating
   d. collect samples from internal organs by needle aspiration
   e. suspend the cadaver by the rear legs so as to accelerate exsanguination and facilitate removal of internal organs

9. *During gross examination of the thoracic organs, you should:*

   a. separate the heart from the lungs for close inspection of each
   b. remove the esophagus, thymus, heart, trachea, lungs, thyroid glands and parathyroid glands sequentially and separately
   c. first remove the heart, with the pericardial sac intact, before removing any other organs
   d. palpate, but not incise, each lung lobe to check for lesions
   e. grasp the tongue, esophagus and trachea, pulling caudally to remove the thoracic organs from the cavity

10. *During gross examination of the abdominal organs, you should:*

   a. check bile duct patency by squeezing the gallbladder
   b. examine the stomach and intestines in their natural position, without severing their mesenteric attachments

c. sever the mesenteric attachments of the intestines and stomach to facilitate examination but not remove these viscera from the cavity
d. place the cadaver in dorsal recumbency to prevent spillage of viscera out of the abdominal cavity
e. first remove the pancreas, to prevent enzymatic contamination, before examining any other abdominal organs

11. During necropsy, the urogenital tract:

a. should be removed after the lateral aspects of the pelvis are cut away
b. of pregnant females should always be examined in its natural position so as to avoid fetal damage
c. should be dissected free individually, with the external and internal genitalia removed first, followed by the bladder, ureters and kidney
d. of females can be removed intact by pulling it caudally through the pelvic canal after dissection around the perineal area
e. should be removed from the abdominal cavity only after ligation of the ureters and urethra

12. During removal of the brain from the cranial cavity,:

a. one saw cut can be made along the midline of the skull, completely through the skull and brain, and each half of the brain pried free
b. saw cuts should be made so the eyes and optic nerve remain attached to the brain
c. the cranial nerves and dural attachments are cut, after which the brain is gently removed with the help of gravity
d. one should always wear a surgical mask to avoid inhaling any aerosolized rabies virus particles that may be present
e. the meninges should be left intact around the brain so that subdural lesions are not overlooked

13. After removal from the cranial cavity, the brain:

a. should be placed whole in a dilute detergent solution for 24 hours before fixation in formalin solution
b. should be immediately sectioned into quadrants, and each portion fixed in 5% chlorhexidine solution
c. should be quick-frozen in liquid nitrogen
d. may be sectioned immediately and then fixed in formalin, or first fixed whole in formalin and later sectioned
e. tends to harden and shrink unless lipids are removed immediately by immersion in absolute isopropyl alcohol

14. In postmortem examination of the spinal cord,:

a. the dorsal aspect of the vertebrae is removed and the spinal cord is examined in its natural position
b. spinal cord samples should be fixed in distilled water rather than in formalin
c. usually only a few 5-mm samples are obtained by punch biopsy because of the difficulty entailed in spinal cord removal
d. the dorsal and ventral nerve roots are severed, and the spinal cord is removed by grasping the meninges
e. little information can be gained because of damage caused by efforts to remove the overlying vertebrae

15. For postmortem microbiologic examination of limb joint fluid,:

a. the unopened joint should be cut free from the limb and then sawed in half along its vertical axis before submersion in a liquid culture medium
b. joint fluid samples are typically of little value because of rapid postmortem bacterial contamination
c. the skin can be reflected from the joint, and a sterile needle and syringe used to aspirate joint fluid
d. the long bones on either side of the joint should be cut, and the intact joint quick-frozen in liquid nitrogen
e. the skin can be reflected from the joint, culture medium injected into the joint with a sterile needle and syringe, and the intact joint submitted to the laboratory

Correct answers are on pages 228-229.

16. *In necropsy of horses, a structure that should be examined for damage by* Strongylus vulgaris *larvae is the:*
    a. stomach wall
    b. cranial mesenteric artery
    c. pericardial sac
    d. guttural pouch
    e. renal pelvis

17. *A structure that the examiner could miss during necropsy in swine unless the entire pharynx is removed is the:*
    a. palatine tonsil
    b. thyroid gland
    c. nasal septum
    d. thymus gland
    e. parotid salivary gland

18. *When submitting tissue samples for histologic examination, a good general rule is to:*
    a. submit sections 2-3 inches thick
    b. freeze tissue samples after fixing them in formalin
    c. use a fixative volume of 10 times the tissue sample volume
    d. use concentrated (100%) formalin solution for optimal tissue fixation and minimal tissue shrinkage
    e. submit 3-foot segments of bowel, with the ends ligated to retain the enclosed ingesta

19. *When used alone, the compound most acceptable for intravenous euthanasia of animals is:*
    a. magnesium sulfate
    b. succinylcholine
    c. strychnine
    d. sodium pentobarbital
    e. pancuronium bromide

20. *A zoonosis that could be transmitted from an infected cadaver to the dissector during necropsy is:*
    a. salmonellosis
    b. lungworm infection
    c. feline infectious peritonitis
    d. bovine leukemia virus infection
    e. Potomac horse fever

For Questions 21 through 25, select the correct answer from the 5 choices below:

a. ergot alkaloid mycotoxicosis
b. strychnine poisoning
c. cyanogenetic plant poisoning
d. warfarin poisoning
e. inorganic arsenic poisoning

21. *Evidenced by intense hyperemia of the gastrointestinal tract.*

22. *Evidenced by rapid onset of rigor mortis.*

23. *Evidenced by dry gangrene of the extremities.*

24. *Evidenced by bright red blood.*

25. *Evidenced by massive hemorrhage into body cavities or the visceral lumina.*

Answers

1. **c** The other species listed are usually necropsied in left lateral recumbency.
2. **b** This decreases the insulating capability of the plumage and faciliates rapid cooling.
3. **a**
4. **b** For some time after death, the rumen continues to function as a fermentation chamber that generates heat as bacteria

continue to multiply and to metabolize nutrients.

5. **d** The history can guide the pathologist in selecting tests for analysis of specific tissues.
6. **b** This is specified by the Code of Federal Regulations, Title 39, Part III amended.
7. **c** Exsanguination is important because excessive blood in tissues or body cavities tends to obscure lesions.
8. **b** Such preliminary observations can help guide later, more specific examinations.
9. **e**
10. **a** If the duct is patent, bile will be seen entering the duodenum.
11. **a**
12. **c** Rough handling can damage the brain.
13. **d**
14. **d**
15. **c**
16. **b** Migrating larvae of *Strongylus vulgaris* can cause endarteritis and subsequent thromboembolism.
17. **a** The tonsil of swine is flat and covered with tiny pits, and could be overlooked on cursory examination.
18. **c** Using a lesser volume of fixative may result in insufficient tissue fixation and consequent sample decomposition.
19. **d** A large dose rapidly induces unconsciousness and respiratory and cardiac arrest.
20. **a** Rubber or latex gloves should be worn during necropsy.
21. **e**
22. **b**
23. **a**
24. **c**
25. **d**

Notes

Notes

Section 23

Nutrition

L.D. Baker, E.A. Moser, R.L. Remillard

Recommended Reading

Blood DC *et al: Veterinary Medicine.* 6th ed. Bailliere Tindall, London, 1983.

Burger JH and JPW Rivers: *Nutrition of the Dog and Cat.* Waltham Symposium 7, Cambridge University Press, New York, 1989.

Cunha T: *Feeding and Nutrition of Horses.* 2nd ed. Academic Press, New York, 1991.

Fraser C: *Merck Veterinary Manual.* 7th ed. Merck, Rahway, NJ, 1991.

Herdt TH: Metabolic diseases of ruminant livestock. *Vet Clin No Am* (Food Anim Pract) 4:213-439, 1988.

Jones B: *Canine and Feline Gastroenterology.* Saunders, Philadelphia, 1986.

Larson BL: *Lactation.* Iowa State University Press, Ames, IA, 1985.

Lewis LD: *Feeding and Care of the Horse.* Lea & Febiger, Philadelphia, 1982.

Lewis L *et al: Small Animal Clinical Nutrition III.* Mark Morris Associates, Topeka, KS, 1987.

Maynard LA *et al: Animal Nutrition.* 7th ed. McGraw-Hill, New York, 1979.

Nutrient Requirements of Domestic Animals. National Academy Press. Washington, DC. Titles in series: Cat 1986, Dog 1985, Dairy Cattle 1989, Beef Cattle 1984, Horses 1989, Sheep 1985, Swine 1988, Goat 1981.

Official Publication, Association of Feed Control Officials. Georgia Department of Agriculture, Atlanta, 1992.

Radostits OM and Blood DC: *Herd Health.* Saunders, Philadelphia, 1985.

Sniffen CS and Herdt TH: Dairy nutrition management. *Vet Clin No Am* (Food Animal Pract) 7:311-632, 1991.

Practice answer sheet is on page 389.

Questions

1. *The approximate energy content of hay is best indicated by:*

   a. stem size
   b. color
   c. smell
   d. number of weeds present
   e. number of leaves present

2. *Which feed has the greatest energy density?*

   a. shelled corn
   b. barley
   c. whole cottonseeds
   d. soybean meal
   e. cottonseed meal

Correct answers are on page 236.

3. *Which of the following is considered a protein supplement?*

   a. shelled corn
   b. corn gluten meal
   c. soybean hulls
   d. oats
   e. barley

4. *Nitrogen required by ruminant tissues is derived from:*

   a. ammonia produced and absorbed through the rumen wall
   b. amino acids produced and absorbed through the rumen wall
   c. amino acids supplied by rumen bacteria in the small intestine only
   d. amino acids supplied by rumen bacteria and rumen undegraded feed protein
   e. amino acids from rumen bacteria and ammonia produced in the rumen

5. *Grass tetany can be prevented by supplementing the diet with:*

   a. molybdenum
   b. calcium
   c. magnesium
   d. potassium
   e. manganese

6. *Feeding concentrates to sheep is beneficial at all of the following times* ***except:***

   a. 1 month after breeding
   b. 1 week before breeding
   c. 1 month before lambing
   d. 1 month after lambing
   e. 1 month before weaning

7. *Urolithiasis in sheep and goats is often related to excessive dietary:*

   a. phosphorus
   b. calcium
   c. potassium
   d. sodium
   e. magnesium

8. *Which horse has the highest energy requirement above that required for maintenance?*

   a. newborn foal
   b. pregnant mare
   c. lactating mare
   d. breeding stallion
   e. pleasure horse ridden on weekends

9. *In horses, intake of excessive protein over requirements can result in all of the following* ***except:***

   a. excessive sweating
   b. bone deformities
   c. ammonia smell in the stall
   d. increased urine volume
   e. increased growth rates

10. *How is 10,000 parts per million expressed as a percentage (parts per hundred)?*

    a. 1.0%
    b. 10.0%
    c. 0.1%
    d. 100.0%
    e. 10,000.0%

11. *Which amino acid is essential for cats but* ***not*** *for dogs?*

    a. valine
    b. threonine
    c. lysine
    d. methionine
    e. taurine

12. *Which of the following are B vitamins?*

    a. tryptophan and thiamin
    b. thiamin and vitamin K
    c. riboflavin and choline
    d. thiamin and pantothenic acid
    e. pantothenic acid and choline

13. *Which vitamin promotes growth and mineralization of bones, and increases calcium absorption?*

a. vitamin A
b. vitamin D
c. thiamin
d. choline
e. niacin

14. *During lactation, the food intake of queens typically:*

a. stays the same
b. increases about 1.5 times
c. increases about 2-3 times
d. increases about 5-6 times
e. increases by about 50%

15. *Newborn dairy calves should receive colostrum for at least the first:*

a. 12 hours of life
b. day of life
c. 3 days of life
d. 2 weeks of life
e. month of life

16. Halogeton *and greasewood are common poisonous plants that grow in the arid and semi-arid saline regions of the western United States. They are toxic to sheep because of their high content of:*

a. copper
b. oxalate
c. calcium
d. selenium
e. ketone bodies

17. *Based on digestive anatomy and physiology, rabbits are classified as:*

a. ruminants
b. carnivores
c. nonruminant herbivores
d. obligate omnivores
e. variable omnivores

18. *What element causes "blind staggers" or "alkali disease" when in dietary excess, and white muscle disease when insufficient in the diet?*

a. calcium
b. copper
c. molybdenum
d. zinc
e. selenium

19. *What species are extremely susceptible to copper toxicosis?*

a. sheep and rabbits
b. pigs and cattle
c. sheep and pigs
d. sheep and cattle
e. cattle and rabbits

20. *To decrease the risk of milk fever in parturient dairy cattle, the diet in the last 2-4 weeks of the dry period should consist of:*

a. the grain and hay ration for lactating cows
b. exclusively legume hay
c. a ration low in calcium and balanced for phosphorus
d. a diet with a high level of cations
e. only sweet feed

21. *In home-cooked diets for dogs and cats, what are the most common nutritional deficits?*

a. protein, fat
b. vitamin A, copper
c. vitamin A, essential fatty acids
d. salt, protein
e. fat, copper

22. *How many cans of dog food (500 kcal metabolizable energy per can) are needed for maintenance of an average 13.6-kg (30-lb) dog?*

a. 2
b. 3
c. 4
d. 5
e. 6

Correct answers are on page 236.

23. *An animal will die most quickly from lack of what nutrient?*

a. water
b. protein
c. carbohydrate
d. fat
e. energy

For Questions 24 through 31, select the correct answer from the 8 choices below.

a. calcium
b. cobalt
c. iodine
d. iron
e. molybdenum
f. selenium
g. thiamin
h. vitamin E

24. *Mineral that should be fed at a ratio of 1:1-2:1 with phosphorus in animal diets.*

25. *Mineral that should be fed at a ratio of 6:1-10:1 with copper in ruminant diets.*

26. *Mineral associated with function of vitamin E.*

27. *Vitamin associated with encephalopathies in ruminants.*

28. *Vitamin associated with steatitis (yellow fat disease).*

29. *Deficiency of this mineral results in a vitamin deficiency in ruminants.*

30. *Mineral that is a major constituent of thyroid hormone.*

31. *A trace mineral, found in limited amounts in milk, that may be deficient in suckling neonates.*

32. *During which period does an animal require the highest dietary energy level?*

a. first trimester of gestation
b. second trimester of gestation
c. third trimester of gestation
d. first half of lactation
e. second half of lactation

33. *In sheep, which nutritional imbalance results in pregnancy toxemia?*

a. deficient energy
b. deficient protein
c. deficient calcium
d. excessive energy
e. excessive protein

34. *Which feeding method is most appropriate for an old, underweight dog?*

a. unlimited access to an unlimited amount of food
b. unlimited access to a limted amount of food
c. limited access to an unlimited amount of food
d. limited access to a limited amount of food
e. forced feeding manually or via gastric tube

35. *Which feeding method is most appropriate for an adult dog of normal weight?*

a. unlimited access to an unlimited amount of food
b. unlimited access to a limited amount of food
c. limited access to an unlimited amount of food
d. limited access to a limited amount of food
e. forced feeding manually or via gastric tube

36. *Which feeding method is most appropriate for a 3-month-old puppy?*

a. unlimited access to an unlimited amount of food
b. unlimited access to a limited amount of food
c. limited access to an unlimited amount of food
d. limited access to a limited amount of food
e. forced feeding manually or via gastric tube

37. Which feeding method is most appropriate for a lactating bitch?

a. unlimited access to an unlimited amount of food
b. unlimited access to a limited amount of food
c. limited access to an unlimited amount of food
d. limited access to a limited amount of food
e. forced feeding manually or via gastric tube

38. Which feeding method is most appropriate for a severely underweight adult dog with a poor appetite, poor body condition, steatorrhea, diarrhea and vomiting?

a. enteral feeding of a liquefied diet via stomach tube
b. parenteral feeding by intravenous infusion
c. voluntary oral consumption
d. parenteral feeding by intraosseous infusion
e. forced feeding of a solid diet by hand

39. Which feeding method is most appropriate for an adult dog of normal body weight and condition, hit by a car this morning and scheduled for femoral fracture repair in 2 days?

a. enteral feeding of a liquefied diet via stomach tube
b. parenteral feeding by intravenous infusion
c. voluntary oral consumption
d. parenteral feeding by intraosseous infusion
e. forced feeding of a solid diet by hand

40. Which feeding method is most appropriate for an adult dog of normal body weight and condition, hit by a car this morning and scheduled for mandibular fracture repair in 2 days?

a. enteral feeding of a liquefied diet via stomach tube
b. parenteral feeding by intravenous infusion
c. voluntary oral consumption
d. parenteral feeding by intraosseous infusion
e. forced feeding of a solid diet by hand

41. Which feeding method is most appropriate for an old, obese cat with anemia, liver disease and complete anorexia for 5 days?

a. enteral feeding of a liquefied diet via stomach tube
b. parenteral feeding by intravenous infusion
c. voluntary oral consumption
d. parenteral feeding by intraosseous infusion
e. forced feeding of a solid diet by hand

For Questions 42 through 50, select the correct answer from the 9 choices below.

a. colitis
b. feline urologic syndrome
c. developmental bone disease
d. food allergy
e. renal disease
f. feline hepatic lipidosis
g. lymphangiectasia
h. megaesophagus
i. obesity

42. The most common nutritional disorder of adult dogs and cats.

43. A low-fat diet is used in treatment.

44. A high-fiber diet is used in treatment.

45. A novel protein source is effective treatment.

46. A magnesium-restricted, urine-acidifying diet is used in treatment.

47. In puppies, avoiding high energy and calcium intake but balancing dietary calcium with phosphorus is recommended for prevention.

48. Feeding in an upright position to avoid regurgitation and aspiration pneumonia is recommended in treatment.

49. Dietary levels of protein, phosphorus and sodium concentrations are decreased in an effort to control serum urea nitrogen levels.

50. Tube feeding a balanced diet is recommended in treatment.

Correct answers are on page 236.

Answers

1. **a** Larger stem sizes reflect forage maturity, higher fiber levels, and lower available energy.
2. **c** This feed contains the greatest amount of fat.
3. **b** This feed contains more than 20% of crude protein.
4. **d**
5. **c**
6. **a**
7. **a**
8. **c**
9. **e**
10. **a** 10,000 ppm = 1.0%.
11. **e** Taurine is an essential amino acid for cats but not for dogs.
12. **d** Thiamin and pantothenic acid are both B vitamins.
13. **b** Vitamin D promotes growth and mineralization of bones, and increases calcium deposition.
14. **c** During lactation, a queen's food intake typically increases 2-3 times.
15. **c** Calves should receive colostrum for a minimum of 3 days and then milk or high-quality milk replacer at about 10% of body weight daily.
16. **b**
17. **c** Rabbits are cecal fermenters.
18. **e** Geographically discrete areas of soil (and hence forage) are characterized by selenium excesses or deficiencies.
19. **a** Sheep and rabbits are very sensitive to copper toxicity. Pig and cattle are moderately resistant to toxicity.
20. **c** The ration should be low in calcium (<50 g/636-kg Holstein cow) and balanced for phosphorus (30 g/636-kg Holstein cow).
21. **b** Most home-cooked diets have high levels of protein and fat.
22. **a** A 13.6-kg dog requires about 900-1000 kcal of metabolizable energy per day.
23. **a** Fat-free muscle is composed of 75-80% water. Water is required for essentially all body functions.
24. **a**
25. **e**
26. **f**
27. **g**
28. **h**
29. **b**
30. **c**
31. **d**
32. **d**
33. **a**
34. **a** This dog should be fed free choice because it is underweight but not anorexic.
35. **b** This dog should be fed a limited daily amount so as to maintain its normal weight.
36. **c** Puppies should be allowed free access to food for about 20 minutes, 3 times a day.
37. **a** Lactating bitches have high energy requirements and so should have unlimited access to food.
38. **b** This dog should be fed intravenously because of small intestinal dysfunction.
39. **c** There is no reason this dog cannot eat voluntarily.
40. **a** This dog should be fed by tube because the mandible is fractured.
41. **a** This cat should be fed by tube because it will not eat voluntarily, but the small intestine remains functional.
42. **i**
43. **g**
44. **a**
45. **d**
46. **b**
47. **c**
48. **h**
49. **e**
50. **f**

Section 24

Parasitology

D.D. Bowman

Recommended Reading

Colville J: *Diagnostic Parasitology For Veterinary Technicians.* American Veterinary Publications, Goleta, CA, 1992.

Georgi JR and Georgi ME: *Canine Clinical Parasitology.* Lea & Febiger, Philadelphia, 1992.

Georgi JR and Georgi ME: *Parasitology for Veterinarians.* 5th ed. Saunders, Philadelphia, 1990.

Foreyt WJ: *Veterinary Parasitology Reference Manual.* 2nd ed. Washington State Univ, Pullman, WA, 1990.

Fraser CM: *The Merck Veterinary Manual.* 7th ed. Merck, Rahway, NJ, 1991.

Ivens VR *et al: Principal Parasites of Domestic Animals in the United States: Biological and Diagnostic Information.* 2nd ed. University of Illinois Publication 52, Urbana, 1988.

Practice answer sheet is on page 391.

Questions

1. *Several littermate Labrador Retriever puppies develop signs of caudal paralysis and polyradiculitis. A likely protozoal cause of this infection is:*

   a. *Giardia duodenalis*
   b. *Neospora caninum*
   c. *Hepatozoon canis*
   d. *Isospora canis*
   e. *Leishmania donovani*

2. *A dog from Arkansas develops severe anemia and icterus. Examination of the blood reveals small organisms within 15% of the red blood cells. The protozoan within the blood cells is most likely to be:*

   a. *Giardia canis*
   b. *Trypanosoma cruzi*
   c. *Sarcocystis capracanis*
   d. *Babesia canis*
   e. *Toxoplasma gondii*

3. *A litter of puppies develops bloody, mucoid diarrhea within a few days after they are moved to the house of their new owner. The most likely cause of diarrhea in these puppies is:*

   a. *Trichodectes canis*
   b. *Hepatozoon canis*
   c. *Toxoplasma gondii*
   d. *Babesia gibsoni*
   e. *Isospora canis*

Correct answers are on pages 249-251.

4. *Routine fecal examination performed on a dog reveals sporocysts of* Sarcocystis cruzi. *The dog most likely acquired this infection from:*

   a. the bite of a tabanid fly
   b. ingestion of a beetle intermediate host
   c. ingestion of a murine paratenic host
   d. ingestion of raw beef
   e. ingestion of sporulated oocysts

5. *A cat that enjoys hunting develops a rapidly progressive disease with signs including anemia and icterus. Death occurs a few days after the onset of clinical signs. Histopathologic examination of the lungs and liver reveals blood vessels filled with very large cells containing parasitic inclusions. The most likely cause of this cat's death is infection with:*

   a. *Aelurostrongylus abstrusus*
   b. *Cytauxzoon felis*
   c. *Leishmania braziliensis*
   d. *Paragonimus kellicotti*
   e. *Eucoleus (Capillaria) aerophila*

6. *You prepare a direct saline smear of a gingival scraping from a cat with periodontal disease that has developed concomitantly with feline immunodeficiency virus infection. Microscopic examination of the smear is most likely to reveal a commensal flagellate of the genus:*

   a. *Trichomonas*
   b. *Giardia*
   c. *Entamoeba*
   d. *Hammondia*
   e. *Sarcocystis*

7. *In a Persian cat with chronic diarrhea, infection with* Giardia duodenalis *(synonym:* Giardia lamblia*) is suspected. An appropriate examination of the feces should include a:*

   a. zinc sulfate centrifugal flotation
   b. modified sugar centrifugal flotation
   c. direct saline smear
   d. sodium nitrate stationary flotation
   e. modified sugar stationary flotation

8. *An Arabian foal with inherited combined immunodeficiency develops diarrhea. Examination of the feces by sugar flotation reveals large numbers of very small oocysts typical of a parasite known to cause diarrhea in immunocompromised hosts. The name of this parasite is:*

   a. *Eimeria leuckarti*
   b. *Cryptosporidium parvum*
   c. *Klossiella equi*
   d. *Trypanosoma brucei*
   e. *Parascaris equorum*

9. *The most likely cause of diarrhea without intestinal blood loss in a 2-week-old calf is:*

   a. *Sarcocystis cruzi*
   b. *Bunostomum phlebotomum*
   c. *Eimeria bovis*
   d. *Toxoplasma gondii*
   e. *Cryptosporidium parvum*

10. *In order of occurrence, the typical pattern of events in the life cycle of a coccidian parasite, such as* Eimeria, *are:*

    a. schizont, schizont, gametocyte, oocyst, sporocyst, sporozoite
    b. oocyst, gametocyte, schizont, schizont, sporozoite, sporocyst
    c. oocyst, sporocyst, sporozoite, gametocyte, schizont, schizont
    d. gametocyte, schizont, schizont, oocyst, sporocyst, sporozoite
    e. schizont, schizont, oocyst, gametocyte, sporocyst, sporozoite

11. *Necropsy of a lamb from a flock that has recently developed severe diarrhea reveals numerous whitish, raised lesions, 3-6 mm in diameter, in the intestinal mucosa. Fecal examinations have not disclosed any parasites present in great numbers; however, saline smears prepared from the lesions reveal hundreds to thousands of small elongate organisms. A likely cause of the diarrhea and the intestinal lesions is:*

    a. *Eimeria ahsata*
    b. *Giardia duodenalis (Giardia lamblia)*
    c. *Isospora canis*

d. *Sarcocystis arieticanis*
e. *Trichuris ovis*

12. *In 5- to 10-day-old piglets, the most likely cause of scours that is unresponsive to antibiotic therapy is:*

a. *Isospora suis*
b. *Eimeria suis*
c. *Trichinella spiralis*
d. *Trichuris suis*
e. *Toxoplasma gondii*

13. *Three parasites that can infect people via ingestion of uncooked or undercooked pork are:*

a. *Toxoplasma gondii, Taenia solium* and *Stephanurus dentatus*
b. *Trichinella spiralis, Taenia solium* and *Hyostrongylus rubidus*
c. *Toxoplasma gondii, Taenia solium* and *Trichinella spiralis*
d. *Trichinella spiralis, Taenia solium* and *Oesophagostomum radiatum*
e. *Toxoplasma gondii, Eimeria deblieki* and *Trichinella spiralis*

14. *Examination of the feces of a clinically normal guinea pig reveals large (100 μ long) ciliate trophozoites and large cysts up to 60 μ in diameter. Similar parasites have also been found in domestic pigs and on rare occasions may have caused disease in dogs. The parasite in question is:*

a. *Entamoeba coli*
b. *Balantidium coli*
c. *Entamoeba histolytica*
d. *Eimeria*
e. *Trichomonas*

15. *Examination of a pig's feces reveals numerous, thin-walled protozoan cysts of several sizes, ranging from 12 to 30 μ in diameter. All of the cysts appear similar, but some contain 1 nucleus, some contain 4 nuclei, and some contain 8 nuclei. These cysts are representative of several species of parasite found in pigs and are classified as:*

a. trichomonads
b. amoebas
c. trypanosomes
d. ciliates
e. coccidia

16. *Which flagellate protozoan is a possible cause of fatal diarrhea in budgerigars and cockatiels?*

a. *Giardia*
b. *Eimeria*
c. *Trichomonas*
d. *Histomonas*
e. *Entamoeba*

17. *A red-tailed hawk housed in a rehabilitation clinic while its broken wing heals is fed pigeons obtained as culls from a nearby pigeon breeder. After about a week in the clinic, the hawk stops eating and begins to lose weight. Examination of the buccal cavity of the hawk reveals yellowish-green plaques in the back of the mouth. Microscopic examination of a direct saline smear of material from one of the plaques reveals numerous flagellate parasites. The probable cause of these plaques is a species of:*

a. *Giardia*
b. *Eimeria*
c. *Trichomonas*
d. *Histomonas*
e. *Entamoeba*

18. *A backyard flock of chickens develops bloody diarrhea that results in death of about 30% of the birds. Examination of some of the birds that die reveals the ceca to be filled with blood and thousands of coccidial oocysts. The species of* Eimeria *responsible for these deaths is most likely:*

a. *Eimeria necatrix*
b. *Eimeria tenella*
c. *Eimeria brunetti*
d. *Eimeria maxima*
e. *Eimeria acervulina*

Correct answers are on pages 249-251.

19. *A mechanical vector of a parasite is one that transmits the parasite:*

a. directly, without development or multiplication of the parasite
b. after internal multiplication of the parasite
c. after required development has occurred
d. after external multiplication of the parasite
e. and is not alive (*eg,* a syringe or needle)

20. *Fecal examinations performed on a closed research colony of Labrador Retrievers that have experienced occasional bouts of diarrhea reveal larvae in a zinc sulfate centrifugal flotation. Additional larvae are found using Baermann analysis. Examination of the larvae reveals that the genital primordium is longer than the larva is wide. Charcoal cultures of the feces reveal longer larvae with an esophagus about one-half the total length of the larva and a tip of the tail that appears notched. These dogs are most likely infected with:*

a. *Rhabditis strongyloides*
b. *Strongyloides stercoralis*
c. *Crenosoma vulpis*
d. *Filaroides hirthi*
e. *Uncinaria stenocephala*

21. *Puppies with hookworm eggs in their feces 2 weeks after birth have typically become infected with* Ancylostoma caninum *by:*

a. ingestion of infective larvae from soil
b. transmammary migration of larvae from the bitch
c. transplacental migration of larvae from the bitch
d. penetration of the skin by infective larvae
e. ingestion of hookworm eggs containing infective larvae

22. *The eggs of* Uncinaria stenocephala *can be differentiated from those of* Ancylostoma *by their:*

a. different shape
b. smaller size
c. larger size
d. embryonated state when passed
e. much thicker shell

23. *Puppies that develop patent* Toxocara canis *infection at the beginning of their fourth week of life have most likely become infected with this parasite by:*

a. ingestion of infective larvae
b. transmammary migration of larvae from the bitch
c. transplacental migration of larvae from the bitch
d. penetration of the skin by infective larvae
e. ingestion of roundworm eggs containing infective larvae

24. *A pet dog obtained originally from a local humane shelter in Illinois develops a weeping, pustular lesion on its right carpus. Microscopic examination of a direct saline smear of the material from the lesion reveals nematode larvae that are over 500 μ long, with a long pointed tail. Surgical exploration of the lesion reveals a white worm about 30 cm in length. The dog probably became infected by drinking water containing the infected intermediate host, a copepod. The parasite causing the lesion is:*

a. *Dipetalonema reconditum*
b. *Dracunculus insignis*
c. *Spirocerca lupi*
d. *Angiostrongylus vasorum*
e. *Dioctophyma renale*

25. *The prepatent period of* Dirofilaria immitis *poses problems in diagnosis of heartworm infection in dogs. By definition, the prepatent period of heartworms is that period between:*

a. the time the mosquito ingests a microfilaria and the time the infective-stage larva is fully developed
b. the time the adult worms have died and the time the microfilariae are ultimately cleared from the blood due to old age and natural death

c. the time a dog has been chemotherapeutically cleared of its microfilariae and the time the microfilariae from the existing adults return to detectable levels in the circulation
d. the time infective-stage larvae are inoculated by a mosquito and the time adult worms first appear in pulmonary vessels
e. the time infective-stage larvae are inoculated by a mosquito and the time microfilariae first appear in the bloodstream

26. *In a large cattery in Oregon, some cats begin vomiting intermittently. Repeated fecal examinations fail to identify any parasites other than a few coccidia and* Giardia *that are not confined only to the vomiting cats. When one of the affected cats dies from other causes, necropsy reveals small nematodes (less than 1 mm long) within a focal lesion about 3 cm in diameter in the stomach. The male worms have a copulatory bursa. The most likely cause of vomiting in these cats is:*

a. *Ancylostoma tubaeforme*
b. *Ollulanus tricuspis*
c. *Strongyloides tumefaciens*
d. *Physaloptera praeputialis*
e. *Gnathostoma spinigerum*

27. *In a cat with coughing and dyspnea, nematode larvae in the feces have dorsally spined tails. This cat is most likely infected with:*

a. *Aelurostrongylus abstrusus*
b. *Crenosoma vulpis*
c. *Ollulanus tricuspis*
d. *Physaloptera praeputialis*
e. *Eucoleus aerophilus (Capillaria aerophila)*

28. *A cat with gastritis, evidenced by vomiting and anorexia, is passing small (45 μ long) thick-shelled larvated eggs in its feces. Gastroscopy reveals pinkish-white worms 3-4 cm long without any marked spines on the head. This cat is most likely infected with:*

a. *Ollulanus tricuspis*
b. *Gnathostoma spinigerum*
c. *Toxocara cati*
d. *Strongyloides tumefaciens*
e. *Physaloptera praeputialis*

29. *The most important route by which kittens become infected with* Toxocara cati *is:*

a. ingestion of a paratenic host
b. transmammary migration of larvae from the queen
c. transplacental migration of larvae from the queen
d. penetration of the skin by infective larvae
e. ingestion of eggs containing infective larvae

30. *A lesion on the lip of a horse does not respond to topical corticosteroids or systemic antibiotics. Ultimately, the horse develops central nervous system signs and is euthanized. Histologic examination of brain tissue reveals large numbers of eosinophils and numerous minute, adult female nematodes. The features of the nematode that allow its identification are its size, the rhabditoid esophagus, and the recurved uterus containing a single egg. The nematode causing this disease is:*

a. *Strongyloides stercoralis*
b. *Strongyloides westeri*
c. *Halicephalobus deletrix*
d. *Habronema muscae*
e. *Draschia megastoma*

31. *Treatment of mares at parturition with large doses of ivermectin can prevent infection of foals with* Strongyloides westeri. *Such anthelmintic intervention is successful probably because:*

a. it prevents passage of infective larvae in the mare's milk
b. it prevents shedding of eggs in the mare's feces, eliminating the stages in the environment that could infect the foal
c. the drug is transferred to the foal in the mare's milk
d. it prevents acquisition of arrested larvae by the mare
e. it kills the infective stages in feces ingested by the foal

Correct answers are on pages 249-251.

32. *After an egg of* Parascaris equorum *is ingested by the host, the larva that hatches:*

a. develops entirely within the intestinal lumen
b. undergoes early development in the intestinal wall before migrating back to the small intestine
c. migrates to the liver and throughout the abdominal cavity before migrating back to the small intestine
d. migrates from the liver to the lungs before returning to the small intestine
e. develops in the colon and then migrates back to the small intestine

33. *A skin lesion on the face of a horse contains large numbers of eosinophils and nematode larvae, and improves markedly after ivermectin therapy. The larvae are probably those of:*

a. *Habronema muscae*
b. *Strongylus vulgaris*
c. *Trichostrongylus axei*
d. *Strongyloides westeri*
e. *Probstmayria vivipara*

34. *Horses become infected with* Draschia megastoma *by:*

a. ingesting infective larvae from pasture
b. ingesting a fly, *Musca domestica,* containing the infective larvae
c. ingesting an earthworm containing the infective larvae
d. the bite of a fly, *Stomoxys calcitrans,* harboring the infective larvae
e. the bite of a tick, *Dermacentor nitens,* harboring the infective larvae

35. *In horses, small strongyles (cyathostomes) can cause disease when present in large numbers or apparently when there is mass emergence of arrested larvae. Where are the hypobiotic larvae (arrested larvae) of these worms located in a parasitized horse?*

a. the lungs
b. the cranial mesenteric arteries
c. caseous nodules in the small bowel
d. the wall of the cecum and colon
e. the wall of the stomach

36. *In horses, the larvae of* Strongylus vulgaris *are the pathogenic stage of this parasite. Damage is caused by migration of larvae within the:*

a. bile canalicidi of the liver
b. islet cells of the pancreas
c. intima of the cranial mesenteric arteries
d. lymphatic vessels in the wall of the small intestine
e. meninges of the spinal cord

37. *Cattle become infected with* Ostertagia ostertagi *by:*

a. ingestion of infective larvae
b. ingestion of infected oribatid mites
c. transmammary migration of infective larvae
d. transplacental migration of infective larvae
e. ingestion of infective larvae encysted in water plants

38. *A winter outbreak of acute parasitic bronchitis in stabled dairy replacement stock is best managed by treatment with ivermectin, fenbendazole or levamisole, and by:*

a. keeping the animals as warm as possible
b. increasing the plane of nutrition
c. exercising the cattle
d. monitoring the output of larvae in the feces
e. removing manure and providing adequate ventilation

39. *As a parasite control measure, the principal objective in administering anthelmintics to all members of a herd or flock is to:*

a. increase the level of nutrition and state of health of host animals by removing the physiologic drain imposed by the parasites
b. decrease the number of parasite eggs distributed in the environment of the host

c. reduce the population of parasites so that the host can develop active immunity in the absence of frank clinical disease
d. totally and permanently eradicate the parasites
e. prevent development of anthelmintic resistance in the parasites

40. *In late winter in Ohio, a group of young cattle develop profuse watery diarrhea, anemia and hypoproteinemia, as evidenced clinically as submandibular edema (bottle jaw). Despite their illness, the cattle continue eating. The parasite most likely responsible for this condition is:*

a. *Fasciola hepatica*
b. *Trichostrongylus axei*
c. *Ostertagia ostertagi*
d. *Nematodirus helvetianus*
e. *Bunostomum phlebotomum*

41. *In a calf that died from severe diarrhea associated with high serum pepsinogen levels, necropsy reveals the rumen, reticulum and omasum to be full of feed, while the remainder of the alimentary tract is virtually empty. The mucosa of the abomasum is covered with grayish white, 3- to 5-mm nodules, each of which contains a small worm. The parasite responsible for this type of lesion in cattle is:*

a. *Hemonchus placei*
b. *Trichostronglyus axei*
c. *Ostertagia ostertagi*
d. *Nematodirus helvetianus*
e. *Bunostomum phlebotomum*

42. *A horse has worms in its eye that are identified as* Thelazia lacrymalis. *Horses become infected with this parasite by:*

a. ingestion of an infected fly, *Musca domestica*
b. ingestion of an infected fly, *Musca autumnalis*
c. ingestion of infective larvae while grazing
d. deposition of infective larvae into the eye by the fly, *Musca autumnalis*
e. deposition of infective larvae into bite wounds by the fly, *Hematobia irritans*

43. *Young beef cattle in Mississippi develop anemia and anasarca during a wet period of the summer. None of the animals shows any signs of diarrhea and some seem constipated. One animal dies and necropsy reveals numerous red and white worms, 20-30 mm long, within the abomasum. The worm most likely responsible for the disease in these cattle is:*

a. *Hemonchus placei*
b. *Trichostrongylus axei*
c. *Ostertagia ostertagi*
d. *Nematodirus helvetianus*
e. *Bunostomum phlebotomum*

44. *In a large confined dairy herd, the cattle are infected with few parasites, including* Strongyloides papillosus *and* Trichuris discolor. *One egg noted in the feces of a few cows is distinguishable from other nematode eggs by its morphologic characteristics. The egg is relatively clear shelled, football shaped (a prolate spheroid) and large (200 μ long), and contains 8-10 large cells (about 25 μ in diameter) and a good deal of empty space on both ends. This is most likely the egg of:*

a. *Hemonchus placei*
b. *Trichostrongylus axei*
c. *Ostertagia ostertagi*
d. *Nematodirus helvetianus*
e. *Bunostomum phlebotomum*

45. *Trichostrongyles parasitizing cattle can be identified by the stages passed in the feces using:*

a. careful measurement of the eggs
b. microscopic examination of first-stage larvae grown in culture
c. microscopic examination of infective larvae grown in culture
d. microscopic examination of the ornamentation of the eggshells
e. microscopic examination of the larva within the eggshell

Correct answers are on pages 249-251.

46. *A calf develops severe bloody diarrhea that proves fatal. At necropsy, the mucosa of the colon is lined with thousands of worms. These worms are pinkish-white and about 2-3 cm long, with a caudal end that is free within the lumen of the bowel, and a thin, hair-like cranial end that is threaded into the colonic mucosa. These worms, which occasionally kill cattle by cecal hemorrhage, are most likely:*

a. *Trichostrongylus axei*
b. *Trichinella spiralis*
c. *Trichuris discolor*
d. *Oesophagostomum radiatum*
e. *Hemonchus placei*

47. *Some people in France eat rare or undercooked horse meat from the United States and develop diarrhea 1-3 days later. The affected individuals then develop myositis and very high eosinophil numbers. Muscle biopsies 4 weeks after the meat was ingested reveal nematode larvae within the striated muscle fibers. The worm most likely responsible for this outbreak of disease is:*

a. *Bunostomum phlebotomum*
b. *Toxocara canis*
c. *Toxocara vitulorum*
d. *Triodontophorus tenuicollis*
e. *Trichinella spiralis*

48. *Three nematodes found in the lungs of sheep are:*

a. *Dictyocaulus, Crenosoma* and *Parelaphostrongylus*
b. *Muellerius, Aelurostrongylus* and *Dictyocaulus*
c. *Muellerius, Metastrongylus* and *Protostrongylus*
d. *Muellerius, Protostrongylus* and *Dictyocaulus*
e. *Muellerius, Oesophagostomum* and *Dictyocaulus*

49. *The concept of "spring rise" refers to:*

a. increased numbers of larvae on pasture in the spring
b. increased development from egg to larvae under spring conditions
c. increased egg output by ewes due to continued development of arrested larvae
d. development of increased *Hemonchus*-specific antibody levels during spring
e. movement of larvae that have overwintered in the soil up onto freshly growing grass in the spring

50. *Larvae that may be found in fresh sheep feces are those of:*

a. *Dictyocaulus, Trichostrongylus* and *Parelaphostrongylus*
b. *Muellerius, Hemonchus* and *Dictyocaulus*
c. *Muellerius, Metastrongylus* and *Protostrongylus*
d. *Muellerius, Protostrongylus* and *Dictyocaulus*
e. *Muellerius, Oesophagostomum* and *Dictyocaulus*

51. *In a large flock of caged chickens, certain rows of pullets have reduced feed consumption. Mortality levels become higher for these rows than the overall average for the facility. In 7-10 days, another area of the cage rows develops similar mortality. Necropsy of the dead birds reveals necrotic enteritis, with eroded, roughened mucosa of the ileum and rectum. The lesion has a superficial appearance similar to the surface of a "turkish towel." Ultimately, you discover that the pathogen is transmitted between rows of cages by a continuous-belt mechanical feed system. The parasite most likely causing this disease is:*

a. *Eimeria brunetti*
b. *Ascaridia galli*
c. *Heterakis gallinarum*
d. *Histomonas meleagridis*
e. *Syngamus trachea*

52. *Pastured swine are anemic and off feed, with occasionally darkened feces. Necropsy reveals small (less than 1 cm long), reddish nematodes within the gastric mucosa. These worms are most likely:*

a. *Trichostrongylus axei*
b. *Hyostrongylus rubidus*
c. *Strongyloides stercoralis*

d. *Ascaris suum*
e. *Ollulanus tricuspis*

53. *A group of swine raised on cement has white "milk spots" on their liver at necropsy and has had previous signs of lung disease (thumps). The worm most likely responsible for these signs is:*

a. *Metastrongylus apri*
b. *Ascaris suum*
c. *Stephanurus dentatus*
d. *Bunostomum phlebotomum*
e. *Strongyloides ransomi*

54. *Scours occurs in 2- to 6-month-old pigs about 3 weeks after they have been moved from confinement to pastures, and does not respond to treatment with antibiotics. A possible cause of the diarrhea is:*

a. *Ascaris suum*
b. *Isospora suis*
c. *Trichinella spiralis*
d. *Trichuris suis*
e. *Stephanurus dentatus*

55. *A nematode that may cause diarrhea in nursing piglets is:*

a. *Oesophagostomum dentatum*
b. *Hyostrongylus rubidus*
c. *Strongylus ransomi*
d. *Metastrongylus apri*
e. *Macracanthorhynchus hirudinaceus*

56. *Occasionally, horses develop lesions on the ventral midline that are characterized by alopecia and depigmentation, and that may respond to ivermectin therapy. These lesions are most likely due to the microfilariae of adult filarids that live within the nuchal ligament. The likely cause of these lesions in horses is:*

a. *Setaria digitata*
b. *Elaeophora schneideri*
c. *Teladorsagia circumcincta*
d. *Onchocerca cervicalis*
e. *Habronema muscae*

57. *Ingestion of infective* Toxocara canis *eggs by a mature bitch is most likely to lead to:*

a. patent infection
b. destruction of the eggs by gastric fluids
c. spurious positive fecal examinations (pseudoparasitism)
d. accumulation of arrested larvae in tissues
e. hepatomegaly and eosinophilia

58. *You are asked to take care of a pet iguana for several weeks, and find that it occasionally passes worms that are white and 1-1.5 cm long. The worms have a short esophagus, with a large round bulb at its base where it joins the intestine, and thick-shelled eggs. These nematodes are most likely members of:*

a. Strongylida (hookworms, trichostrongyles, strongyles)
b. Rhabditida (*Strongyloides* and relatives)
c. Oxyurida (pinworms)
d. Ascaridida (ascarids)
e. Spirurida (*Gnathostoma*, other spirurids, filarids)

59. *Kittens can become infected with* Alaria marcianae *soon after birth. The mode of transmission of this trematode parasite to kittens is unusual in that:*

a. there is transmammary transmission
b. there is transplacental transmission
c. the life cycle of this trematode is direct
d. cercariae penetrate the skin directly
e. it uses a frog as an intermediate host

60. *In Florida, a cat with hepatic insufficiency has biliary obstruction. During corrective surgery, flukes are found within the bile duct. The trematode causing this disease is identified as* Platynosomum fastosum. *Cats become infected by this parasite by eating:*

a. ants
b. snails
c. fish
d. lizards
e. mice

Correct answers are on pages 249-251.

61. *Cattle become infected with* Dicrocoelium dendriticum, *the lanceolate fluke of the bile duct, by:*

a. ingesting metacercariae on vegetation
b. ingesting infected snails
c. ingesting infected ants
d. cercariae penetrating the skin
e. the bite of a mosquito

62. *Outbreaks of clinical* Fasciola hepatica *infection may occur during periods of drought because:*

a. sheep are forced to eat unpalatable aquatic vegetation that may be covered with infected ants
b. sheep are forced to eat unpalatable aquatic vegetation that may contain encysted metacercariae
c. sheep are forced to graze close to ant hills
d. sheep may enter bodies of water and be penetrated by cercariae
e. *Fasciola hepatica* causes disease only in malnourished sheep

63. *Examination of a dog's feces reveals a large (120 μ long), ovoid, brown-shelled egg with a marked operculum and containing several developing cells. The parasite from which this egg came is most likely:*

a. *Heterobilharzia americana*
b. *Paragonimus kellicotti*
c. *Spirometra mansonoides*
d. *Diphyllobothrium latum*
e. *Taenia pisiformis*

64. *Radiographs of the lungs of a cat show circular lesions about 2-3 cm in diameter in the distal lobes. Examination of the feces reveals brown, operculate eggs. This cat is probably infected with:*

a. *Platynosomum fastosum*
b. *Paragonimus kellicotti*
c. *Alaria marcianae*
d. *Clonorchis sinensis*
e. *Cryptocotyle lingua*

65. *Adult taeniid tapeworms are found in dogs, cats and people. The life cycle of taeniid cestodes is characterized by the requirement of:*

a. an annelid intermediate host, such as an earthworm
b. a molluskan intermediate host, such as a snail
c. an arthropod intermediate host, such as an insect
d. a mammalian intermediate host
e. a fish intermediate host

66. *A dog in Minnesota is passing operculate eggs identified as those of the tapeworm,* Diphyllobothrium latum. *This dog was most likely infected by ingesting:*

a. fish
b. beef
c. pork
d. mutton
e. mice

67. *Cats become infected with* Dipylidium caninum *by ingesting fleas containing cysticercoids. The fleas become infected with this cestode by ingesting:*

a. cysticerci in circulating blood
b. tapeworm eggs in larval fleas
c. tapeworm eggs in young adult fleas
d. mesocercariae in circulating blood
e. infected oribatid mites

68. *Cats become infected with* Taenia taeniaeformis *by ingesting infected:*

a. fleas
b. fish
c. earthworms
d. rodents
e. snails

69. *Necropsy of a horse reveals the intestine to contain a very large number of white tapeworms at the ileocecal valve, though no eggs were detected in the feces before necropsy. This parasite is most likely:*

a. *Taenia hydatigena*
b. *Echinococcus granulosus*
c. *Moniezia expansa*
d. *Anoplocephala perfoliata*
e. *Thysanosoma actinoides*

70. *You find a large cyst (8 cm in diameter) in the lung of a cow in Utah. The cyst contains thousands of microscopic tapeworm scolices. This cyst respresents a:*

a. sparganum
b. cysticerus
c. coenurus
d. hydatid
e. cysticeroid

71. *At necropsy of a dog, you find a tapeworm with no hooks on its proboscis. The segments are small and have no lateral genital opening, and gravid segments contain a central and single thick-walled mass of eggs. This tapeworm is a species of:*

a. *Echinococcus*
b. *Taenia*
c. *Dipylidium*
d. *Hymenolepis*
e. *Mesocestoides*

72. *A 12-year-old Pomeranian dog is losing mats of hair on its back, near the base of the tail. You examine the lesion and discover 50-100 maggots in and on the skin. The fly causing this lesion is most likely:*

a. *Musca*
b. *Stomoxys calcitrans*
c. a calliphorid
d. *Hypoderma lineatum*
e. a cuterebrid

73. *A puppy adopted from a local shelter is infested with lice, which have a head about as wide as the abdomen. These lice are:*

a. anopluran lice
b. mallophagan lice
c. *Linognathus setosus*
d. human lice
e. very difficult to treat

74. *The stage of the flea that becomes infected with the dog tapeworm,* Dipylidium caninum, *lives off the host in soil or bedding. Before becoming an adult, the flea goes through a pupal stage, and the adult flea emerges from the pupal case. The life cycle of fleas is said to involve:*

a. incomplete metamorphosis
b. simple metamorphosis
c. partial metamorphosis
d. complex metamorphosis
e. continuous metamorphosis

75. *Adult fleas of dogs and cats usually prefer to be:*

a. in the bedding of the host
b. on the host
c. in the soil
d. in small cracks in the carpet or floor
e. within the ear canal

76. Ixodes dammini *was described as a new species in 1979. This tick is the vector of Lyme disease (borreliosis) in the northeastern United States. The final host of this tick is typically the white-tailed deer (*Odocoileus virginiana*). The larva of this tick typically feeds on:*

a. cattle
b. rabbits
c. lizards
d. white-footed mice (*Peromyscus leucopus*)
e. white-tailed deer

77. *A nymphal* Ixodes *can be differentiated from a nymph of other genera of hard ticks by its:*

a. elongated third palpal segments
b. spur at the base of the tarsal segment of the first pair of legs
c. 3 pair of legs
d. pre-anal groove on its ventral surface
e. spur on the caudal aspect of the tarsal segment of the last pair of legs

Correct answers are on pages 249-251.

78. *Mites in the ear of a dog are typically:*

a. *Sarcoptes scabiei*
b. *Notoedres cati*
c. *Otodectes cynotis*
d. *Lynxacarus radovskyi*
e. *Pyemotes tritici*

79. *Small, dandruff-like flakes in the hair of a dog appear to move. Examination of the apparent dandruff reveals it to be comprised of mites. This "walking dandruff" is associated with infestation by:*

a. *Sarcoptes scabiei*
b. *Myocoptes musculinus*
c. *Cheyletiella yasguri*
d. *Chirodiscoides caviae*
e. *Pyemotes tritici*

80. *Dogs typically acquire* Demodex *infestations from:*

a. association with infested dogs
b. the bitch as pups while nursing
c. wild rodents
d. birds
e. contact with infested people

81. *Microscopic examination of skin scrapings from a cat with localized dermatitis on its face reveals large numbers of small sausage-shaped mites. These mites are most likely:*

a. *Demodex cati*
b. *Notoedres cati*
c. *Lynxacarus radovskyi*
d. *Cheyletiella blakei*
e. *Sarcoptes scabiei*

82. *Face flies (*Musca autumnalis*) on horses are best controlled by:*

a. applying insecticides to the horse's face
b. applying insecticides to the horse's face, in conjunction with use of fly veils
c. feeding a larvicide (tetrachlorovinphos) to nearby cattle
d. feeding a larvicide (tetrachlorovinphos) to the horses
e. feeding a larvicide (tetrachlorovinphos) to the horses and nearby cattle

83. *Horses in a herd develop ventral midline dermatitis that disappears each winter. The shelter where they are fed in the evening is near a stand of rather open forest. After other measures fail, you suggest placing a slowly revolving fan on one end of the shelter. The fan is an overwhelming success during the next spring and summer. Your decision to suggest the fan was based on a guess as to the causative agent from your knowledge of the flight behavior of:*

a. mosquitos
b. tabanids
c. black flies
d. biting midges (Heleids, Ceratopogonids)
e. deer flies

84. *Horses with stomach bots can be treated with ivermectin or dichlorvos after the first killing frost. One waits until after the killing frost because:*

a. by then larvae have completed their migration through the spinal canal
b. the cold weather kills the eggs of *Gasterophilus intestinalis* that are attached to hairs
c. the cold weather kills the egg-laying adult flies
d. there are no drugs that eliminate the stages developing within the buccal tissues of horses
e. by then larvae have completed their migration through the liver

85. Damalinia equi *is a louse found on horses. The eggs of this louse are most likely to be found:*

a. in the feces
b. glued to the hairs
c. in water containers within the box stall
d. in the bedding of the box stall
e. in soil surrounding the stable

86. Oestrus ovis *overwinters as:*

a. third-stage larvae in the frontal sinuses of sheep
b. second-stage larvae in the frontal sinuses of sheep
c. adults in lofts and attics
d. eggs deposited on vegetation in sheep pastures
e. first-stage larvae in the nasal cavity and as pupae in soil

87. Tick paralysis occurs in a tick-infested animal when the ticks inject a:

a. neural toxin
b. neurotropic virus
c. rickettsial agent
d. toxigenic bacterium
e. substance that induces anaphylaxis

88. An old sow that cannot walk because of severe arthritis has large numbers of very large lice at the base of its ears and on the back of its neck. The lice on this pig are most likely of the genus:

a. *Hematopinus*
b. *Damalinia*
c. *Linognathus*
d. *Solenopotes*
e. *Trichodectes*

89. Ear canker in rabbits is typically caused by:

a. *Psoroptes cuniculi*
b. *Sarcoptes scabiei*
c. *Chorioptes ovis*
d. *Cheyletiella blakei*
e. *Otodectes cynotis*

90. A budgerigar that develops greatly thickened ceres and feet is found to be infested with skin-dwelling mites. The mites that typically cause this condition are of the genus:

a. *Sarcoptes*
b. *Psoroptes*
c. *Chorioptes*
d. *Knemidokoptes*
e. *Myobia*

Answers

1. **a** Another possible cause is *Toxoplasma gondii.*

2. **d** This organism should be differentiated from *Hemobartonella.*

3. **e** Other species of *Isospora* would also be likely causes of these signs.

4. **d** Bradyzoites (chronic cyst stages) of this parasite are found mainly in striated muscle cells of cattle.

5. **b** Cats acquire fatal infections with this parasite from tick bites; the sylvatic cycle is tick-bobcat-tick.

6. **a** Trichomonads of a nonpathogenic nature can be found in the mouth of many animals, including people.

7. **c** Another approach would be a fecal ELISA, but these have not yet been verified for use in domestic animals.

8. **b** Immunosuppressed horses, not unlike dogs, cats and people, can develop severe diarrhea due to cryptosporidiosis.

9. **e** In certain housing situations, it is not uncommon for 100% of calves to be infected by the third week of life. *Cryptosporidium muris,* another mammalian parasite, also is found in cattle, but usually in older animals. The oocysts of *C parvum* are 5 μ, and those of *C muris* are 7 μ.

10. **a**

11. **a** Disease is likely to occur before oocysts are being shed in the feces. Diagnosis requires examination of the intestinal mucosa of dead animals.

12. **a** *Eimeria* species are seldom pathogenic in pigs. Other parasites that can induce diarrhea in nursing pigs are *Cryptosporidium* and *Strongyloides.*

13. **c**

14. **b** The large size of this parasite typically raises concern, but it often does not cause disease. A similar protozoan parasite of cattle, *Buxtonella sulcata,* is similar in that its discovery often initially raises questions about possible pathogenicity.

15. **b** Pigs have many nonpathogenic amoebas that may be detected on fecal examination.

16. **a**

17. **c** Hawks sometimes become infected with this parasite from their prey, such as pigeons, and occasionally develop severe diarrhea.

18. **b** *Eimeria tenella* causes the classic cecal lesions. Lesions caused by the different species of coccidia parasitizing chickens are sufficiently distinct to allow recognition of the causative species from the lesions in the intestinal tract. Thus, due to the nature of the industry and the ease with which different species can be identified by lesion appearance, a diagnosis is often made by necropsy of several animals.

19. **a**

20. **b** *Strongyloides stercoralis* and *Filaroides* are the 2 most likely possibilities in a closed colony. The larvae of *Filaroides* are sluggish and typically are not recovered by Baermann analysis; also, they would not proliferate in a charcoal culture due to their different life history. *Crenosoma vulpis* also produces larvae, but typically is not transmitted in closed colonies and would not proliferate in charcoal cultures. *Rhabditis strongyloides* is found in skin. *Uncinaria stenocephala* produces eggs that would be found in the feces.

21. **b**

22. **c**

23. **c** Transplacentally acquired *Toxocara canis* larvae can be pathogenic *in utero* or after parturition.

24. **b**

25. **d** The diagnostic dilemma is that there are no detectable microfilariae and antigen tests do not begin to detect infection until several weeks to months after the mosquito bite.

26. **b**

27. **a**

28. **e**

29. **b**

30. **c** This rare infection with a free-living nematode is of interest as a curiosity and as a representative case of facultative parasitism, that is, when an organism becomes parasitic only when it has the opportunity.

31. **a**

32. **d**

33. **a** Dermal habronemiasis is caused by the larvae of these worms; fortunately, the lesions respond very well to ivermectin therapy.

34. **b**

35. **d**

36. **c**

37. **a** *Ostertagia ostertagi,* like most other trichostrongyles and strongyles, has a direct life cycle.

38. **e** The larvae can develop in the manure pack. Ventilation is good for the cattle.

39. **b**

40. **c**

41. **c**

42. **d**

43. **a** The white reproductive organs of the female can be seen through the red translucent body spiralling about the intestine, giving the worm a "barber pole" appearance.

44. **d** Eggs of the other very large tricho-strongylid, *Marshallagia marshalli,* differ from those of *Nematodirus* in having more parallel sides and being less pointed at the poles; also, this was not offered as a choice.

45. **c** This is the only sure way of identifying the species of parasite involved on the basis of a fecal sample.

46. **c**

47. **e** It is difficult to imagine how the horse was originally infected, but the scenario is a real one.

48. **d**

49. **c** It may also be called the periparturient rise.

50. **d**

51. **a** Species of coccidia of chickens, other than *E tenella,* can produce small bowel disease.
52. **b**
53. **b** The "thumps" is associated with lung migration.
54. **d**
55. **c** Transmammary transmission may lead to signs very early in life.
56. **d**
57. **d**
58. **c**
59. **a** This is unusual for a trematode.
60. **d**
61. **c**
62. **b**
63. **b** The egg of *Heterobilharzia* has no operculum and contains a developed miracidium when passed in the feces. The eggs of *Spirometra* and *Diphyllobothrium* are very similar and resemble those of *Paragonimus;* however, with experience, they can be distinguished from eggs of *Paragonimus* by their smaller size, lighter-colored shell, and often less demarcated operculum.
64. **b**
65. **d**
66. **a**
67. **b** Flea larvae that feed on undigested blood passed in the feces of the adult fleas and detritus in the environment are attracted to the egg balls of *Dipylidium caninum* that are passed in the feces of dogs and cats. Tapeworm larvae in the larval, pupal and adult fleas do not become infective until adult fleas have been on the mammalian host for a couple of days.
68. **d** A taeniid tapeworm has a mammalian intermediate host.
69. **d**
70. **d**
71. **e**
72. **c**
73. **b**
74. **d**
75. **b** The belief that fleas constantly jump on and off their hosts is a commonly held misconception. Once fleas get on a dog or cat, they tend to stay on the host.
76. **d**
77. **d** The larvae, nymphs and adults of *Ixodes* can all be recognized by the pre-anal groove. This structure is not present in any other ticks. Due to the public awareness of Lyme disease, of which species of *Ixodes* are primary vectors, this characteristic is useful in identifying a tick as a possible vector when it is brought to the clinic for identification.
78. **c**
79. **c**
80. **b**
81. **a**
82. **c** The maggots develop in cattle feces.
83. **d** Midges are very weak fliers.
84. **c**
85. **b**
86. **e** Larvae gaining access to the nasal sinuses of sheep in late spring or early summer leave the nose in the fall and overwinter in the soil. Any larvae deposited in late summer await spring within the nasal passages.
87. **a** A tick injects a considerable volume of saliva at the feeding site; this saliva contains toxin(s) capable of producing paralysis. One tick is sufficient in the case of small animals and people, whereas several or many may be required in cattle. In Australia, there is a species of ixodid tick capable of causing severe paralysis that requires treatment with a specific antitoxin and supportive therapy.
88. **a** This is the only louse typically found on pigs.
89. **a**
90. **d**

Notes

Section 25

Pharmacology and Pharmacy Procedures

L.E. Davis, S. Hudson Duran

Recommended Reading

Booth NH and McDonald LE: *Veterinary Pharmacology and Therapeutics.* 6th ed. Iowa State University Press, Ames, 1988.

Brumbaugh G and Davis LE: Clinical pharmacology. *Vet Clin No Am* (Equine Pract) 3:1-254, 1987.

Davis LE, in Zaslow IM: *Veterinary Trauma and Critical Care.* Lea & Febiger, Philadelphia, 1984.

Davis LE: *Handbook of Small Animal Therapeutics.* Churchill Livingstone, New York, 1985.

Gilman AG *et al: Goodman and Gilman's The Pharmacological Basis of Therapeutics.* 8th ed. Pergamon Press, New York, 1990.

Hinchcliff KW and Jernigan AD: Applied pharmacology and therapeutics I. Vet Clin No Am (Food Animal Pract) 7:633-814, 1991.

Hinchcliff KW and Jernigan AD: Applied pharmacology and therapeutics II. *Vet Clin No Am* (Food Animal Pract) 8:1-168, 1992.

Johnston D: *The Bristol Veterinary Handbook of Antimicrobial Therapy.* 2nd ed. Veterinary Learning Systems, Trenton, NJ, 1987.

Koterba A *et al: Equine Clinical Neonatology.* Lea & Febiger, Philadelphia, 1990.

Plumb D: *Veterinary Drug Handbook.* Pharma Vet Publishing, White Bear Lake, MN, 1991.

Short CE: *Principles and Practice of Veterinary Anesthesia.* Williams & Wilkins, Baltimore, 1987.

USP – Dispensing Information. Drug Information for the Health Care Professional. US Pharmacopeial Convention, Rockville, MD, 1992.Bennett K: *Compendium of Veterinary Products.* 1st ed. North American Compendiums, Port Huron, MI, 1991.

Veterinary Pharmaceuticals and Biologicals 92/93. 8th ed. Veterinary Medicine Publishing, Lenexa, KS, 1993.

Practice answer sheet is on page 393.

Correct answers are on pages 263-267.

Questions

1. *Approved veterinary drugs are:*

   a. drugs whose use for certain diseases in certain species has been approved by the Food and Drug Administration
   b. drugs prescribed by veterinarians
   c. drugs that may be purchased at a retail pharmacy
   d. drugs that may be purchased at a feed store
   e. drugs used in human medicine

2. *All of the following are examples of extra-label use of a veterinary drug* ***except:***

   a. the drug is used only as indicated on the label
   b. the drug is used for a species other than those indicated on the label
   c. the route of administration is different than that indicated on the label
   d. the disease treated is different than those indicated on the label
   e. the dosage interval is different than that indicated on the label

3. *Extra-label use of veterinary drugs is legal only if:*

   a. a farmer asks for at least a week's supply of medication
   b. a producer insists on ordering the medication over the phone
   c. a dairyman must treat his herd for a respiratory problem
   d. there is a cheaper human drug than the available veterinary product
   e. there is a valid veterinarian-client-patient relationship, with the animal's medical diagnosis established

4. *All doses charted in an animal's medication records should be expressed in:*

   a. milliliters (ml)
   b. cubic centimeters (cc)
   c. milligrams (mg), grams (g) or units (U)
   d. number of capsules
   e. number of tablets

5. *A 7% solution of chloral hydrate contains:*

   a. 7 g in 10 ml
   b. 7 g in 100 ml
   c. 7 g in 1000 ml
   d. 7 mg in 100 ml
   e. 7 mg in 1000 ml

6. *A milliequivalent (mEq) is calculated by dividing the milligram (mg) molecular weight by the valence, which gives mg/mEq. If potassium chloride (KCl) has a molecular weight of 74.5, how many milliequivalents are in 1 gram of KCl?*

   a. 74.5 mEq
   b. 7.45 mEq
   c. 13.4 mEq
   d. 20 mEq
   e. 134 mEq

7. *A vial of sodium penicillin G powder contains 5 million units. If you add 18 milliliters (ml) of sterile water to the vial, the concentration will be 250,000 units/ml. What volume of powder was originally in the vial?*

   a. 4 ml
   b. 2 ml
   c. 1 ml
   d. 20 ml
   e. 5 ml

8. *By law, veterinary technicians are permitted to dispense veterinary drugs to clients:*

   a. provided the client has been in the clinic for a prior visit
   b. only if the technician is familiar with the drug
   c. only if the veterinarian is away and has given general permission
   d. only if the technician is over 21 years of age
   e. only in the presence and under the direct supervision of a licensed veterinarian

9. The veterinarian asks you to dispense an external parasiticide to a client. In what type of container should the insecticide be dispensed?

a. the original container, with a safety cap
b. a clear glass bottle, appropriately labeled
c. an amber glass bottle, appropriately labeled
d. a plastic 1-gallon container
e. a plastic container with a wide mouth

10. What is the osmolarity of an isotonic solution?

a. 750 mOsm/L
b. 300 mOsm/L
c. 1000 mOsm/L
d. 200 mOsm/L
e. 150 mOsm/L

11. United States Pharmacopeia (USP) Standards state that drugs used in human medicine must contain ± 10% of the amount of those ingredients indicated on the label. USP standards for veterinary drugs are:

a. ± 10%
b. ± 5%
c. ± 15%
d. ± 20%
e. ± 25%

12. Aminoglycoside antibiotics, such as gentamicin and amikacin, are used in veterinary medicine to treat infections caused by Gram-negative bacteria. Types of toxicities associated with these drugs are:

a. nephrotoxicity, ototoxicity and neurotoxicity
b. nephrotoxicity, hepatotoxicity and cardiotoxicity
c. cardiotoxicity, bone marrow suppression and immunosuppression
d. neurotoxicity, cardiotoxicity and bone marrow suppression
e. immunosuppression, hepatotoxicity and neurotoxicity

13. Gentamicin and amikacin are antibiotics with a narrow therapeutic index, meaning the dosage must be carefully controlled so as to prevent toxicity. The safest way to monitor the response to these antibiotics is to:

a. measure levels in serum to make sure they are within the safe range
b. give very low dosages
c. use these drugs for no more than 1 day
d. use these drugs for 3 days, withhold the drugs for another 3 days, then resume treatment for 3 more days
e. keep the animal well nourished while the drugs are being given

14. A dog has a serum creatinine level of 3 mg/dl. The veterinarian asks you to begin ampicillin therapy at 25 mg/kg body weight. How often should you give the drug?

a. every 4-6 hours
b. every 6-8 hours
c. every 8-10 hours
d. every 1-2 hours
e. every 12-18 hours

15. What key words should you look for when purchasing fluids for intravenous injection?

a. sterile, distilled
b. distilled, bacteriostatic
c. sterile, pyrogen free
d. autoclaved, distilled
e. bactericidal, irradiated

*16. Lactated Ringer's Injection USP is **not** compatible with:*

a. calcium chloride
b. potassium chloride
c. sodium chloride
d. sodium bicarbonate
e. potassium acetate

*17. A horse has an allergic reaction to xylazine. Another drug that should **not** be administered to this animal is:*

a. ketamine
b. acepromazine
c. thiamylal sodium
d. guaifenesin
e. detomidine

Correct answers are on pages 263-267.

18. If you wish to prepare 1000 ml of a 5% guaifenesin solution in 5% dextrose, how much of each ingredient will the solution contain?

a. 100 grams of dextrose and 100 grams of guaifenesin
b. 5 grams of dextrose and 5 grams of guaifenesin
c. 50 grams of dextrose and 50 grams of guaifenesin
d. 10 grams of dextrose and 10 grams of guaifenesin
e. 0.5 grams of dextrose and 0.5 grams of guaifenesin

19. Current laws state that the label on medications dispensed for use in food animals must contain all of the following information ***except:***

a. name of the veterinarian dispensing the drug
b. identification (name or number) of the animal being treated
c. withdrawal time if the animal is to be slaughtered for meat
d. withdrawal time if the animal's milk is used for food
e. last treatment date of the animal

20. The half-life of a drug is the time it takes for:

a. the drug to be totally eliminated from the body
b. the drug to kill half of the bacteria causing an infection
c. drug concentrations in the body to be reduced by one-half
d. half of a usual course of therapy
e. half of the recommended dosage to resolve disease

21. All of the following drugs have narrow therapeutic indexes (safety margins) ***except:***

a. theophylline
b. penicillin
c. gentamicin
d. digoxin
e. phenobarbital

22. Cimetidine and ranitidine are:

a. antacids used for reflux esophagitis
b. anthelmintics used for hookworm infections
c. antibiotics used against Gram-positive bacteria
d. H_2 antagonists used for gastrointestinal ulcers
e. injectable laxatives

23. The more water soluble a drug is, the higher its accumulation in:

a. fatty tissues
b. the brain
c. bone or teeth
d. the liver and spleen
e. serum or plasma

24. In addition to its main use, cimetidine is also used to treat:

a. keratoconjunctivitis sicca (dry eye)
b. congestive heart failure
c. malignant melanoma
d. endocrine alopecia
e. lungworm infection

25. Gentamicin should ***not*** *be used in:*

a. food animals soon to be slaughtered for food
b. nursing foals
c. dogs with marginal cardiopulmonary function
d. cats with dilative cardiomyopathy
e. horses with periodic ophthalmia

26. A lipophilic (fat-loving) drug tends to accumulate in:

a. teeth
b. serum
c. urine
d. plasma
e. soft tissues

27. In horses, H_2 antagonists are:

a. commonly associated with penile prolapse in stallions

b. poorly absorbed when given orally
c. not effective when given intravenously
d. not effective because of inactivation by enzymes
e. not effective because of the unique alimentary tract of horses

28. In dogs, digoxin has an elimination half-life of:

a. 30-112 minutes
b. 14-56 hours
c. 7-15 days
d. 72-96 hours
e. 21-30 days

29. When given by injection, oxytetracycline should be given:

a. with calcium products
b. very slowly intravenously
c. by any convenient route
d. with blood products
e. very rapidly as an intravenous bolus

30. Diethylstilbestrol, chloramphenicol and dimetronidazole are all:

a. illegal for use in food animals
b. potent antibiotics that must be used cautiously in neonates
c. antineoplastics that must be carefully handled to avoid human contamination
d. anthelmintics that may contaminate pastures when passed in the feces of horses
e. approved only for use in dogs

31. Atropine has all of the following clinical uses ***except:***

a. antispasmodic
b. inhibit salivation
c. bronchoconstriction
d. diagnosis of sinus node dysfunction
e. treatment of sinus bradycardia

32. Aminophylline, prednisone and terbutaline are used in combination to treat:

a. infections with Gram-positive bacteria
b. intestinal malabsorption
c. squamous-cell carcinoma
d. chronic obstructive pulmonary disease
e. diabetes insipidus

33. The anticoagulant heparin can be added to saline to make a solution used to flush intravenous catheters, so as to prevent obstruction by blood clots. How much heparin should be added to each milliliter of saline to make such a flushing solution to be used in adult animals?

a. 1 unit per ml
b. 2 units per ml
c. 3 units per ml
d. 5 units per ml
e. 10 units per ml

34. Whole blood, plasma and blood substitutes should:

a. be kept at room temperature for 24 hours before use
b. be given in the same intravenous line as other medications
c. not be used to dilute any drugs
d. be mixed with calcium products before use
e. be given with dextrose solutions

35. Antineoplastic agents, such as vincristine and doxorubicin, should be:

a. cautiously handled so as to avoid human and environmental contamination
b. mixed with calcium solutions and infused as a bolus intravenous injection
c. prepared at least 24 hours before intended use so as to allow precipitation of contaminants
d. used only when the prognosis for recovery is poor
e. used only in animals less than 3 years of age

Correct answers are on pages 263-267.

36. Amprolium is used to treat:

a. heartworm infection
b. coccidiosis
c. congestive heart failure
d. laminitis
e. otitis externa

37. When given orally once a month for heartworm prevention in dogs, the recommended dosage of ivermectin is:

a. 200 μg/kg
b. 2 μg/kg
c. 300 μg/kg
d. 6 μg/kg
e. 50 mg/lb

38. After administration of hetacillin potassium, the drug is metabolized and appears in tissue and blood as:

a. ampicillin and amoxicillin
b. hetacillin and carbenicillin
c. ampicillin and hetacillin
d. amoxicillin and penicillin
e. penicillin and carbenicillin

39. Strong tincture of iodine USP is comprised of:

a. 2% iodine in water
b. 2% iodine in alcohol
c. 7% iodine in water
d. 7% iodine in alcohol
e. 15.6% iodine in water

40. Xylazine hydrochloride is classified as:

a. an alpha-1 adrenergic agonist
b. an alpha-2 adrenergic antagonist
c. an alpha-2 adrenergic agonist
d. a beta-1 adrenergic agonist
e. a beta-2 adrenergic agonist

41. The approved sedative most commonly used for chemical restraint of deer and elk is:

a. morphine
b. meperidine
c. butorphanol
d. pentazocine
e. xylazine

42. Yohimbine is classified as:

a. an alpha-1 adrenergic agonist
b. an alpha-1 adrenergic antagonist
c. an alpha-2 adrenergic agonist
d. an alpha-2 adrenergic antagonist
e. a beta-1 adrenergic agonist

*43. Epinephrine should **not** be given with any of the following medications **except**:*

a. dextrose 5% injection USP
b. sodium bicarbonate
c. warfarin sodium
d. ascorbic acid
e. Hetastarch

44. A dog is having a seizure. The drug of choice to immediately stop the seizure is:

a. phenytoin per os
b. acepromazine intramuscularly
c. xylazine intravenously
d. diazepam intravenously
e. ketamine intramuscularly

45. In dogs, primidone is metabolized to:

a. phenobarbital
b. diazepam
c. xylazine
d. ketamine
e. acepromazine

46. The half-life of phenylbutazone in horses is 4-6 hours. What is the half-life of phenylbutazone in cattle?

a. 1-3 hours
b. 6-16 hours
c. 18-27 hours
d. 30-37 hours
e. 40-55 hours

47. *Records on use of controlled substances in a veterinary practice should be maintained by:*

a. a veterinary technician with a license in that state
b. a clerk with experience in inventory control
c. a hospital administrator with a key to the controlled substances cabinet
d. an office manager
e. a veterinarian registered with the Drug Enforcement Administration

48. *Concerning a veterinarian's dispensing of medication to hospital staff members for use in treating themselves, which statement is most accurate?*

a. It is permitted if they present a prescription written by a physician.
b. It is permitted if the drugs are used on the premises.
c. It is permitted if they have been employed by the hospital for at least 3 years.
d. It is permitted if they are blood relatives.
e. It is not permitted under any circumstances.

49. *Concerning the legality of dispensing outdated drugs (after the date of expiration indicated on the label), which statement is most accurate?*

a. It is permitted within 1 month after the date of expiration.
b. It is permitted within 2 months after the date of expiration.
c. It is permitted within 3 months after the date of expiration.
d. It is permitted within 6 months after the date of expiration.
e. It is not permitted under any circumstances.

50. *A drug that is a direct respiratory stimulant is:*

a. epinephrine
b. norepinephrine
c. doxapram
d. ketamine
e. calcium

51. *Magnesium hydroxide, an ingredient in some antacids, can be given orally in treatment of:*

a. constipation
b. diarrhea
c. emesis
d. nausea
e. indigestion

52. *Which drug used in dogs and cats to treat gastric ulcers is **not** absorbed?*

a. cimetidine
b. ranitidine
c. neomycin
d. sucralfate
e. omeprazole

53. *According to the Controlled Substances Act of 1970, anabolic steroids have some potential for abuse, and therefore are classified as:*

a. Schedule I
b. Schedule II
c. Schedule III
d. Schedule IV
e. Schedule V

54. *Oxfendazole is an anthelmintic in the same class of drugs as:*

a. fenbendazole
b. levamisole
c. ivermectin
d. pyrantel pamoate
e. trichlorfon

55. *A client calls and says she left the container of diethylcarbamazine citrate oral liquid in her car for 3 weeks during the summer. Concerning the potency of the drug after such storage, which statement is most accurate?*

a. It has probably lost potency.
b. It has probably gained potency.
c. It will regain any lost potency if placed in the refrigerator.
d. It will lose any excessive potency if placed in the refrigerator.
e. It is probably unaffected and can be used without concern.

Correct answers are on pages 263-267.

56. *Veterinary prescription medications should be dispensed in:*

a. white envelopes with a self-sealing adhesive flap
b. brown envelopes with a gummed flap sealed by moistening
c. child-proof amber vials and bottles
d. transparent plastic cups with a pop-off top
e. transparent plastic bags with a "zip-lock" closure

57. *All of the following are nonsteroidal anti-inflammatory drugs* ***except:***

a. phenylbutazone
b. aspirin
c. flunixin
d. dexamethasone
e. dipyrone

58. *Which of the following is the most potent glucocorticoid?*

a. dexamethasone
b. prednisone
c. prednisolone
d. methylprednisolone
e. hydrocortisone

59. *Glucocorticoids are* ***contraindicated*** *in all of the following conditions* ***except:***

a. first trimester of gestation
b. last trimester of gestation
c. systemic fungal infections
d. corneal ulcers
e. trauma or shock

60. *What is the main adverse effect of phenylbutazone?*

a. pulmonary edema
b. crystals in the urine
c. gastric ulcers
d. cardiac decompensation
e. dryness of the mouth

61. *Which glucocorticoid is metabolized to prednisolone?*

a. dexamethasone
b. prednisone
c. betamethasone
d. hydrocortisone
e. cortisone

62. *The veterinarian asks you to give a dog sucralfate for treatment of a gastric ulcer. Which drug enhances healing of gastric ulcers, when given with sucralfate?*

a. cimetidine
b. ranitidine
c. famotidine
d. antacids
e. no other drug

63. *Enrofloxacin should be used with caution when treating:*

a. young dogs
b. dogs with infections by Gram-negative bacteria
c. dogs with marginal cardiopulmonary functions
d. brachycephalic dogs
e. dolichocephalic dogs

64. *In dogs, overdosage of ivermectin can produce all of the following* ***except:***

a. tremors
b. ataxia
c. mydriasis
d. weight loss
e. degenerative joint disease

65. *Cloxacillin sodium is an antibiotic that is effective against:*

a. lecithinase-producing micrococci
b. *E coli*
c. penicillinase-producing staphylococci
d. *Proteus*
e. collagenase-producing enterobacteria

66. ***In horses, the nonsteroidal antiinflammatory drug flunixin meglumine is most beneficial when used to treat:***

a. renal disease
b. colic
c. heart disease
d. gastric ulcers in foals
e. endocrine-related skin disease

67. ***The major toxicity associated with flunixin meglumine is:***

a. ototoxicity
b. liver toxicity
c. renal toxicity
d. glaucoma
e. gastrointestinal ulcers

68. ***Isoxsuprine is a peripheral vasodilating agent used in horses used to treat:***

a. infections with Gram-negative bacteria
b. septicemia
c. navicular disease
d. glaucoma
e. chronic obstructive pulmonary disease

69. ***Dobutamine, a drug used for treatment of heart failure, is classified as:***

a. a beta-1 adrenergic antagonist
b. an alpha-1 adrenergic agonist
c. an alpha-2 adrenergic agonist
d. a beta-1 adrenergic agonist
e. a histamine type-2 antagonist

70. ***A dehydrated animal is best treated by intravenous infusion of:***

a. dextrose 15% injection USP
b. dextrose 10% injection USP
c. dextrose 20% injection USP
d. dextrose 50% injection USP
e. acetated Ringer's injection USP

71. ***One gram of dextrose contains 3.4 calories. How many calories are contained in 1 liter of 5% dextrose?***

a. 170 calories
b. 2000 calories
c. 50 calories
d. 500 calories
e. 1000 calories

72. ***Because of the likelihood of adverse reaction, solutions of B vitamins should never be administered:***

a. intramuscularly
b. orally
c. subcutaneously
d. as an intravenous bolus
e. by slow intravenous infusion after dilution in 1-2 liters of fluid

73. ***The diuretic of choice to combat pulmonary edema in an animal with congestive heart failure is:***

a. thiazide
b. chlorothiazide
c. aldosterone
d. furosemide
e. ethacrynic acid

74. ***Tiletamine hydrochloride is an injectable anesthetic closely related to:***

a. acepromazine
b. diazepam
c. ketamine
d. guaifenesin
e. xylazine

75. ***Therapeutic drug monitoring involves:***

a. periodic physical examination of animals that have been treated with drugs
b. testing of animals for possible anaphylactic reaction before treatment with a drug
c. measurement of serum or plasma levels of a drug to maintain levels in the optimal range
d. close visual observation of animals in the first 8 hours after a drug is administered
e. periodically obtaining tissue or exudate specimens for culture during a course of drug therapy

Correct answers are on pages 263-267.

76. *An example of a long-acting insulin is:*

a. semi-lente insulin
b. lente insulin
c. insulin injection USP
d. protamine zinc insulin
e. isophane insulin

77. *The cathartic whose action is limited to the colon is:*

a. castor oil
b. magnesium sulfate
c. cascara sagrada
d. docusate
e. liquid petrolatum

78. *How many grams of potassium permanganate are required to prepare 1 gallon of a 1:3000 solution?*

a. 0.3
b. 1.3
c. 3
d. 13
e. 30

79. *Five grains are equivalent to how many grams?*

a. 0.75
b. 0.075
c. 300
d. 0.325
e. 7.50

80. *You wish to dilute strong tincture of iodine (7%) with 70% ethanol to prepare 4 oz of tincture of iodine USP (2%) for use on small animals. How much ethanol and 7% iodine must be used?*

a. 3 fl oz of ethanol and 1 fl oz of 7% iodine
b. 50 ml of ethanol and 45 ml of 7% iodine
c. 160 ml of ethanol and 80 ml of 7% iodine
d. 86 ml of ethanol and 34 ml of 7% iodine
e. 45 ml of ethanol and 55 ml of 7% iodine

81. *The most rapid recovery of consciousness would be expected after discontinuing administration of:*

a. methoxyflurane
b. halothane
c. diethyl ether
d. nitrous oxide
e. enflurane

82. *Chronic administration of which drug may lead to clinical signs of thiamin deficiency?*

a. trimethoprim
b. amprolium
c. chlortetracycline
d. levamisole
e. metronidazole

83. *The breed of dog that exhibits an idiosyncratic reaction to ivermectin is the:*

a. Great Dane
b. Golden Retriever
c. Dalmatian
d. Cocker Spaniel
e. Collie

84. *Lactated Ringer's solution should **not** be mixed with:*

a. calcium chloride
b. potassium chloride
c. sodium chloride
d. sodium bicarbonate
e. potassium acetate

85. *What is the drug of choice for topical treatment of an infected thermal burn?*

a. neomycin ointment
b. petrolatum
c. povidone-iodine solution
d. tannic acid spray
e. silver sulfadiazine cream

86. Burrow's solution is employed in wet dressings because of its:

a. emollient effect
b. depilatory action
c. demulcent effect
d. astringent action
e. effect on pigmentation

87. Drugs used to treat newborn animals must be carefully selected because:

a. neonates are unable to metabolize drugs
b. neonates have poorly developed drug receptors
c. correct dosage ranges have not been determined
d. neonates have poorly developed excretory organs
e. neonates absorb drugs poorly from the intestine

88. Sulfonamides act against bacteria by:

a. inhibiting cell wall synthesis
b. interfering with bacterial metabolism
c. inhibiting protein synthesis
d. interfering with membrane function
e. impairing protein synthesis

89. The principal danger associated with use of nitrous oxide during inhalation anesthesia is:

a. explosion
b. cardiac arrhythmia
c. metabolic alkalosis
d. hypoxia
e. hemolysis

90. Paralysis of the retractor penis muscle caused by phenothiazine tranquilizers has been observed in:

a. bulls
b. boars
c. stallions
d. rams
e. bucks

Answers

1. **a** Approved drugs are those for which experimental data document safety and efficacy for a particular disease in certain species.
2. **a** Extra-label use involves use of an approved drug in a manner not consistent with the drug's label.
3. **e** A veterinary drug may be used in an extra-label fashion only when a proper veterinarian-client-patient relationship exists, with a medical diagnosis established, and when there is no approved drug available to treat the disease properly. Animals so treated must be easily identified and/or kept separate from the rest of the herd.
4. **c** All records of the medication should be cited in metric units of the total dose given. For example, 500 mg of flunixin (not 10 ml).
5. **b** A 7% solution contains 7 g/dl. Remember, percent is parts (in this case, grams) per 100.
6. **c** There are 13.4 milliequivalents (mEq) in 1 gram (1000 mg) of potassium chloride. The equation is
$$\text{mEq} = \frac{\text{mg}}{\text{molecular weight/valence}}$$
7. **b** First divide the initial amount (5 million units) by the final amount (250,000 units/ml). 5,000,000 ÷ 250,000 = 20 ml. Then subtract the volume of diluent added (18 ml). 20 – 18 = 2 ml of powder originally in the vial.
8. **e** Veterinary technicians are permitted to dispense drugs only in the presence of a licensed veterinarian.
9. **a** All insecticides should be dispensed in the original container, with all EPA information on the label and in a safety-cap container or spray container.

10. **b** An isotonic solution has an osmolarity of 300 mOsm/L, which is the same osmotic pressure as for body fluids. A solution with an osmolarity less than 300 mOsm/L is hypotonic and could cause lysis of red blood cells. A solution with an osmolarity greater than 300 mOsm/L is hypertonic.

11. **d**

12. **a** Aminoglycosides can produce nephrotoxicity, ototoxicity and neurotoxicity.

13. **a** The safest way to monitor patients receiving aminoglycosides is to obtain serum samples and measure peak and trough levels to make sure drug levels are within the safe, therapeutic range.

14. **e** Ampicillin is eliminated primarily by the kidneys and normally administered every 6 hours for 7-10 days. If an animal has a serum creatinine value of 3 mg/dl (normal, 1-2 mg/dl), this indicates reduced renal function, so the drug should be given less frequently, as it is not being eliminated at a normal rate. A good rule of thumb is: serum creatinine x normal dosage interval = adjusted dosage interval. 3 x 6 = 18 hours.

15. **c** Only fluids that are sterile and pyrogen free should be given intravenously.

16. **d** Lactated Ringer's USP contains calcium chloride. Mixing with sodium bicarbonate forms an insoluble precipitate, calcium carbonate.

17. **e** Detomidine and xylazine are chemically related. Horses that have an adverse reaction to xylazine may also react to detomidine.

18. **c** A 5% dextrose-5% guaifenesin solution contains 5 grams of dextrose and 5 grams of guaifenesin per 100 ml, which is equal to 50 grams of each per 1000 ml.

19. **e** Current laws require that labels of drugs dispensed for food animals state the name of the veterinarian dispensing the medication, date of dispensing, name of product dispensed, withdrawal dates, and identification of the animal being treated. If the drug is being used in an unapproved (extra-label) manner, the Food Animal Residue Avoidance Data Bank (FARAD) should be consulted for extended withdrawal information.

20. **c** The half-life of a drug is the time it takes for the drug concentration to decrease by one-half. Usually in animals, 99% of the drug is cleared from the animal's body in 10 half-lives.

21. **b** Theophylline, phenobarbital, digoxin, amikacin and gentamicin all have narrow safety ranges and could cause adverse reactions and toxicities if serum levels are not monitored. Penicillin has a larger margin of safety.

22. **d** Cimetidine and ranitidine are H_2 antagonists that block gastric acid secretion, which aids treatment of ulcers. Because there are no H_2 antagonists approved for veterinary use, these drugs can only be used in accordance with extra-label laws.

23. **e** Water-soluble drugs, such as gentamicin, tend to remain in the serum or plasma and are often used for Gram-negative septicemia.

24. **c** Cimetidine acts as an immunostimulant and is sometimes used to treat melanomas in horses and dogs.

25. **a** Gentamicin should not be used in food animals because residues accumulate in the kidney and may persist for 12-18 months after administration.

26. **e** A lipophilic drug has an affinity for such areas as soft tissue, the outer layers of the lungs, and bone.

27. **b** Cimetidine, ranitidine and famotidine are poorly absorbed in horses and require large oral doses to achieve therapeutic results. Initial therapy should be administered intravenously.

28. **b** Digoxin has a variable half-life in dogs, ranging from 14 to 56 hours. Serum levels of the drug should be monitored after initiation of therapy and at least once a month during therapy.

29. **b** Oxytetracycline chelates (binds) calcium. The vehicles used in some oxytetracycline products, such as propylene glycol, can cause anaphylaxis if these drugs are given by rapid intravenous injection. Because of their pH or vehicles, some products cannot be given intramuscularly.

30. **a** Diethylstilbestrol, chloramphenicol and dimetronidazole may pose health hazards if consumed in meat or milk from treated animals.

31. **c** Atropine causes bronchodilation.

32. **d** Aminophylline (a bronchodilator), prednisone (an antiinflammatory glucocorticoid) and terbutaline (a selective beta-2 adrenergic agonist) can be given in combination to treat chronic obstructive pulmonary disease.

33. **e** Heparinized saline is commonly prepared at a concentration of 10 units/ml. A commercial preparation of heparin is available 1000 units/ml. To prepare a sterile solution, add 1 ml of heparin to 100 ml of sodium chloride injection 0.9% USP. In neonates, a concentration of 1 unit/ml is often used.

34. **c** Whole blood, plasma and blood substitutes should not be used as diluents of any drugs, and can be infused only by piggyback with sodium chloride injection 0.9% USP.

35. **a** Antineoplastic agents can pose a threat to human health if not handled properly. EPA guidelines, including disposal of medical waste, should be observed. This may require that you attend a continuing education class on safe preparation of drugs used in cancer therapy.

36. **b**. Amprolium is used in prevention and treatment of coccidiosis caused by *Eimeria bovis* and *E zurnii* in calves.

37. **d** The ivermectin dosage for heartworm prevention in dogs is very small (6 μg/kg). There are 1000 μg in 1 mg. Certain breeds of dogs, such as Collies, are more sensitive to ivermectin, though the dosage used for heartworm prevention should be safe, as it is extremely low.

38. **c** Hetacillin potassium is chemically related to ampicillin. Some of the drug is metabolized to ampicillin, while some remains as hetacillin.

39. **d** Strong tincture of iodine USP is a 7% tincture, which has an alcohol base. It is commonly used to dip the umbilical cord of newborn calves. Mild tincture of iodine is a 2% solution and can be used to dip the umbilical cord of foals.

40. **c** Xylazine is an alpha-2 adrenergic agonist. It stimulates alpha-2 receptors and is a sedative/analgesic with muscle relaxant properties.

41. **e** Xylazine is an alpha-2 adrenergic agonist that is approved for use in dogs, cats, horses, deer and elk.

42. **d** Yohimbine is an alpha-2 adrenergic antagonist and can be used to reverse xylazine.

43. **a** Epinephrine is usually given by intravenous bolus injection. If it must be diluted, it should be added to dextrose 5% injection USP.

44. **d** Diazepam is the drug of choice for rapid control of seizures. Other anticonvulsants can be used for maintenance therapy, such as primidone, phenobarbital and phenytoin. All of these drugs require monthly monitoring of serum levels to ensure accurate dosage.

45. **a** Primidone is converted to phenobarbital and other active metabolites, and is monitored in the serum as phenobarbital.

46. **e** The half-life of phenylbutazone in horses is 4-6 hours and 40-55 hours in cattle. Dosages should never be extrapolated from one species to another; toxicities and deaths may occur from overdosing. Phenylbutazone can be used in an extra-label manner in food animals. The Food Animal Residue Avoidance Databank (FARAD) should be called to check for extended withdrawal dates.

47. **e** A veterinarian registered with the DEA and prescribing controlled substances should keep accurate records.

48. **e** A veterinarian is not permitted to dispense any drugs for use in people. Severe penalties are associated with this offense.

49. **e** Only drugs that are in date (not expired) and stored in proper containers at the proper temperature may be legally dispensed by or on prescription of a licensed veterinarian.

50. **c** Doxapram has a direct stimulatory effect on the medullary respiratory center.

51. **a** Magnesium hydroxide is often found in antacids and is also used as a laxative. When added to magnesium hydroxide, the constipating antacid aluminum hydroxide seems to provide a balanced antacid.

52. **d** Sucralfate is an alkaline aluminum complex of sucrose sulfate that acts locally rather than systemically. It forms a barrier at the ulcer site and protects the ulcer from further damage caused by pepsin, acid or bile.

53. **c** Anabolic steroids, such as boldenone, stanozolol, nandrolone, testosterone, chorionic gonadotropin and any growth stimulants, are currently Schedule-III controlled substances due to their potential for abuse.

54. **a** Fenbendazole and oxfendazole are benzimidazole anthelmintics.

55. **a** Diethylcarbamazine citrate, used for heartworm prevention in dogs, decomposes when exposed to temperatures over 30 C (86 F) and when exposed to light. Always dispense this drug in an amber bottle.

56. **c** Any medication that could be ingested by a child should be dispensed in amber safety-cap vials or bottles.

57. **d** Dexamethasone is a glucocorticoid and not a nonsteroidal antiinflammatory; however, it does have antiinflammatory activity.

58. **a** Dexamethasone is a fluorinated prednisolone glucocorticoid. Fluorination of the drug molecule gives the greatest antiinflammatory effects.

59. **e** Glucocorticoids are contraindicated in all pregnant animals. Deformities may occur in the first trimester, and abortions may occur in the last trimester, particularly with the longer-acting glucocorticoids, such as methylprednisolone, dexamethasone, betamethasone and triamcinolone. Fungal infections and corneal ulcers may worsen with glucocorticoid treatment.

60. **c** The major toxicity associated with phenylbutazone is gastric ulcers. The dosage should be tapered to small amounts or the drug should be used for short periods only, as it accumulates.

61. **b** Prednisone is metabolized to prednisolone by the liver.

62. **e** Sucralfate requires an acidic environment to be effective. All of the other drugs listed increase the pH of the stomach and decrease the efficacy of sucralfate.

63. **a** Enrofloxacin is contraindicated in small and medium-sized dogs 2-8 months of age, and in large-breed dogs of all ages. Changes in articular cartilage have been noted when the drug was given at 2-5 times recommended doses for 30 days, though clinical signs have only been seen at 5 times the recommended dose.

64. **e** Excessive ivermectin dosages may produce tremors, ataxia, mydriasis and weight loss when administered to dogs. Collie breeds seem to be more sensitive to toxicities.

65. **c** Cloxacillin sodium is a penicillin that is effective against penicillinase-producing staphylococci. Other drugs in that category are oxacillin, dicloxacillin, and antibiotics combined with clavulanate sodium or clavulanic acid.

66. **b** Flunixin meglumine is the nonsteroidal antiinflammatory of choice for colic, as it has analgesic and antiinflammatory effects while not decreasing gastrointestinal motility. It also may improve hemodynamics in animals with septic shock.

67. **e** Flunixin meglumine causes severe irritation of the gastrointestinal tract in dogs, and should be used with great caution in horses with gastrointestinal ulcers. The dosage and frequency of administration may also need to be adjusted in dehydrated horses. Prophylactic treatment with ranitidine or sucralfate may be helpful in preventing gastric ulcers.

68. **c** Isoxsuprine causes direct vascular smooth muscle relaxation, primarily in skeletal muscles, and raises distal limb temperatures significantly in horses with navicular disease.

69. **d** Dobutamine is a direct beta-1 adrenergic agonist that is used as a rapid-acting injectable positive inotropic agent for short-term treatment of heart failure. It must be diluted in sodium chloride or dextrose 5% injection and infused continuously intravenously because of its short half-life.

70. **e** Acetated Ringer's injection is the fluid of choice. Hypertonic dextrose solutions would act as an osmotic diuretic and further dehydrate the animal.

71. **a** Dextrose normally has 4 kilocalories per gram; however, hydrous dextrose is used to prepare 5% dextrose injection. It has 3.4 calories per gram. 3.4 calories x 50 grams per liter of dextrose equals 170 calories.

72. **d** B vitamins must never be administered by direct intravenous injection, as anaphylactic reactions can result in death due to massive release of histamine.

73. **d** Furosemide is the diuretic of choice for congestive heart failure. It is approved for use in dogs, cats, horses and cattle. The response is very rapid and the drug may be effective in animals nonresponsive to other diuretics.

74. **c** Tiletamine hydrochloride is an injectable anesthetic closely related to ketamine. It is commercially available in combination with zolazepam hydrochloride and is approved for use in dogs.

75. **c** Therapeutic drug monitoring involves measuring the amount of drug in the serum or plasma of the diseased animal to achieve the best therapeutic dosage, with the least toxicity.

76. **d** Protamine zinc insulin is slowly absorbed from the injection site.

77. **c** Cascara is an anthraquinone glycoside that is inactive until it is hydrolyzed by bacterial enzymes found in the colon. The other drugs listed act either in the small intestine or throughout the bowels.

78. **b** One gallon equals approximately 4000 ml. A 1:3000 solution is equivalent to 0.03%. 4000 x 0.0003 = 1.3 g of potassium permanganate.

79. **d** 5 gr x 65 mg/gr = 325 mg or 0.325 g.

80. **d** 4 oz x 30 ml/oz = 120 ml total, comprised of 5 parts 70% ethanol and 2 parts 7% tincture.

81. **d** Nitrous oxide has very low solubility in blood.

82. **b** Amprolium is a thiamin antagonist used to control coccidiosis.

83. **e** Some Collies develop blindness, coma and death in response to ivermectin.

84. **d** Lactated Ringer's solution contains calcium chloride. Mixing Ringer's solution with sodium bicarbonate forms the insoluble precipitate, calcium carbonate.

85. **e** This preparation was developed specifically for burn patients.

86. **d** This solution of aluminum subacetate is used to treat acute, oozing skin lesions.

87. **a** The microsomal enzyme system is not developed at birth in domestic animals.

88. **b** Sulfonamides compete with paraaminobenzoic acid in synthesis of folic acid.

89. **d** Nitrous oxide is an inert gas, but it may replace oxygen in the inspired gas mixture and cause hypoxia.

90. **c** Phenothiazines relax the retractor muscle, but in some individuals this effect is prolonged, leading to paraphimosis.

Notes

Notes

Section **26**

Physical Restraint

T.F. Sonsthagen

Recommended Reading

Fowler ME: *Restraint and Handling of Wild and Domestic Animals.* Iowa State University Press, Ames, IA, 1978.

Harkness JE and Wagner JE: *The Biology and Medicine of Rabbits and Rodents.* 3rd ed. Lea & Febiger, Philadelphia, 1989.

Pratt PW: *Medical Nursing for Animal Health Technicians.* American Veterinary Publications, Goleta, CA, 1985.

Sonsthagen TF: *Restraint of Domestic Animals.* American Veterinary Publications, Goleta, CA, 1991.

Practice answer sheet is on page 395.

Questions

1. *Which restraint instrument can cause broken bones, strangulation and death if used improperly in physical restraint?*
   a. cat bag
   b. nose lead
   c. twitch
   d. capture pole
   e. restraint gloves

2. *Because of their bellows-like breathing, which of the following animals should be held loosely if grasped around the thorax?*
   a. cats
   b. small dogs
   c. birds
   d. ferrets
   e. hamsters

3. *If a bird is presented to you in a cage containing perches, toys, and water and food dishes, what is the best procedure for capturing the bird?*
   a. throw a towel over the bird and grasp it
   b. turn the lights down and reach in behind the bird
   c. talk gently and coax the bird to stand on your finger
   d. remove all paraphernalia from the cage, then reach in behind the bird
   e. reach in, approaching the bird from the front, so it will not be frightened

Correct answers are on page 272.

4. *To collect a blood sample from the cephalic vein of a dog or cat, you should place the animal in:*

   a. a sitting position and lift the head to expose the ventral aspect of the neck
   b. lateral recumbency and steady the uppermost back leg
   c. a sitting position and steady a front leg
   d. a sitting position and steady the pinna
   e. lateral recumbency and lift the uppermost rear leg out of the way to expose the medial surface of the other rear leg

5. *For oral administration of liquid medication to a dog or cat, you should:*

   a. tilt the head up slightly and roll the lips over the canine teeth to open the mouth
   b. tilt the head straight up toward the ceiling and open the mouth using the index finger of the other hand
   c. leave the head in a horizontal position, administer the liquid between the lips, and stroke the throat
   d. tilt the head straight up toward the ceiling, administer the liquid between the lips, and stroke the throat
   e. tilt the head slightly down and open the mouth

6. *Of the following steps to place a cat in a cat bag, which should be first?*

   a. close the zipper
   b. place the cat inside of the bag
   c. hook the bag around the cat's neck
   d. place the cat in the center of the bag
   e. place the open bag on a table

7. *In prolonged attempts to capture a sheep or pig in a paddock or pen, it is extremely easy to cause:*

   a. abortions
   b. limb fractures
   c. bladder rupture
   d. hyperthermia
   e. death from shock

8. *In applying a chain twitch to a horse, the twitch should be:*

   a. placed on the upper lip and tightened as much as possible
   b. placed on the upper lip and tightened but with intermittent pressure
   c. placed on the lower lip and tightened as much as possible
   d. placed on the ear and tightened to some extent but with intermittent pressure
   e. chain twitches should be avoided because they cannot be applied safely

9. *What is the piece of restraint equipment most commonly used in horses?*

   a. halter
   b. twitch
   c. hobbles
   d. cradle
   e. whip

10. *When disturbed by attempts at physical restraint, a horse's initial response usually is:*

    a. kicking
    b. biting
    c. rearing
    d. vocalizing
    e. running

11. *When restraining a foal for treatment or diagnostic procedures, you should:*

    a. lead the mare out of eyesight from the foal
    b. keep the mare nearby, within eyesight of the foal
    c. leave the mare with the foal, but heavily sedate the mare
    d. pick the foal up off the ground so it cannot run away
    e. heavily sedate the foal so it does not traumatize itself

12. *Which piece of restraint equipment usually remains permanently attached to bulls used for breeding?*

    a. halter
    b. nose lead
    c. nose ring

d. hobbles
e. bull staff

13. Which animals have the strongest instinct to remain in a group when threatened?

a. sheep
b. goats
c. pigs
d. chickens
e. cattle

For Questions 14 through 18, select the correct answer from the 5 choices below.

a. bowline
b. sheet bend
c. halter tie
d. bowline on a bight
e. clove hitch

14. The knot used to tie together 2 ropes of different size.

15. The knot that can be used for breeding hobbles.

16. The knot used to secure a lead rope to a stationary object.

17. The knot used to secure a rope to a vertical bar without slippage.

18. A non-slip knot that is safe to place around an animal's neck.

19. In tail jacking a cow, you grasp the tail:

a. by the end and pull it to one side as far as possible
b. at the base and elevate it dorsally and to the right
c. by the end and elevate it dorsally and to the left
d. at the end and elevate it dorsally, directly on the midline
e. at the base and elevate it dorsally, directly on the midline

20. When carrying a rabbit, it is important to support its hindquarters so the animal does not:

a. scratch you with its hind feet
b. struggle and possibly fracture its spine
c. injure its ear
d. jump out of your arms
e. reflexively defecate and urinate

21. After securing a mouse by the tail, the head and body can then be restrained by:

a. twirling the mouse until it is dizzy and then quickly grasping the scruff of the neck
b. placing the mouse on a smooth surface, pulling caudally on the tail, and then quickly grasping the scruff of the neck
c. grasping loose skin along the back and moving the grasp cranially
d. placing the mouse on a grate or sloping surface, pulling caudally on the tail, and then quickly grasping the scruff of the neck
e. quickly grasping the scruff of the neck while the mouse is suspended by the tail

For Questions 22 through 25, select the correct answer from the 5 choices below.

a. V-trough
b. stocks
c. stanchion
d. tilt table
e. squeeze chute

22. Apparatus usually used to restrain beef cattle.

23. Apparatus used to restrain horses.

24. Apparatus used to restrain pigs weighing up to 80 lb.

25. Apparatus ideal in restraining a bull for hoof trimming.

Correct answers are on page 272.

Answers

1. **e** Restraint gloves decrease your tactile perception to the extent that you could cause strangulation, broken bones and ultimately death.
2. **c** The lungs of birds cannot inflate if the thorax is grasped too tightly.
3. **d** Removing all paraphernalia reduces the chance of the bird's injuring itself in attempts to escape.
4. **c** The cephalic vein is on the cranial surface of the front leg.
5. **c** The head should remain horizontal and the mouth closed. Stroking the throat induces swallowing.
6. **e** Place the open bag on the table.
7. **d** The insulation of a sheep's heavy wool coat and a pig's layer of body fat can lead to overheating if the animal is chased excessively.
8. **b** The twitch is placed on the upper lip, with pressure applied intermittently to keep the horse's attention on the twitch and to preserve circulation to the lip.
9. **a** The halter is the main tool of restraint for horses.
10. **e** Running is a horse's first instinct when threatened. If it cannot run away, it will fight.
11. **b** The foal and mare should remain within eyesight of each other. If not, both will fret and struggle to be reunited.
12. **c** Nose rings are permanently inserted through the nasal septum of bulls.
13. **a** Sheep have the strongest herding instinct.
14. **b**
15. **d** When this knot is tied in the middle of a long rope, it forms a non-slip noose that can go around the animal's neck. The long ends can be wrapped around the rear legs and secured so the mare cannot kick.
16. **c** This quick-release knot should be the only knot used to tie a lead rope to a stationary object.
17. **e** A clove hitch will not slip, even when one end is pulled.
18. **a**
19. **e** The tail should be grasped at the base and elevated straight up. Moving the tail toward one side or holding the tail by the end can damage the tail.
20. **b** Rabbits carried without support of the rear legs can struggle to the extent that they fracture their spine.
21. **d** A mouse will instinctively grasp a grate with their forefeet. You can then quickly grasp it by the scruff of the neck.
22. **e** A squeeze chute is usually used to restrain beef cattle. Dairy cattle usually are restrained in stanchions.
23. **b** Stocks are used to protect the veterinarian or technician while working on a horse.
24. **a** Pigs weighing up to 80 pounds can be placed on on their back in a V-trough.
25. **d** A tilt table is ideal for trimming cattle hooves. The animal is led to the side of the tabletop, which is in a vertical position. After the animal is strapped to it, the table is then moved to a horizontal position so that the animal is in lateral recumbency.

Section 27

Physiology

J.E. Breazile, T. Colville

Recommended Reading

Berne RM and Levy MN: *Physiology.* Mosby, St. Louis, 1988.
Bone JF: *Animal Anatomy and Physiology.* 3rd ed. Prentice-Hall, Englewood Cliffs, NJ, 1988.
Cunningham JG: *Textbook of Veterinary Physiology.* Saunders, Philadelphia, 1991.
Frandson RD and Spurgeon TL: *Anatomy and Physiology of Farm Animals.* 5th ed. Lea & Febiger, Philadelphia, 1992.
Patton HD *et al: Textbook of Physiology.* 21st ed. Saunders, Philadelphia, 1989.
Reece WO: *Physiology of Domestic Animals.* Lea & Febiger. Philadelphia, 1991.
Ruckebusch Y *et al: Physiology of Small and Large Domestic Animals.* Decker, Philadelphia, 1991.
Swenson MJ: *Dukes' Physiology of Domestic Animals.* 10th ed. Comstock Publishing, Ithaca, NY, 1984.
West JB: *Best and Taylors' Physiological Basis of Medical Practice.* 12th ed. Williams & Wilkins, Baltimore, 1991.

Practice answer sheet is on page 397.

Questions

1. *Which type of joint movement decreases the angle between 2 bones?*

   a. abduction
   b. adduction
   c. extension
   d. flexion
   e. pronation

2. *Which cardiac chamber receives blood from the systemic veins?*

   a. left atrium
   b. pulmonary trunk
   c. right atrium
   d. sinus venosus
   e. vena cava

3. *The second heart sound is produced by closure of which heart valves?*

   a. aortic and mitral
   b. mitral and pulmonary
   c. mitral and tricuspid
   d. pulmonary and aortic
   e. pulmonary and tricuspid

Correct answers are on pages 279-281.

4. *The first heart sound is produced by closure of which heart valves?*

a. aortic and mitral
b. mitral and pulmonary
c. mitral and tricuspid
d. pulmonary and aortic
e. pulmonary and tricuspid

5. *Which vessel normally carries blood with a high level of carbon dioxide?*

a. aorta
b. carotid artery
c. pulmonary vein
d. umbilical vein
e. vena cava

For Questions 6 through 9, select the correct answer from the 5 choices below.

a. aortic valve
b. mitral valve
c. pulmonary valve
d. semilunar valve
e. tricuspid valve

6. *Which cardiac valve prevents backflow of blood into the right ventricle during ventricular diastole?*

7. *Which cardiac valve prevents backflow of blood into the right atrium during ventricular systole?*

8. *Which cardiac valve prevents backflow of blood into the left ventricle during ventricular diastole?*

9. *Which cardiac valve prevents backflow of blood into the left atrium during ventricular systole?*

10. *Which organ is **not** essential to life?*

a. esophagus
b. heart
c. liver
d. pancreas
e. spleen

11. *The most numerous blood cell is the:*

a. basophil
b. eosinophil
c. erythrocyte
d. lymphocyte
e. monocyte

12. *Which blood cell has phagocytosis as its main function?*

a. basophil
b. eosinophil
c. erythrocyte
d. monocyte
e. thrombocyte

13. *A muscle that increases the angle between 2 bones is known as:*

a. an abductor
b. an adductor
c. a circumductor
d. an extensor
e. a flexor

14. *Inspiration of air into the lungs is produced by contraction of the:*

a. abdominal oblique muscles
b. diaphragm
c. internal intercostal muscles
d. rectus abdominis muscles
e. sternal muscles

15. *Most of the filtering, humidifying and warming of inspired air occurs in the:*

a. larynx
b. nares
c. nasal passages
d. pharynx
e. trachea

16. *Which of the following is **not** a function of the respiratory system?*

    a. acid-base regulation
    b. olfaction
    c. phonation
    d. prehension
    e. temperature regulation

17. *Oxygen and carbon dioxide are transferred between inspired air and blood in the lung by the process of:*

    a. flow down the pressure gradient
    b. diffusion
    c. ion pumping
    d. nitrogenation
    e. osmosis

18. *Which organ has endocrine functions and also produces many digestive enzymes?*

    a. kidney
    b. liver
    c. pancreas
    d. spleen
    e. thymus

19. *Stimulation of the parasympathetic portion of the autonomic nervous system causes:*

    a. dilation of airways in the lung
    b. dilation of the pupil of the eye
    c. increased gastrointestinal function
    d. increased blood pressure
    e. increased heart rate

20. *Stimulation of the sympathetic portion of the autonomic nervous system causes all of the following **except**:*

    a. dilation of airways in the lung
    b. dilation of the pupil of the eye
    c. increased gastrointestinal function
    d. increased heart rate
    e. piloerection

21. *The part of the central nervous system that initiates conscious movements of the body is the:*

    a. brachial plexus
    b. brainstem
    c. cerebellum
    d. cerebrum
    e. spinal cord

22. *Concerning neurons, which statement is **least** accurate?*

    a. They cannot replicate themselves.
    b. They are the basic functional unit of the nervous system.
    c. They cannot regenerate damaged processes.
    d. They contain no blood vessels.
    e. They have a very high oxygen requirement.

23. *Damage to which part of the nervous system is most likely to produce instant death in an animal?*

    a. brachial plexus
    b. brainstem
    c. cerebellum
    d. cerebrum
    e. spinal cord

24. *The portion of the central nervous system that serves to coordinate and smooth out, but not initiate, movements is the:*

    a. brachial plexus
    b. brainstem
    c. cerebellum
    d. cerebrum
    e. spinal cord

25. *Which structure is the most important direct link between the nervous and endocrine systems?*

    a. hypothalamus
    b. parathyroid gland
    c. pituitary gland
    d. thyroid gland
    e. thalamus

Correct answers are on pages 279-281.

26. *Which hormone is produced by the anterior pituitary gland?*

a. antidiuretic hormone
b. calcitonin
c. luteinizing hormone
d. oxytocin
e. progesterone

27. *Which hormone is released by the posterior pituitary gland?*

a. adrenocorticotropic hormone
b. calcitonin
c. luteinizing hormone
d. oxytocin
e. prolactin

28. *Which hormone is produced by the corpus luteum of the ovary?*

a. estrogen
b. luteinizing hormone
c. oxytocin
d. progesterone
e. prolactin

29. *The hormone necessary for maintenance of pregnancy is:*

a. estrogen
b. oxytocin
c. progesterone
d. prolactin
e. testosterone

30. *Which hormone is produced by a developing follicle in the ovary?*

a. estrogen
b. follicle-stimulating hormone
c. luteinizing hormone
d. progesterone
e. testosterone

31. *Which endocrine gland releases the hormone that causes milk letdown from the mammary gland?*

a. adrenal cortex
b. anterior pituitary gland
c. ovary
d. posterior pituitary gland
e. thyroid gland

32. *Hormones of the adrenal medulla are released under the influence of:*

a. adrenocorticotropic hormone
b. adrenomedullotropic hormone
c. the parasympathetic nervous system
d. the somatic nervous system
e. the sympathetic nervous system

For Questions 33 through 36, select the correct answer from the 5 choices below.

a. chemical
b. electromagnetic
c. mechanical
d. thermal
e. vestibular

33. *The kinesthetic (movement, position) sense reacts to which general type of stimuli?*

34. *The visual (sight) sense reacts to which general type of stimuli?*

35. *The gustatory (taste) sense reacts to which general type of stimuli?*

36. *The auditory (hearing) sense reacts to which general type of stimuli?*

37. *Rotary motion of the head is detected by which sensory structure?*

a. cochlea
b. malleus
c. organ of Corti
d. semicircular canal
e. vestibule

38. Accommodation for near and far vision is accomplished by contraction or relaxation of muscles in the:

a. ciliary body
b. conjunctiva
c. iris
d. limbus
e. retina

39. The kidney helps control water balance in the body under the influence of:

a. adrenocorticotropic hormone
b. antidiuretic hormone
c. calcitonin
d. oxytocin
e. parathormone

40. Spermatogenesis takes place in the:

a. epididymis
b. prostate gland
c. seminal vesicles
d. seminiferous tubules
e. vas deferens

41. In dogs, seminal fluid is produced by the:

a. bulbourethral glands and prostate gland
b. prostate gland, seminal vesicles and bulbourethral glands
c. prostate gland and seminal vesicles
d. prostate gland
e. seminal vesicles

42. After spermatogenesis, spermatozoa are stored until ejaculation in the:

a. bulbourethral glands
b. epididymis
c. seminal vesicles
d. seminiferous tubules
e. vas deferens

43. During which stage of the estrous cycle do females allow males to copulate?

a. anestrus
b. diestrus
c. estrus
d. metestrus
e. proestrus

44. What is the correct sequence of development of ovarian structures in a normal cycle?

a. corpus albicans, corpus luteum, corpus hemorrhagicum
b. corpus hemorrhagicum, graafian follicle, corpus luteum
c. corpus luteum, graafian follicle, corpus hemorrhagicum
d. graafian follicle, corpus hemorrhagicum, corpus lutuem
e. graafian follicle, corpus luteum, corpus hemorrhagicum

45. Fertilization of an ovum by a spermatozoon normally occurs in the:

a. cervix
b. oviduct
c. uterus
d. vagina
e. vulva

46. The process of capacitation of spermatozoa normally occurs in the:

a. cervix
b. epididymis
c. oviduct
d. testes
e. vas deferens

47. Milk letdown in the mammary gland is stimulated by:

a. adrenocorticotropic hormone
b. growth hormone
c. oxytocin
d. progesterone
e. prolactin

Correct answers are on pages 279-281.

48. *Which anterior pituitary hormone stimulates spermatogenesis in males?*

a. estrogen
b. follicle-stimulating hormone
c. growth hormone
d. luteinizing hormone
e. prolactin

49. *Which hormone is responsible for the signs of "heat" in a female animal?*

a. estrogen
b. follicle-stimulating hormone
c. oxytocin
d. progesterone
e. prolactin

50. *In which portion of the ruminant digestive system does the majority of microbial fermentation take place?*

a. abomasum
b. cecum
c. duodenum
d. omasum
e. rumen

51. *Blood:*

a. contains cells and plasma
b. is not important for CO_2 transport
c. consists of cells and serum
d. has no excretory function
e. consists of mostly cells

52. *The major determinant of blood viscosity is the:*

a. specific gravity of plasma
b. plasma protein concentration
c. lipoprotein concentration
d. hematocrit
e. number of white blood cells

53. *Circulating blood volume is regulated primarily by control of:*

a. total body water volume
b. intracellular water volume
c. systemic arterial blood pressure
d. central venous pressure
e. plasma protein concentration

54. *The feature that is essential for venous return from dependent body parts is:*

a. muscle pumps
b. foot or hoof pumps
c. respiratory pumps
d. venous valves
e. postcapillary blood pressure

55. *In ruminants, saliva plays an important role in recycling:*

a. ammonia
b. urea
c. sodium
d. potassium
e. chloride

56. *In ruminants, eructation results in passage of rumen gases:*

a. out through the nose
b. out through the mouth
c. out through the nose and mouth
d. into the lung
e. into the omasum

57. *The elastic recoil of lung tissue is primarily attributable to:*

a. connective tissues
b. pneumocytes
c. bronchiolar walls
d. surfactant
e. blood vessels

58. *Blood cells that are in the blood but not circulating are said to be in the:*

a. extravasated pool
b. marginated pool

c. occult pool
d. sequestered pool
e. limited pool

59. Concerning delivery of oxygen to tissues by arterial blood, which statement is most accurate?

a. All of the oxygen in arterial blood is delivered.
b. Most of the oxygen is delivered.
c. It is enhanced by exercise.
d. It is inhibited at high altitude.
e. It is diminished during periods of fever.

60. The proportion of body weight represented by total body water content in an extremely obese animal is:

a. about 60%
b. greater than 60%
c. greater than 90%
d. as much as 75%
e. as low as 40%

Answers

1. **d** None of the other joint movements listed produces this effect.
2. **c** Blood from the systemic veins enters the right atrium on its way to the lungs.
3. **d** The second heart sound is produced by closure of the 2 ventricular outflow valves (pulmonary and aortic).
4. **c** The first heart sound is produced by closure of the 2 atrioventricular valves (mitral and tricuspid).
5. **e** All of the other vessels normally carry oxygen-rich blood.
6. **c** The pulmonary valve closes during ventricular diastole, sealing the right ventricle off from the pulmonary artery.
7. **e** The tricuspid valve is the right artrioventricular valve.
8. **a** The aortic valve closes during ventricular diastole, sealing the left ventricle from the aorta.
9. **b** The mitral valve is the left atrioventricular valve.
10. **e** Only the spleen can be removed without causing death of the animal.
11. **c** All of the other cells listed are white blood cells that are much less numerous.
12. **d** Monocytes function mainly as macrophages.
13. **d** An extensor muscle increases the angle between 2 bones at a joint.
14. **b** Only contraction of the diaphragm has the effect of increasing the volume of the thoracic cavity, which causes air to be drawn into the lungs.
15. **c** The large surface area, extensive venous plexus, and active cilia of the nasal passages significantly condition inspired air.
16. **d** Prehension is the act of grasping.
17. **b** The gases diffuse from an area of high concentration to an area of low concentration through the thin alveolar and capillary walls.
18. **c** The pancreas is both an endocrine gland, producing insulin and glucagon, and an exocrine gland, producing a variety of digestive enzymes.
19. **c** The parasympathetic nervous system is the "business as usual system" that helps support basic body functions, such as digestion.
20. **c** The sympathetic nervous system is the "fight or flight" system that prepares the body for intense short-term activity.
21. **d** The cerebrum is the only portion of the nervous system that can initiate conscious body movements. The others serve to transmit and/or modify nerve impulses that produce movements.

22. **c** Severed neuron processes (axons and dendrites) can regenerate if the severed ends are carefully aligned.

23. **b** The brainstem contains control centers for many basic body functions, such as respiration and cardiovascular function. Damage to those control centers results in rapid death.

24. **c** The cerebrum initiates movements of the body. The cerebellum "filters" the impulses from the cerebrum and generally "fine tunes" them.

25. **a** The hypothalamus has extensive links to the brain and produces releasing and inhibiting factors that influence the anterior pituitary gland. It also produces hormones that are stored and released by the posterior pituitary gland.

26. **c** All of the other hormones listed are produced in other endocrine glands.

27. **d** Oxytocin is produced in the hypothalamus and transmitted along specialized nerve fibers to the posterior pituitary gland for storage and release.

28. **d** The corpus luteum develops from a ruptured follicle after ovulation and produces the hormone progesterone necessary for maintenance of pregnancy.

29. **c** Progesterone, produced by the corpus luteum of the ovary, supports pregnancy by helping prevent premature expulsion of the developing embryo from the uterus.

30. **a** Developing follicles produce increasing amounts of estrogen as they grow. Rising serum estrogen levels produce the signs of "heat" and prepare the animal for breeding and conception.

31. **d** Oxytocin, the hormone that produces milk letdown, is produced in the hypothalamus and transported to the posterior pituitary gland along nerve fibers for storage and release.

32. **e** Adrenal medullary hormones (epinephrine, norepinephrine) are part of the "fight or flight" response of the sympathetic nervous system.

33. **c** The kinesthetic (movement, position) sense receives information from mechanical receptors in muscles and joints.

34. **b** The visual sense (sight) converts light waves (electromagnetic radiation) into nerve impulses.

35. **a** The gustatory sense (taste) reacts to chemical substances in the mouth.

36. **c** The auditory sense (hearing) converts mechanical vibrations of air molecules (sound waves) into nerve impulses.

37. **d** The semicircular canals in each inner ear are arranged in different planes, so one or more is stimulated by rotary motion of the head in any direction.

38. **a** Muscles of the ciliary body cause stretching and relaxation of the lens of the eye.

39. **b** Antidiuretic hormone is secreted when the body becomes dehydrated. It increases water resorption from the kidney tubules.

40. **d** The seminiferous tubules are long U-shaped tubes in the testes where spermatozoa are produced before moving into the epididymis for storage. The other structures listed are part of the system that transports spermatozoa during ejaculation and produces the components of semen.

41. **d** The prostate gland is the only accessory sex gland in dogs.

42. **b** The other structures listed are involved in spermatogenesis or production of semen components.

43. **c** Estrus is the "heat" period when the female is sexually receptive to the male.

44. **d** Rupture of a graafian follicle (ovulation) results in formation of a corpus hemorrhagicum, which soon evolves into a corpus luteum.

45. **b** The fertilized ovum must undergo cleavage in the oviduct for several days before it is ready to implant in the uterus.

46. **c** Spermatozoa normally arrive in the oviduct before the ovum does. During their "waiting period," they undergo changes that enable them to more readily fertilize the ovum. These changes are collectively termed capacitation.

47. **c** Oxytocin causes contraction of myoepithelial cells around mammary gland alveoli and small ducts, squeezing milk into the large mammary ducts and sinuses.

48. **b** Though it is named for its effect in the female, follicle-stimulating hormone promotes spermatogenesis in the male.

49. **a** Estrogen, produced by the developing follicle(s) in the ovary, helps prepare the female animal physiologically and behaviorally for breeding. The resulting signs of "heat" act as a signal to the male.
50. **e** The rumen is a large "vat" in which various kinds of microorganisms break down plant materials to allow absorption of nutrients.
51. **a**
52. **d**
53. **e**
54. **d**
55. **b**
56. **d**
57. **d**
58. **b**
59. **c**
60. **e**

Notes

Notes

Section 28

Preventive Medicine

P.C. Bartlett, C.N. Carter, J.D. Hoskins

Recommended Reading

Hoskins JD: The puppy's first veterinary examination. *Vet Technician* 12:521-528, 1991.

Hoskins JD: Clinical evaluation of the kitten. *Vet Technician* 12:121-131, 1991.

Hoskins JD *et al,* in McCurnin DM: *Clinical Textbook for Veterinary Technicians.* 2nd ed. Saunders, Philadelphia, 1990.

Practice answer sheet is on page 399.

Questions

1. *Dogs or cats being prepared for shipment or entering a boarding facility should be vaccinated how many weeks before the event?*

   a. 16-18 weeks
   b. 12-14 weeks
   c. 8-10 weeks
   d. 4-6 weeks
   e. 1-2 weeks

2. *Rabies vaccine is **not** recommended for dogs younger than what age?*

   a. 7 months
   b. 6 months
   c. 5 months
   d. 4 months
   e. 3 months

3. *What is the youngest age at which puppies and kittens can be safely treated with insecticides for fleas and ticks?*

   a. 1 week
   b. 1 month
   c. 2 months
   d. 3 months
   e. 4 months

Correct answers are on pages 289-290.

4. *At what age should most kittens first be presented for initial immunizations?*

   a. 4-6 weeks
   b. 8-10 weeks
   c. 12-14 weeks
   d. 16-20 weeks
   e. 24-30 weeks

5. *At what age should most puppies first be presented for initial immunizations?*

   a. 2-4 weeks
   b. 8-10 weeks
   c. 12-16 weeks
   d. 16-20 weeks
   e. 24-30 weeks

6. *Feline leukemia virus vaccine can be safely administered to kittens as young as:*

   a. 2 weeks of age
   b. 3 weeks of age
   c. 4 weeks of age
   d. 5 weeks of age
   e. 6 weeks of age

7. *Cheyletiellosis most commonly affects what area on cats?*

   a. chin
   b. legs
   c. ventral thorax
   d. back
   e. eyelids

8. *The passive antibodies transferred from immune dams to the fetus during gestation may make puppies and kittens unresponsive to vaccination for what period at the beginning of life?*

   a. 3-6 weeks
   b. 6-8 weeks
   c. 2-3 weeks
   d. 6-7 days
   e. 10-12 days

9. *The most common cause of vaccination failure in young dogs and cats is:*

   a. disease at the time of vaccination
   b. the presence of maternal antibodies
   c. ineffective vaccine
   d. human error in mixing or administering the vaccine
   e. congenital or acquired immunodeficiency

10. *Which of the following is most likely to cause vaccination failure?*

    a. attenuation of the vaccine components
    b. storage at refrigeration temperatures
    c. no disinfectant used on needles or syringes
    d. wrong strain or type of microbe used to make the vaccine
    e. mixing with a sterile diluent

11. *Which of the following is* ***least*** *likely to contribute to vaccination failure?*

    a. vaccination of an anesthetized patient
    b. fever or hypothermia
    c. general debilitation
    d. very young or very old age
    e. use of glucocorticoids or cytotoxic agents

12. *Human errors that may cause vaccination failure include all of the following* ***except****:*

    a. vaccinating during estrus
    b. improper mixing of vaccine
    c. incorrect route of administration
    d. storing vaccine at very warm temperatures
    e. vaccinating too frequently

13. *Which genetic engineering technique is* ***not*** *used in production of vaccines?*

    a. genetic manipulation to construct mutants of a virus, bacterium, parasite or cancer cell
    b. production of vaccines against the pathogen's vector
    c. removal of pathogenic genes that affect the pathogen's multiplication properties
    d. insertion of fragments of DNA material into immunogenic proteins of a virus, bacterium, parasite or cancer cell

e. production of vaccines containing mutant strains of the pathogen

14. Concerning disease in cats, which statement is most accurate?

a. Feline infectious peritonitis occurs most commonly in middle-aged cats.
b. Temperature-sensitive feline infectious peritonitis vaccine provides protection against coronavirus challenge in healthy cats.
c. Male cats are affected more frequently with feline infectious peritonitis than are female cats.
d. Feline infectious peritonitis virus is resistant to most household detergents and disinfectants.
e. Natural infection with feline enteric coronaviruses results in production of antibody that can be serologically distinguished from that produced by infection with feline infectious peritonitis virus.

15. At what age should puppies be given canine distemper-measles vaccine?

a. 4-6 weeks
b. 6-12 weeks
c. 14-18 weeks
d. 20-24 weeks
e. 24-32 weeks

16. What approximate percentage of maternal antibodies is transferred from the dam to the fetus via the placenta and to puppies and kittens via colostrum?

a. 100% colostral and 0% transplacental
b. 95-99% colostral and 1-5% transplacental
c. 50% colostral and 50% transplacental
d. 1-5% colostral and 95-99% transplacental
e. 0% colostral and 100% transplacental

17. A 9-week-old kitten has a serous ocular discharge and mild sneezing. The kitten is still eating and, according to the owner, very active. In conjunctival scrapings stained with Giemsa stain, epithelial cells contain intracytoplasmic inclusions. The most likely cause of disease in this kitten is infection with:

a. feline leukemia virus
b. calicivirus
c. *Chlamydia*
d. rhinotracheitis virus
e. *Toxoplasma*

18. The intranasal vaccine against feline viral rhinotracheitis and feline calicivirus infection may cause adverse effects in young kittens. After vaccine administration, these adverse effects are usually observed within:

a. 36-48 hours
b. 4-7 days
c. 10-14 days
d. 14-21 days
e. 12-24 hours

19. Concerning canine adenovirus type 1 in dogs, which statement is ***least*** *accurate?*

a. It causes ocular lesions.
b. It causes renal lesions.
c. The vaccine protects susceptible dogs against infectious canine hepatitis and infectious tracheobronchitis.
d. It causes virus shedding in urine.
e. The vaccine is approved for intranasal use.

20. Concerning Bordetella *infection in dogs, which statement is most accurate?*

a. *Bordetella bronchiseptica* cannot reside within the trachea and bronchi of asymptomatic dogs.
b. *Bordetella bronchiseptica* vaccine administered by the parenteral route is not recommended for male and female dogs used for breeding.
c. *Bordetella bronchiseptica* vaccine given by the intranasal route is not recommended for puppies as young as 2-4 weeks of age.
d. *Bordetella bronchiseptica* is naturally spread from dog to dog by aerosol.
e. *Bordetella bronchiseptica* is naturally spread from dog to dog by contaminated feces.

Correct answers are on pages 289-290.

21. *A 20-week-old puppy has a serous nasal discharge, depression, inappetence and diarrhea of 2 days' duration. The total white blood cell count is 10,500 cells/μl (normal range, 6000-17,000 cells/μl), with 7500 segmented neutrophils/μl (normal range, 3000-11,500 cells/μl). Which virus is most likely involved?*

    a. canine leukemia virus
    b. canine parvovirus-2
    c. canine coronavirus
    d. canine herpesvirus
    e. canine rotavirus

22. *Canine coronavirus vaccine is labeled by the manufacturer for first recommended use in puppies as young as:*

    a. 7-10 days
    b. 2-3 weeks
    c. 10-12 weeks
    d. 4-6 weeks
    e. 14-20 weeks

23. *The indirect fluorescent antibody test (IFA) and the enzyme-linked immunosorbent assay (ELISA) detect feline leukemia virus (FeLV) infection in affected cats of all ages. To confirm FeLV infection in a 12-week-old kitten before FeLV vaccination, what diagnostic test is most appropriate to conduct in a veterinary hospital?*

    a. virus isolation and identification
    b. ELISA for gp70 antigen
    c. IFA for feline oncornavirus cell membrane antigen
    d. Western immunoblotting technique on serum
    e. ELISA for p27 antigen

24. *At what age can puppies safely begin receiving heartworm preventive?*

    a. 1-2 weeks
    b. 24-30 weeks
    c. 12-16 weeks
    d. 6-8 weeks
    e. 4-5 weeks

25. *Hookworm infection in dogs can be prevented by regular administration of:*

    a. fenbendazole, piperazine or praziquantel
    b. cythioate, pyrantel pamoate or clotrimazole
    c. thiacetarsamide, ivermectin or dichlorvos
    d. diethylcarbamazine, oxibendazole or milbemycin
    e. amprolium, sulfadimethoxine or fenthion

26. *In the United States, which drug is approved for treatment of hookworm infection in cats?*

    a. fenbendazole
    b. pyrantel pamoate
    c. thenium closylate
    d. ivermectin
    e. no drug has been approved for treatment of hookworm infection in cats

27. *Which drug is used for treating giardiasis in dogs and cats?*

    a. milbemycin oxime
    b. metronidazole
    c. fenbendazole
    d. nitroscanate
    e. febantel-praziquantel

28. *Antemortem inspection is necessary in livestock presented for slaughter because:*

    a. without antemortem inspection there is no way to determine the nutritional state of the slaughtered animal
    b. certain diseases are manifested in the live animal but show no gross lesions on necropsy
    c. antemortem inspection allows inspection personnel to collect specimens (blood, urine, biopsy) from questionable animals to allow for more specific diagnoses
    d. it is required by certain religious groups
    e. proper animal identification is needed before death

29. Outbreaks of chronic, noninfectious disease can be difficult to investigate because:

a. they have a short incubation period
b. affected people cite different sources as the cause of disease
c. affected animals have usually been exposed to multiple predisposing causes
d. specific diagnostic tests are often not available, as opposed to infectious diseases, for which serologic and other laboratory tests are available
e. affected animals or people usually die of other, unrelated causes

30. What quality tests are required on an individual farm's milk supply?

a. total bacterial count, somatic cell count, drug residue, cooling temperature
b. total bacterial count, somatic cell count, drug residue
c. total bacterial count, somatic cell count
d. total bacterial count, drug residue
e. tests are required on truckloads, not on milk from an individual farm

31. Staphylococcus aureus *food intoxication in people is most likely to occur from:*

a. consumption of infected poultry
b. contamination of raw meat products in the slaughterhouse
c. a cook's sneezing into the food during preparation
d. inclusion of raw milk products in food
e. contamination from infected pets

32. What species is a major reservoir of rabies in the United States?

a. rats
b. fox
c. pigs
d. cats
e. bats

33. In the United States, most cases of scabies in people are caused by contact with:

a. dogs
b. cats
c. horses
d. cattle
e. other people

34. Concerning vaccination of wild animals against rabies, which statement is most accurate?

a. Rabies vaccines are now available and approved for use in pet raccoons and skunks.
b. Any wild animal can be vaccinated against rabies, as long as it has been adequately domesticated by its owner.
c. There are no licensed rabies vaccines approved for use in wild animals, with the exception of ferrets.
d. Rabies vaccines licensed for use in dogs can be used on pet coyotes, foxes and wolves.
e. The AVMA does not consider rabies in wild animals to be a real threat in the United States and, therefore, vaccination is optional.

35. What is the appropriate management of a dog or cat that bites a person?

a. the animal should be immediately euthanized, regardless of ownership status and the animal's head sent to the local state health department for rabies examination
b. the animal should be confined and observed for 10 days; if any signs of illness arise, a veterinarian should evaluate the animal and report to the health department; if signs of rabies emerge, the animal should be humanely killed and the head sent to the local or state health department for rabies examination
c. the animal should be immediately given a rabies booster, confined and observed for 30 days
d. the animal should be simply observed for 10 days and released after examination by a licensed veterinarian
e. a copy of the bite report must be given to the local or state health department

Correct answers are on pages 289-290.

36. *Only modified-live vaccines have been shown to protect dogs against distemper. Which of the following best describes the most reasonable vaccination regimen against canine distemper in a puppy that received adequate colostrum?*

a. vaccinate at 3- to 4-week intervals, beginning at 5-8 weeks of age, until the animal is 12 weeks of age
b. vaccinate at 3- to 4-week intervals, beginning at 12 weeks of age, until the animal is 20 weeks of age
c. vaccinate at 4- to 5-week intervals, beginning at 4 weeks of age, until the animal is 16 weeks of age
d. vaccinate at 4- to 5-week intervals, beginning at 6 weeks of age, until the animal is vaccinated for rabies
e. vaccinate at 8-week intervals, beginning at 8 weeks of age, for a total of 3 vaccinations

37. *A new client with a kitten is asking questions about feline distemper (feline panleukopenia). Which of the following is **least** appropriate in advising this client?*

a. Two modified-live-virus or 3 inactivated vaccine doses should be given at 3- to 4-week intervals, beginning at 8-9 weeks of age.
b. Boosters should be given every 2 years if modified-live-virus products are used and annually if inactivated products are used.
c. Inactivated vaccines should be used in pregnant, immunosuppressed or diseased animals, and in kittens less than 4 weeks of age.
d. Modified-live-virus products must not be used in kittens less than 4 weeks of age because of the risk of cerebellar degeneration.
e. Immune serum can give some protection for unvaccinated kittens in the face of exposure.

38. *Concerning prevention and control of borreliosis (Lyme disease), which statement is most accurate?*

a. Many commercially available vaccines provide good protection.
b. Immunomodulating drugs work well in preventing borreliosis and should be used when exposure to ticks is probable.
c. Lifetime prophylactic administration of oxytetracycline to outdoor dogs and people in high-risk occupations provides excellent protection.
d. It may take up to 24 hours of tick feeding before the *Borrelia* organism is secreted in the tick's saliva.
e. No progress has been made in developing a borreliosis vaccine, as no species have been found to generate an active immune response.

39. *Concerning control of dermatophytosis in a cattery, which statement is **least** accurate?*

a. Infected animals should be segregated from all others during treatment.
b. Sanitizing materials and grooming instruments used on infected cats must be kept separate from those used on uninfected cats so as to prevent cross contamination.
c. Handlers must change clothes and first work with uninfected cats before working with infected cats.
d. Treatment should include clipping, topical antifungal rinses and systemic griseofulvin or ketoconazole until cultures are negative.
e. Large doses of corticosteroids can help prevent severe onychomycosis.

40. *Trichobezoars (hairballs) are a common problem in cats. How are they best prevented in cats?*

a. give mineral oil directly per os or in the animal's food each day
b. train the cat not to groom
c. give enzymes that dissolve any hair material in the gastrointestinal tract
d. give petrolatum-based lubricants per os and encourage frequent grooming by the client
e. palpate the animal regularly to detect trichobezoars and perform surgery before they cause problems

41. *How do children contract toxocariasis?*

a. by ingestion of raw meat

b. by direct contact with dogs infected with roundworms
c. by ingestion of roundworm eggs in dog feces
d. by inhaling aerosol from infected animals
e. by ingestion of uncooked or undercooked chicken eggs

42. *Visceral larva migrans in people is caused by:*

a. *Toxoplasma*
b. *Toxocara*
c. *Ancylostoma*
d. *Hypoderma*
e. *Dermacentor*

43. *Rabies vaccine is **not** recommended for dogs younger than what age?*

a. 7 months
b. 6 months
c. 5 months
d. 4 months
e. 3 months

44. *The passive antibodies transferred from immune dams to the fetus during gestation may make puppies and kittens unresponsive to vaccination for what period at the beginning of life?*

a. 3-6 weeks
b. 6-8 weeks
c. 2-3 weeks
d. 6-7 days
e. 10-12 days

45. *Human errors that may cause vaccination failure include all of the following **except**:*

a. vaccinating during estrus
b. improper mixing of vaccine
c. incorrect route of administration
d. storing vaccine at very warm temperatures
e. vaccinating too frequently

46. *At what age can puppies safely begin receiving heartworm preventive?*

a. 1-2 weeks
b. 24-30 weeks
c. 12-16 weeks
d. 6-8 weeks
e. 4-5 weeks

Answers

1. **e** This is adequate time before shipment or entering a boarding facility for a dog or cat.
2. **e** This is the recommendation of the World Health Organization and other governing agencies.
3. **e** It is safest to wait until this age.
4. **b** This is the most common age for initial presentation.
5. **b** This is the most common age for initial presentation.
6. **e** Kittens 6 weeks of age and older can be safely vaccinated.
7. **d** This is the most common site for this mite.
8. **c** The maternal antibodies passed *in utero* can be present in the first 2 weeks of life.
9. **b**
10. **d** The vaccine may contain the wrong strain or type of agent needed for protection of the animal.
11. **a** The other factors listed are more likely to reduce the effectiveness of vaccination.
12. **a** Estrus has no effect on immunization.
13. **c**
14. **b**
15. **b** Check the label of the commercial product.
16. **b**
17. **c** Finding cytoplasmic inclusions confirms chlamydial infection.
18. **b**

19. **e**
20. **d**
21. **c** The white blood cell count is normal in canine coronavirus infection but is decreased in canine parvovirus-2 infection.
22. **d** Check the label of the commercial product.
23. **e** This is the basis of such test kits as Assure, Virachek and Flex II.
24. **d** As soon as puppies begin eating solid food, they can safely begin receiving heartworm preventive.
25. **d** Check the label of the commercial products listed.
26. **e**
27. **b**
28. **b**
29. **e**
30. **a**
31. **c** This organism rarely comes from an animal source.
32. **e**
33. **e** People can get scabies from animals, but these cases are usually not severe. Most cases of scabies in people involve the human variety of mite.
34. **c** Because there are no vaccines licensed for wild animals, the AVMA strongly encourages that states pass laws prohibiting ownership of wild animals and wild animals crossbred to domestic dogs and cats as pets.
35. **b** The 10-day observation period ensures that animals that may have exposed human beings to rabies virus are promptly identified, as virus is shed in the saliva no more than a few days before the onset of clinical signs.
36. **a** Most commercially available vaccines overcome maternal immunity by 12 weeks. Colostrum-deprived pups should be vaccinated beginning at 2-3 weeks of age.
37. **b** Boosters should be given annually, regardless of use of modified-live or attenuated products, though modified-live-virus products probably provide longer immunity.
38. **d** Borreliosis vaccine has been effective against experimental challenge. Prompt removal of ticks appears to be an effective preventive measure.
39. **e** One study reveals that in 69.9% of all households with dermatophyte-infected cats, at least one person also became infected.
40. **d** Hairballs are sometimes found secondary to other, more serious ailments. In cats with chronic hairball problems, diagnostics should be performed to rule out primary gastric disease.
41. **c**
42. **b**
43. **e** This is the recommendation of the World Health Organization and other governing agencies.
44. **c** The maternal antibodies passed *in utero* can be present in the first 2 weeks of life.
45. **a** Estrus has no effect on immunization.
46. **d** As soon as puppies begin eating solid food, they can safely begin receiving heartworm preventive.

Section **29**

Principles of Disease

R.D. Hunt

Recommended Reading

Cheville NF: *Cell Pathology*. 2nd ed. Iowa State University Press, Ames, 1983.
Cotran RS *et al: Pathologic Basis of Disease.* 4th ed. Saunders, Philadelphia, 1989.
Jones TC and Hunt RD: *Veterinary Pathology.* 5th ed. Lea & Febiger, Philadelphia, 1983.
Jubb KVF *et al: Pathology of Domestic Animals.* 3rd ed. Academic Press, New York, 1985.
Slauson DO and Cooper BJ: *Mechanisms of Disease – A Textbook of Comparative General Pathology.* Williams & Wilkins, Baltimore, 1982.
Thomson RG: *Special Veterinary Pathology.* Decker, Philadelphia, 1988.

Practice answer sheet is on page 401.

Questions

1. *Tissue specimens mailed to a laboratory for histopathologic examination should be submitted:*

   a. intact in formalin or other fixative
   b. frozen
   c. as thin slices in formalin or other fixative
   d. fresh
   e. in physiologic saline

2. *If a necropsy must be delayed for 24 or more hours, it is best to:*

   a. freeze the body
   b. maintain the body at near-normal body temperature
   c. refrigerate the body
   d. not do a necropsy
   e. maintain the body at above-normal body temperature

3. *Which of the following diseases is* ***not*** *characterized by vesicles?*

   a. pemphigus vulgaris
   b. infectious myxomatosis of rabbits
   c. cowpox
   d. sarcoid in horses
   e. foot and mouth disease

Correct answers are on pages 296-297.

4. *Gout is characterized by tissue deposits of:*

a. silicon
b. urates
c. calcium carbonate
d. lipofuscin
e. biliverdin

5. *The single most differentiating feature of malignant neoplasms is their:*

a. ability to metastasize
b. large size
c. anaplastic microscopic appearance
d. origin from epithelial tissues
e. tendency to regress

6. *Histamine is produced by:*

a. mast cells
b. fibroblasts
c. T cells
d. neutrophils
e. macrophages

7. *Which cellular change is* **not** *reversible?*

a. fatty change
b. glycogenolysis
c. atrophy
d. karyorrhexis
e. potassium loss

8. *Fat necrosis is characterized by formation of:*

a. calcium soaps
b. oxalate crystals
c. amyloid
d. hyalin
e. lipofuscin

9. *Atrophy is characterized by:*

a. increased size of an organ or cells
b. karyomegaly
c. decreased size of an organ or cells
d. karyolysis
e. postmortem autolysis

10. *Chronic inflammation is:*

a. characterized by a short course
b. characterized by a long course
c. usually restricted to the central nervous system
d. very rare in animals
e. characterized by pus

11. *Which cell type most characterizes granulomatous inflammation?*

a. fibroblasts
b. neutrophils
c. mast cells
d. endothelial cells
e. epithelioid cells

12. *Macrophages, Langhans' giant cells and epithelioid cells are derived from:*

a. myeloblasts
b. monocytes
c. mast cells
d. megakaryocytes
e. melanoblasts

13. *Metaplasia is characterized by replacement of:*

a. differentiated tissue with another type of undifferentiated tissue
b. undifferentiated tissue with another type of differentiated tissue
c. differentiated tissue with another type of differentiated tissue
d. undifferentiated tissue with another type of undifferentiated tissue
e. aplastic tissue with neoplastic tissue

14. *Hypertrophy of an organ can result from cellular:*

a. hyperplasia
b. dysplasia

c. metaplasia
d. aplasia
e. hypoplasia

15. Benign neoplasms:

a. tend to metastasize
b. are often encapsulated
c. are most often caused by viruses
d. are characterized by marked cellular pleomorphism
e. of no clinical concern

16. Infarcts are:

a. restricted to the heart
b. caused by interference with blood supply
c. any well-demarcated area of necrosis
d. reversible
e. restricted to the kidney

17. Necrosis is:

a. reversible
b. a postmortem tissue change
c. irreversible
d. synonymous with autolysis
e. limited to viral infections

18. Endotoxin is:

a. a polysaccharide component of the wall of Gram-negative bacteria
b. a polysaccharide component of the wall of Gram-positive bacteria
c. a polysaccharide released from endothelial cells
d. responsible for endometrial necrosis
e. used to treat ectoparasites

19. Diapedesis refers to:

a. bilateral laminitis
b. escape of erythrocytes from congested blood vessels
c. twinning
d. emigration of leukocytes in inflammation
e. bilateral footrot

20. Which feature would allow you to differentiate an area of liquefaction necrosis in a kidney from postmortem autolysis?

a. presence of bacteria
b. size of the lesion
c. presence of acute inflammation in surrounding tissue
d. absence of acute inflammation in surrounding tissue
e. presence of karyorrhexis

21. Under conditions of hypoxia, cells:

a. shrink, lose water, lose potassium and gain sodium
b. shrink, lose water, lose sodium and gain potassium
c. swell, gain water, lose sodium and gain potassium
d. swell, gain water, lose potassium and gain sodium
e. usually remain normal in size and composition

22. Tissue necrosis heals by way of:

a. emigration of neutrophils
b. regeneration and/or scarring
c. liquefaction
d. bacterial enzymes
e. interferons

23. Viral inclusion bodies are:

a. cytoplasmic or nuclear in location
b. restricted to the nucleus
c. restricted to the cytoplasm
d. seen in all viral diseases
e. composed of lead acetate

24. Abnormally high serum levels of indirect bilirubin indicate:

a. toxic jaundice
b. hemolytic anemia
c. obstructive jaundice
d. primary photosensitization
e. myelophthisic anemia

Correct answers are on pages 296-297.

25. *Hypertrophy is characterized by:*

a. increased size and number of cells
b. increased number of cells
c. decreased size of cells
d. increased size of cells
e. decreased number of cells

26. *Fat necrosis is often a feature of:*

a. acute hepatitis
b. a high-calorie diet
c. acute pancreatitis
d. acute splenitis
e. shipping fever

27. *The injurious effects of radiation are greatest on:*

a. cells of fully differentiated tissues
b. cells with a high rate of replication
c. neurons
d. cells of highly vascularized tissues
e. fibroblasts

28. *An acute inflammatory response is dependent upon:*

a. neutrophils
b. macrophages
c. blood vessels
d. eosinophils
e. bacteria

29. *In acute inflammation, various chemical mediators initiate and sustain the acute inflammatory response. All of the following are important mediators of acute inflammation* **except**:

a. histamine
b. serotonin
c. bradykinin
d. complement
e. collagenase

30. *Neutrophils and macrophages ordinarily do not phagocytize invading bacteria until:*

a. the bacteria have died
b. the cells are activated
c. the bacteria have been opsonized
d. fever has developed
e. the cells degranulate

31. *The breeds predisposed to ventricular septal defects are the:*

a. Boxer and Cocker Spaniel
b. Chihuahua and Pekingese
c. Great Dane and Bull Mastiff
d. English Bulldog and Keeshond
e. Irish Setter and English Foxhound

32. *The most common oral neoplasm of cats is the:*

a. fibrosarcoma
b. malignant melanoma
c. squamous-cell carcinoma
d. chondrosarcoma
e. histiocytoma

33. *In addition to affecting dogs, canine distemper virus is an important cause of disease in:*

a. raccoons and seals
b. cats and rabbits
c. ferrets and porpoise
d. skunks and coyotes
e. mink and gerbils

34. *Ethylene glycol poisoning in cats and* Halogeton gloveratus *poisoning in sheep are both characterized by:*

a. urate nephrosis
b. oxalate nephrosis
c. centrilobular hepatic necrosis
d. peripheral lobular hepatic necrosis
e. disseminated intravascular coagulation

35. A rise in serum alkaline phosphatase activity could indicate disease of the:

a. skeleton or liver
b. skeleton or kidneys
c. liver or kidneys
d. heart or liver
e. skeleton or lungs

*36. Edema may result from any of the following **except**:*

a. hyperproteinemia
b. lymphatic obstruction
c. increased capillary and venous blood pressure
d. renal insufficiency
e. allergic reaction

37. In response to histamine, fluid leaks from the vascular tree are:

a. exclusively from arterioles
b. exclusively from venules
c. exclusively from capillaries
d. from both arterioles and venules
e. from both arterioles and capillaries

*38. Characteristics of chronic inflammation include all of the following **except**:*

a. infiltration of macrophages
b. fibrosis
c. long duration
d. marked hyperemia
e. infiltration of lymphocytes

*39. Reddening of the skin or other tissue may indicate any of the following **except**:*

a. hyperemia
b. congestion
c. acute inflammation
d. hemorrhage
e. arterial thrombosis

40. The most important event in the pathogenesis of thrombosis is:

a. blood stasis
b. endothelial injury
c. hypercoagulability
d. hypercalcemia
e. hyperviscosity

*41. An embolus may have any of the following features **except**:*

a. composed of air
b. composed of fibrin
c. composed of neoplastic cells
d. can lead to infarction
e. attached to the endothelium

*42. All of the following are pathologic features of malignant neoplasms **except**:*

a. anaplasia
b. slow growth rate
c. metastasis
d. large number of mitoses
e. cellular pleomorphism

43. In general, most neoplasms are:

a. restricted to older animals
b. of monoclonal origin
c. caused by viruses
d. restricted to young animals
e. of polyclonal origin

*44. Features of tetralogy of Fallot include all of the following **except**:*

a. ventricular septal defects
b. aorta overriding the venticular defect
c. patent ductus arteriosus
d. obstruction of right ventricular outflow
e. right ventricular hypertrophy

45. Urticaria is characterized by multifocal:

a. epidermal ulceration and serous effusion
b. dermal hyperemia and edema
c. epidermal vesiculation
d. dermal vesiculation
e. epidermal erosions without serous effusion

Correct answers are on pages 296-297.

*46. Concerning macrophages, which statement is **least** accurate?*

a. They differentiate into epithelioid cells.
b. They are derived from circulating monocytes.
c. They can phagocytize bacteria.
d. They release factors that stimulate blood vessel growth.
e. They can synthesize collagen.

47. In which tissue is repair limited by lack of effective replication of parenchymal cells?

a. epidermis
b. myocardium
c. liver
d. bone marrow
e. pancreas

48. Which feature can be used to help differentiate a postmortem clot from an antemortem venous thrombus?

a. A postmortem clot has lines of Zahn.
b. A postmortem clot is infiltrated with leukocytes.
c. A postmortem clot is infiltrated with fibroblasts.
d. A postmortem clot is usually recanalized.
e. A postmortem clot is not attached to the vessel wall.

49. A hematoma is defined as:

a. a malignant neoplasm of erythroid cells
b. a benign neoplasm of erythroid cells
c. a roughly spherical confined hemorrhage
d. hemorrhage into the peritoneal cavity
e. hemorrhage into the pericardium

*50. Which of the following is **not** a feature of necrotic cells?*

a. karyorrhexis
b. pyknosis
c. karyolysis
d. karyomegaly
e. absence of a nucleus

Answers

1. c
2. c
3. d
4. b
5. a
6. a
7. d
8. a
9. c
10. b
11 e
12. b
13. c
14. a
15. b
16. b
17. c
18. a
19. b
20. c
21. d
22. b
23. a
24. b
25. d
26. c
27. b
28. c

29. **e**
30. **c**
31. **d**
32. **c**
33. **a**
34. **b**
35. **a**
36. **a**
37. **b**
38. **d**
39. **e**
40. **b**
41. **e**
42. **b**
43. **b**
44. **c**
45. **b**
46. **e**
47. **b**
48. **e**
49. **c**
50. **d**

Notes

Notes

Section 30

Reproduction

T.J. Burke, S.M. Dennis, M. Drost, B.E. Eilts, F.L. Frye, M.B. Paster, R.C. Tubbs, C.S.F. Williams, S.D. Van Camp

Recommended Reading

Almond GW and Dial GD: Pregnancy diagnosis in swine: Principles, application, and accuracy of available techniques. *JAVMA* 191:858-870, 1987.

Blood DC and Radostits OM: *Veterinary Medicine.* 7th ed. Bailliere Tindall, London, 1989.

Burke TJ: *Small Animal Reproduction and Infertility.* Lea & Febiger, Philadelphia, 1986.

Clark LK: The model herd: A basis for troubleshooting reproductive failure in swine. *Vet Med* 85:1251-1258, 1990.

Connor JF: Reproductive problems in swine breeding herd: Making the field diagnosis. *Vet Med* 84:218-227, 1989.

Cooper JE and Jackson OF: *Diseases of the Reptilia.* Academic Press, New York, 1981.

Dial GD *et al,* in Leman AD *et al: Diseases of Swine.* 7th ed. Iowa State University Press, Ames, 1992.

Epple A and Stetson MH: *Avian Endocrinology.* Academic Press, New York, 1980.

Feldman EC and Nelson RW: *Canine and Feline Endocrinology and Reproduction.* Saunders, Philadelphia, 1987.

Frandson RD and Spurgeon TL: *Anatomy and Physiology of Domestic Animals.* 5th ed. Lea & Febiger, Philadelphia, 1992.

Frye FL: *Biomedical and Surgical Aspects of Captive Reptile Husbandry.* 2nd ed. Krieger Publishing, Melbourne, FL, 1991.

Ginther OJ: *Reproductive Biology of the Mare: Basic and Applied Aspects.* Cross Plains, WI, 1992.

Haibel GK: Advances in sheep and goat medicine. *Vet Clin No Am* (Food Animal Pract) 6:577-583, 1990.

Hughes JP: *Reproduction in the Mare.* Veterinary Learning Systems, Trenton, NJ, 1983.

Johnston SD and Romagnoli SE: Canine reproduction. *Vet Clin No Am* (Small Animal Pract) 21:421-640, 1991.

Kilgour R and Dalton C: *Livestock Behaviour.* Granada Publishing, St. Albans, UK, 1984.

Kirkbride CA: *Laboratory Diagnosis of Livestock Abortion.* 3rd ed. Iowa State University Press, Ames, 1990.

Marcus LC: *Veterinary Biology and Medicine of Captive Amphibians and Reptiles.* Lea & Febiger, Philadelphia, 1981.

McDonald LE: *Veterinary Endocrinology and Reproduction.* 4th ed. Lea & Febiger, Philadelphia, 1989.

Morrow DA: *Current Therapy in Theriogenology.* 2nd ed. Saunders, Philadelphia, 1986.

Paster M: Avian reproductive endocrinology. *Vet Clin No Am* (Small Anim Pract) 21:1343-1357, 1991.

Peaker M: *Avian Physiology.* Zoologic Soc London, 1975.

Roberts SJ: *Veterinary Obstetrics and Genital Diseases.* 3rd ed. David & Charles, North Pomfret, VT, 1986.

Tubbs RC: Factors that influence the weaning-to-estrus interval in sows. *Comp Cont Ed Pract Vet* 12:105-115, 1990.

Tubbs RC and Leman AD: Swine reproduction. *Vet Clin No Am* (Food Animal Pract) 8:1 *et seqq,* 1992.

Varner DD *et al: Diseases and Management of Breeding Stallions.* American Veterinary Publications, Goleta, CA, 1991.

Welty JC and Baptista L: *Excretion, Reproduction and Photoperiodism: The Life of Birds.* 4th ed. Saunders, Philadelphia, 1988.

Practice answer sheet is on page 403.

Questions

1. *The ejaculate of male dogs consists of 3 fractions. Concerning the fractions of canine ejaculates, which statement is* ***least*** *accurate?*

   a. The second fraction is the sperm-rich fraction.
   b. A pause often occurs between the semen fractions being collected.
   c. The most voluminous fraction is the third fraction.
   d. The third fraction consists mainly of prostatic fluid.
   e. The first fraction emitted should be collected to ensure adequate sperm motility.

2. *Blood in the canine ejaculate may be associated with any of the following* ***except:***

   a. prostatitis
   b. urethritis
   c. seminal vesiculitis
   d. orchitis
   e. ruptured blood vessel on the surface of the penis

3. *Semen is most often collected from dogs by:*

   a. electroejaculation
   b. rectal massage
   c. penile massage
   d. prostatic stimulation
   e. magnetic resonance impulsing

4. *In transvaginal artificial insemination in the bitch, using fresh semen, semen should be deposited into the:*

   a. uterus
   b. vestibule
   c. cervical body
   d. cranial vagina
   e. oviduct

5. *An initial rise in plasma progesterone levels in a bitch indicates that:*

   a. ovulation has occurred and it is too late to breed the bitch
   b. ovulation is imminent and the bitch should be bred in the next few days
   c. the bitch is pregnant
   d. the bitch is due to whelp within 3 days
   e. the bitch has entered proestrus and should be bred immediately

6. *Erection persists in some male dogs after mating because hair adheres to the penis and the preputial orifice is inverted as the penis is withdrawn. Concerning this condition, which statement is most accurate?*

   a. This is an emergency condition and should receive prompt care to prevent permanent damage to the penis.
   b. This condition is usually self-correcting and resolves with rest.
   c. This condition is known as phimosis.
   d. Treatment should include tranquilization to increase blood pressure.
   e. Atropine is indicated to alleviate this condition, as erection is a sympathetic nervous system response and atropine is a sympatholytic drug.

7. *In managing breeding of dogs, several "rules of thumb" have proven valuable. Concerning dog breeding, which statement is* ***least*** *accurate?*

   a. Matings in which the male does not become "tied" to the female, by locking of the bulbis glandis in the vagina, are as fertile as those in which a "tie" does occur.

b. Bitches should be bred on the first, third and fifth days of standing heat if vaginal smears and/or progesterone determinations are not available.

c. Bitches should be introduced to the male's territory to maximize the chance of successful mating.

d. Breeding on the 11th and 13th day or the 12th and 14th day after the bloody vulvar discharge is detected may not be adequate for all bitches to conceive.

e. Bitches are most fertile between 3 and 5 years of age.

8. *Pseudopregnancy is a common clinical complaint in dogs. It is usually characterized by mammary development, lactation, nesting and possibly adoption of kittens or inanimate objects as surrogate puppies. It usually occurs within 60 days of the previous heat. Concerning pseudopregnancy in dogs, which statement is most accurate?*

a. Pseudopregnancy is caused by abnormal hormone imbalance in the bitch.

b. Repeated pseudopregnancy can lead to pyometra.

c. Pseudopregnancy can occur after ovariohysterectomy performed 1-2 months after the previous heat.

d. Pseudopregnancy must be treated with hormones.

e. Bitches experiencing pseudopregnancy are permanently infertile.

9. *Various hormones have been used to control estrus in dogs and cats. Concerning drugs used in estrual animals, which statement is **least** accurate?*

a. Megestrol acetate can be used to prevent or suppress heat in dogs.

b. Mibolerone can be used to prevent but not suppress heat in dogs.

c. Megestrol acetate can be used to suppress or postpone heat in cats.

d. Mibolerone should not be used in cats because it can be nephrotoxic and hepatotoxic.

e. Estrogens are safe and effective for inducing fertile heat in dogs.

10. *Hormones used to control estrus and prevent or terminate pregnancy in dogs can have potentially harmful side effects. Concerning such use of hormones, which statement is **least** accurate?*

a. Mibolerone should not be given to a pregnant bitch because it may maculinize the female pups.

b. Megestrol acetate should not be given to bitches in advanced estrus because pyometra may result.

c. Overdoses of estrogen used to treat mismating can lead to anemia, reduced platelet numbers and hemorrhaging in bitches.

d. Use of prostaglandins to treat pyometra or terminate pregnancy in bitches can have fatal results if the bitch is overdosed or if the bitch has a heart condition.

e. Testosterone can be safely administered to prepubertal bitches to increase growth and muscle mass without affecting reproductive cycles and fertility.

11. *Dystocia (difficult or abnormal birth) can be related to maternal or fetal factors. Which condition is **least** likely to cause dystocia in a bitch?*

a. dead puppy blocking the birth canal

b. uterine inertia

c. a single-puppy litter

d. previous pelvic fracture

e. a multiple-puppy litter

12. *In most bitches, the entire estrous cycle spans:*

a. 4-7 months

b. 21 days

c. 7 days

d. 28 days

e. 63 days

Correct answers are on pages 311-313.

13. In dogs, gestation lasts approximately:

a. 21 days
b. 30 days
c. 63 days
d. 90 days
e. 115 days

14. In a vaginal smear of a bitch in standing heat, what is the predominant epithelial cell type?

a. parabasal cell
b. noncornified small intermediate cell
c. cornified, large intermediate and superficial cell
d. red blood cell
e. white blood cell

*15. Which of the following is **not** an indication for cesarean section in a queen?*

a. pregnancy lasting more than 67 days
b. period of more than 4 hours since delivery of the previous kitten
c. foul-smelling, hemorrhagic vulvar discharge
d. constant straining to deliver a kitten
e. nonodoriferous, brownish vulvar discharge after delivery of the second kitten

*16. Concerning reproduction in cats, which statement is **least** accurate?*

a. Cats ovulate in response to vaginal stimulation.
b. In the Northern Hemisphere, cats are polyestrous from late January to fall.
c. In a nonpregnant cat, the corpus luteum produces progesterone for 10 days between heats.
d. Cats that have been bred but that are not pregnant may develop pseudopregnancy and show signs of pregnancy.
e. Cats that have been bred but that are not pregnant cease cycling for several months.

*17. In cats, classic signs of estrus include all of the following **except**:*

a. vocalization, rear-leg treading
b. mounting of the male by the female
c. rubbing and rolling
d. elevated hindquarters (lordosis), tail deflected
e. attraction of male cats

*18. In cats, normal signs of copulation, but not necessarily conception, include all of the following **except**:*

a. the male's biting queen's neck while holding the queen between his front legs
b. the queen's crying out and turning to strike at the tom as he dismounts
c. the queen's rolling and licking at her vulva in a frenzied manner
d. the queen's rejecting the tom for 20-60 minutes
e. draining of white blood-flecked mucus from the queen's vulva

*19. Concerning reproduction in cats, which statement is **least** accurate?*

a. The estrous cycle lasts about 14 days.
b. Cats remain in standing heat (estrus) about 3-6 days if not bred.
c. Corpora lutea formed after sterile matings last 60-90 days.
d. Progesterone is produced for 20-44 days after matings with a vasectomized tom.
e. Nonbred queens go through a period of "nonestrus," but not diestrus, between heats.

20. In queens, pregnancy lasts approximately:

a. 21 days
b. 65 days
c. 90 days
d. 120 days
e. 150 days

21. Concerning cytologic examination of feline vaginal smears, which statement is most accurate?

a. Smears should not be collected because this may alter the duration of heat.
b. Cellular changes are similar to those in bitches.
c. Papanicolaou, new methylene blue and Diff-Quik stains are not acceptable for staining vaginal smears.
d. Queens in anestrus have a high percentage of anuclear, flat, cornified cells in vaginal smears.
e. Spermatozoa cannot be seen in vaginal smears from cats bred 2 hours previously.

22. *Signs of queening (parturition) in cats include all of the following* ***except:***

a. fall in rectal temperature in the first stage of labor
b. nesting behavior
c. increased appetite
d. frequent licking of the vulva
e. straining

23. *The contraceptive method of choice for an adult queen whose owner does* ***not*** *intend to breed her is:*

a. ovariohysterectomy
b. progesterone injection
c. estrogen injection
d. androgen implants
e. prostaglandin suppositories

24. *Concerning anesthesia of a cat for cesarean section, which statement is* ***least*** *accurate?*

a. Impingement of the large, pregnant uterus on the diaphragm can reduce the functional residual capacity of the lungs, leading to decreased oxygen reserves.
b. Oxygen uptake is increased during pregnancy and labor.
c. Anesthetics decrease arterial blood pressure, and placing a cat in dorsal recumbency can cause hypotension.
d. Fetal hypoxia can delay respiration in kittens after delivery.
e. Even though fetal drug metabolism is limited, most anesthetics are safe for cesarean section because they do not cross the placenta.

25. *Concerning vaccination of queens and bitches during pregnancy, which statement is most accurate?*

a. Modified-live-virus vaccines should not be given to pregnant females.
b. Modified-live-virus rabies vaccine is safe in pregnant dogs but not in pregnant queens.
c. Modified-live-virus canine distemper vaccine is safe in pregnant dogs.
d. Modified-live-virus panleukopenia vaccine is safe in pregnant queens.
e. Modified-live-virus feline viral rhinotracheitis vaccine is acceptable for use in pregnant cats.

26. *The embryonic vesicle is highly mobile within the mare's uterine lumen during certain days after ovulation. During which days does this mobility occur?*

a. days 1-6 postovulation
b. days 11-15 postovulation
c. days 20-30 postovulation
d. days 45-60 postovulation
e. days 60-90 postovulation

27. *Most mares pass the placenta within 1-2 hours after foaling. Concerning placental retention in mares, which statement is* ***least*** *accurate?*

a. Mares that retain the placenta for 3 or more hours after foaling should be seen by a veterinarian within 6 hours after foaling.
b. Oxytocin injection may help a mare pass the placenta.
c. Strong traction should be applied to the placenta to speed its passage.
d. Placental retention can lead to metritis and laminitis.
e. Placental retention may be life threatening in mares.

Correct answers are on pages 311-313.

*28. A flexible fiberoptic endoscope can be used to examine the uterine lumen in mares for evidence of adhesions and endometrial cysts. Concerning uterine endoscopy in mares, which statement is **least** accurate?*

a. The endoscope is passed through the cervix and into the uterus manually by a transvaginal approach.
b. The uterus must be inflated with air or another gas to adequately visualize the internal lining of the uterus.
c. Once in the uterus, the endoscope can be directed by rectal palpation and manipulation of the scope within the uterus.
d. The endoscope should be disinfected with a chemical that is effective against *Streptococcus*, as this is a major cause of uterine infection in mares.
e. Most flexible endoscopes are designed to withstand sterilization in an autoclave.

29. Body condition scoring is a method for assessing the mare's nutritional status. Concerning assessment of body condition in mares, which statement is most accurate?

a. Body weight tapes are more accurate than condition scoring for assessing a pregnant mare's nutritional status.
b. Using a scale to weigh a mare at monthly intervals is an accurate method for assessing a pregnant mare's condition.
c. Body condition scoring is a visual and manual method for assessing the amount of body fat on a mare.
d. Mares with a high condition score (8 or 9 out of 9) have impaired breeding efficiency.
e. Condition scoring is not as accurate as weighing to assess nutritional status because it does not take into account the weight of the foal and fetal fluids.

*30. Proper teasing of mares is an important part of breeding when the stallion is not running with mares. Concerning teasing of mares, which statement is **least** accurate?*

a. A common, very effective method for teasing is introduction of the mare to the stallion with a sturdy barrier separating them.
b. Mares in heat usually elevate the tail, stand with the rear feet wide apart, squat, urinate frequently, "wink" the clitoris and fail to kick or strike at the stallion.
c. Mares in diestrus show active resistance. They switch their tail, squeal, pin their ears back and strike or kick at the teaser horse.
d. Mares with a foal at their side do not cycle until after the foal is weaned and not need be teased.
e. Nonpregnant, cycling mares should be teased at least every other day until they are successfully bred.

*31. Mares are seasonal breeders. Concerning reproductive cycling in mares, which statement is **least** accurate?*

a. Mares respond to decreasing day length (photoperiod) by starting to ovulate.
b. Mares have irregular cycles in the spring and fall transition periods as they enter or leave the breeding season.
c. Mares can be made to begin cycling by exposing them to light for 16 hours a day starting in December (Northern Hemisphere).
d. Most mares stop cycling and enter anestrus during the winter.
e. Mares in anestrus are frequently nonresponsive to stallions.

*32. A fertile stallion is required for an efficient broodmare program. Concerning fertility in stallions, which statement is **least** accurate?*

a. Colts reach puberty at about 18 months of age.
b. The stallion's ejaculate is composed of 3 fractions; the second fraction is sperm rich.
c. The gel fraction of the ejaculate should be filtered and excluded before evaluating semen or using it for artificial insemination.
d. The volume of a normal stallion's ejaculate is 5-20 milliliters.
e. Most people recommend using an aliquot of semen containing at least 500 million sperm to inseminate a mare.

33. *Semen collection from stallions requires special equipment and training. Concerning stallion semen collection and evaluation, which statement is* ***least*** *accurate?*

a. Stallions can be trained to mount dummy or phantom mares.
b. The outer jacket of the artificial vagina used to collect semen from stallions should be filled with water at 50-55 C to achieve an internal lining temperature of 45-50 C at collection.
c. The artificial vagina should be lubricated with a sterile but not bactericidal water-soluble lubricant, as bactericidal lubricants may contain spermicidal chemicals.
d. Disposable liners inside the artificial vagina are advantageous because they prevent spread of disease between stallions, facilitate sanitation and eliminate the risk of spermicidal soap residues contacting the semen.
e. Stallion semen is not photosensitive and is resistant to cold shock.

34. *Pregnancy in horses lasts approximately:*

a. 63 days
b. 115 days
c. 280 days
d. 330 days
e. 540 days

35. *A mare in heat should be bred:*

a. on day 2 of standing heat and every other day until she goes out of heat
b. daily for 7 consecutive days, regardless of the signs exhibited
c. once, regardless of the duration of estrual signs
d. only in the middle of heat
e. only on the first day of heat

36. *The average duration of estrus in mares is:*

a. 15 days
b. 21 days
c. 3 days
d. 5 days
e. 30 days

37. *In most mares, the entire estrous cycle spans:*

a. 6 days
b. 4-10 days
c. 21-22 days
d. 28 days
e. 35 days

38. *Embryo transfer in cattle requires mastery of a number of techniques. Which of the following is* ***not*** *an essential part of embryo transfer technology in beef cattle?*

a. artificial insemination
b. superovulation
c. heat detection
d. uterine flushing
e. semen collection

39. *Concerning embryo transfer in cattle, which statement is most accurate?*

a. The donor cow and recipient cow should have had their heats within 4 days of each other.
b. Nonsurgical embryo transfer is the method of choice because it produces the highest pregnancy rate.
c. A major advantage of freezing embryos is that it reduces the cost of trying to keep a large number of recipients on hand and it also makes international transport possible.
d. Superovulation is produced by multiple injections of estrogen and progesterone.
e. For best results, fresh embryos should be transferred within 15 minutes of collection.

40. *In most cows, the entire estrous cycle spans:*

a. 7-10 days
b. 10-15 days
c. 18-23 days
d. 24-36 days
e. 40-45 days

Correct answers are on pages 311-313.

41. *In Holstein cows, standing heat (estrus) lasts:*

a. 7-10 hours
b. 16-18 hours
c. 24-36 hours
d. 48-72 hours
e. 3-5 days

42. *In cows, ovulation occurs:*

a. at the onset of heat
b. at the end of heat
c. a few hours after the end of heat
d. at varying times, depending on the duration of heat
e. within 6 hours after coitus

43. *Signs of estrus in cows include all of the following* ***except:***

a. restlessness and bellowing
b. standing to be ridden by other cows
c. clear, stringy vaginal mucus
d. low serum progesterone level
e. lordosis, tail flagging and clitoral "winking"

44. *In cows, a dark, bloody, mucous vulvar discharge at the time of estrus indicates:*

a. the best time to artificially inseminate the cow
b. that the vagina was damaged during breeding
c. that the cow has aborted
d. that the cow did not conceive at the most recent breeding
e. that the cow has ovulated and it is too late to breed her

45. *Concerning estrus detection in cows, which statement is most accurate?*

a. Observing cows for 20 minutes a day is adequate.
b. Cows should be observed for heat while grouped before milking or while eating after milking.
c. Low milk progesterone levels indicate that the cow is in heat and should be bred.
d. Most cows in heat show signs between 6 AM and 6 PM.
e. Cow should be observed for heat twice a day at about 12-hour intervals and should be bred artificially 12 hours after heat is first detected.

46. *In Holstein cows, pregnancy lasts approximately:*

a. 90 days
b. 120 days
c. 150 days
d. 280 days
e. 330 days

47. *In cows, definitive indications of pregnancy include all of the following* ***except:***

a. rectal palpation of the amniotic vesicle in the uterus
b. rectal palpation of cotyledons in the uterus
c. an enlarged uterus
d. rectal palpation of the fetus
e. "slipping" of the fetal membranes in the uterus on rectal palpation

48. *Unlike primates, which exhibit a menstrual cycle, dogs, cats, ruminants and horses experience estrous cycles. The stage of the estrous cycle associated with standing heat and acceptance of the male for breeding is:*

a. proestrus
b. estrus
c. diestrus
d. metestrus
e. anestrus

49. *The hormone necessary for maintenance of pregnancy in domestic animals is:*

a. follicle-stimulating hormone
b. testosterone
c. progesterone
d. estrogen
e. prostaglandin

50. *Ovulation occurs after and in response to copulation in:*

a. mares
b. cows
c. bitches
d. queens
e. sows

51. *Females of most domestic species can be artificially inseminated with fresh or frozen semen. Depositing the semen at the correct site is important so as to achieve acceptable pregnancy rates. Which of the following* ***least*** *accurately correlates the species, type of semen used, and correct site of semen deposition?*

a. mare, fresh semen, uterus
b. cow, thawed frozen semen, vagina
c. sow, fresh semen, cervix or uterus
d. bitch, thawed frozen semen, uterus
e. goat doe, frozen semen, cervix or uterus

52. *Twin pregnancies may be advantageous in some species but not in others. Concerning twinning, which statement is* ***least*** *accurate?*

a. One twin should be eliminated early in pregnancy in mares because both twins are rarely carried to term or survive after foaling.
b. In ewes, twinning is considered desirable.
c. In dairy cattle, twinning is not desirable because if they are of opposite sexes, the female is likely to be infertile (freemartin).
d. In beef cattle, twinning may be desirable when the producer's goal is to maximize a cow's calf production.
e. In goats, twinning is rare and should be discouraged, as one is usually an unthrifty runt.

53. *In most sows, the entire estrous cycle spans:*

a. 15 days
b. 21 days
c. 30 days
d. 60 days
e. 115 days

54. *The average duration of estrus in sows is:*

a. 12-16 hours
b. 7-10 days
c. 48-72 hours
d. 8-10 hours
e. 24-36 hours

55. *In sows, ovulation occurs:*

a. early in estrus
b. toward the end of estrus
c. 12 hours after estrus
d. 12 hours before diestrus
e. 36 hours after proestrus

56. *In sows, gestation lasts approximately:*

a. 115 days
b. 150 days
c. 90 days
d. 210 days
e. 63 days

57. *After farrowing, sows return to fertile heat:*

a. in 9 days
b. in 21 days
c. the next season
d. a few days after weaning the litter
e. in 60 days

58. *In sows, signs of estrus include all of the following* ***except:***

a. standing to be ridden by the boar
b. assuming a rigid "sawhorse" stance with manual pressure applied to the back
c. "perked up" ears
d. mounting of the male by the sow
e. salivation, champing and grunting

59. *Boars are different from the males of other domestic species in all of the following ways* ***except:***

a. spiral tip on the penis
b. sigmoid flexure of the penis located cranial to the scrotum
c. tapioca-like gel fraction in the ejaculate
d. small volume of highly concentrated semen
e. preputial diverticulum may interfere with protrusion of the penis

Correct answers are on pages 311-313.

60. What type of reproductive cycle is exhibited by most domestic breeds of goats and sheep?

a. seasonally polyestrous
b. polyestrous throughout the year
c. monestrous
d. seasonally monestrous, with 2 seasons per year
e. irregularly polyestrous

61. In dairy goats, the entire estrous cycle spans:

a. 7 days
b. 16 days
c. 21 days
d. 28 days
e. 42 days

62. In domestic sheep, the entire estrous cycle spans:

a. 7 days
b. 16 days
c. 21 days
d. 28 days
e. 42 days

63. In does (goats) and ewes, pregnancy lasts approximately:

a. 100 days
b. 150 days
c. 210 days
d. 280 days
e. 330 days

64. During the breeding season, the scrotal circumference of normal fertile rams:

a. increases
b. decreases
c. remains the same
d. varies with the interval since the previous breeding
e. is directly related to environmental temperatures

*65. Which of the following is **not** an accurate way to detect pregnancy in ewes?*

a. return to heat
b. Doppler ultrasonic examination
c. real-time ultrasonographic examination
d. abdominal radiography
e. serum progesterone assay at 14-16 days postbreeding

*66. In goat does, signs of estrus include all of the following **except**:*

a. rapid tail wagging in the presence of a buck
b. following a rag that has been rubbed on a buck's head
c. vulvar swelling and reddening
d. grayish-white mucus on the floor of the vagina
e. mounting of the buck by the doe

*67. When using a marking harness on a ram running with the flock to detect matings, several things must be taken into consideration. Concerning this practice, which statement is **least** accurate?*

a. The ambient temperature must be considered and the appropriate ink used to ensure marking and prevent loss of the crayon.
b. The color of the ink should be changed every 2 weeks so as to tell new breedings from old.
c. The width and intensity of the marking must be evaluated so as to differentiate mounting attempts from actual breedings.
d. The size of the ram's chin must be sufficient to accept the chin-ball marker.
e. Regular examination of the flock and recording of the identification of females bred are essential for identifying infertile or problem breeders.

*68. The female of which species is **not** an induced ovulator?*

a. rabbits
b. cats

c. ferrets
d. llamas
e. cattle

69. *Concerning reproduction in llamas, which statement is **least** accurate?*

a. When not erect, the penis points caudally.
b. Female llamas lie down sternally for mating.
c. Copulation averages 20-30 minutes in duration.
d. Most pregnancies occur in the left uterine horn.
e. The estrous cycle of llamas lasts 21 days.

70. *Concerning reproduction in domestic rabbits, which statement is **least** accurate?*

a. Female rabbits reach breeding maturity at 4-7 months of age.
b. Rabbits are nonseasonal breeders.
c. Heat lasts 14-16 days in does and is recurrent unless they become pregnant.
d. Gestation lasts 64 days.
e. The vulva of young does is a slit-like opening and the male's penis is a rounded protrusion.

71. *As compared with that of mammals, the reproductive system of chickens is unique in all of the following ways **except:***

a. only the left oviduct develops in hens
b. all of the follicles are ovulated from the left ovary
c. the oviduct is the main portion of the reproductive tract
d. the "uterus" is modified into a "shell gland"
e. fertilization takes place in the oviduct

72. *Concerning reproduction in albino rats, which statement is **least** accurate?*

a. Heat occurs at 5-day intervals.
b. Ovulation is induced by copulation.
c. Gestation lasts an average of 21 days.
d. Heat lasts 13-15 hours.
e. Puberty is reached at 70-100 days of age.

73. *Concerning reproduction in gerbils, which statement is **least** accurate?*

a. Gerbils reach sexual maturity at 10-12 weeks of age.
b. Pregnancy lasts 24-26 days.
c. They usually have only 2 offspring per litter.
d. Weaning can occur after 21 days of age.
e. They are polyestrous, nonseasonal breeders.

74. *Concerning iguanas, which statement is **least** accurate?*

a. Iguanas live 40-60 years.
b. Male iguanas are larger than females.
c. Iguana eggs hatch after 80 days if the ambient temperature is about 30 C.
d. Baby iguanas do not eat for the first few days after hatching.
e. Male iguanas have a brighter coloration than females during the breeding season.

75. *Determining the gender of cage birds ("sexing"), especially young birds, is difficult. Concerning gender determination of cage birds, which statement is **least** accurate?*

a. In general, the head and beak of male birds is larger than those of females.
b. Mature male canaries are brightly colored and have a pronounced swelling around the cloaca that becomes greatly distended during breeding.
c. Most mature budgerigars have a bright blue cere, but this does not hold true for pied, albino and lutino males.
d. Laparoscopy is a time-consuming and inaccurate technique for sexing birds.
e. Fecal steroid analysis, plasma hormone analysis, and genetic techniques are being developed for sexing of birds.

Correct answers are on pages 311-313.

76. *Concerning reproduction in nonhuman primates, which statement is **least** accurate?*

a. Apes and monkeys have menstrual cycles, rather than estrous cycles.
b. Ape chorionic gonadotropin test kits are available for detecting pregnancy in gorillas; however, human chorionic gonadotropin kits available for at-home pregnancy tests in women can also be used on gorillas.
c. The gender of chimpanzees can be identified at birth.
d. In chimpanzees, gestation lasts about 1 month longer than in women.
e. Lactation causes amenorrhea (lack of menstruation) or delays return to cycling in most nonhuman primates.

77. *Female ferrets must be allowed to breed or be treated with human chorionic gonadotropin so as to prevent:*

a. toxicity from estrogen unovulated follicles
b. pyometra from progesterone produced by multiple corpora lutea
c. endometriosis produced by lack of negative hormonal feedback
d. persistent anestrus from ovarian exhaustion
e. masculinization from ovarian exhaustion

78. *Which dog breed normally exhibits only 1 estrus per year?*

a. German Shepherd
b. Miniature Poodle
c. Basset Hound
d. Basenji
e. Great Dane

79. *Which of the following is **least** likely to terminate standing heat in a queen?*

a. mating with a fertile tom
b. mating with an infertile tom
c. injection of 0.25 mg of estradiol cypionate
d. oral administration of 5 mg of megestrol acetate daily for 10 days
e. obtaining a deep vaginal sample for culture, using a sterile swab

80. *In vaginal cytology, which cell predominates during standing heat (estrus) in the bitch?*

a. parabasal epithelial cell
b. uncornified epithelial cell
c. superficial epithelial cell
d. erythrocyte
e. polymorphonuclear cell

81. *Estrogen is the predominant hormone during:*

a. pregnancy
b. anestrus
c. diestrus
d. metestrus
e. estrus

82. *A definitive sign of estrus in cows is:*

a. mucous vulvar discharge
b. ruffled hair on the tailhead
c. a large follicle on the ovary
d. vulvar swelling
e. standing to be mounted

83. *The most common cause of poor reproductive performance in cows on large dairy farms is:*

a. anestrus
b. cystic follicles
c. improper semen handling and poor artificial insemination technique
d. poor estrus detection
e. uterine infections

84. *In the Northern Hemisphere, mares normally have estrous cycles:*

a. in the spring
b. in the fall
c. in the winter
d. at any time of the year
e. in the fall and winter

85. *Rectal palpation of a mare in estrus is most likely to reveal:*

a. a flaccid uterus and a cervix with tone
b. a uterus with tone and a flaccid cervix
c. a flaccid uterus and a flaccid cervix
d. a uterus with tone and a cervix with tone
e. an edematous uterus and a cervix with tone

86. *You collect semen from a stallion once, and then again an hour later. As compared with the first ejaculate, the second ejaculate is likely to have:*

a. half the volume and the same number of spermatozoa
b. the same volume and half as many spermatozoa
c. the same volume and twice the number of spermatozoa
d. half the volume and half the number of spermatozoa
e. the same volume and the same number of spermatozoa

87. *The most important factor influencing the time of onset of puberty in gilts is:*

a. environment
b. housing
c. nutrition at the time of expected onset of puberty
d. transport
e. exposure to a mature boar near the time of expected onset of puberty

88. *Ewes lambing in the spring typically do not return to estrus for at least 6 weeks after lambing. This delay is attributable to the suppressive effects of:*

a. grazing on spring pastures with low energy content
b. cool ambient temperatures
c. incomplete uterine involution
d. suckling and photoperiod
e. overwinter parasite burden

89. *In goats, gestation lasts:*

a. 3 months
b. 3 months, 3 weeks and 3 days
c. 4.5 months
d. 5 months
e. 6 months

90. *Concerning the reproductive tract of female birds, which statement is most accurate?*

a. The left ovary is more well developed than the right ovary.
b. The right ovary is more well developed than the left ovary.
c. The ovaries are equally well developed throughout life.
d. The ovaries periodically hypertrophy and atrophy on alternate sides throughout life.
e. The ovaries become especially active during molting.

Answers

1. **e**
2. **c**
3. **c**
4. **d**
5. **b**
6. **a**
7. **a**
8. **c**
9. **e**
10. **e**
11. **e**
12. **a**
13. **c**
14. **c**
15. **e**
16. **c**

17. **b**
18. **e**
19. **c**
20. **b**
21. **b**
22. **c**
23. **a**
24. **e**
25. **a**
26. **b**
27. **c**
28. **e**
29. **c**
30. **d**
31. **a**
32. **d**
33. **e**
34. **d**
35. **a**
36. **d**
37. **c**
38. **e**
39. **c**
40. **c**
41. **b**
42. **c**
43. **e**
44. **e**
45. **e**
46. **d**
47. **c**
48. **b**
49. **c**
50. **d**
51. **b** Semen should be deposited in the uterus of cows.
52. **e**
53. **b**
54. **c**
55. **b**
56. **a**
57. **d**
58. **d**
59. **d** Boars ejaculate a large volume of semen with a low concentration of spermatozoa.
60. **a**
61. **c**
62. **b**
63. **b**
64. **a**
65. **a**
66. **e**
67. **d**
68. **e**
69. **e**
70. **d** Gestation lasts 28-36 days in domestic rabbits.
71. **e** As in mammals, fertilization takes place in the oviduct of chickens.
72. **b**
73. **c**
74. **a** Iguanas live up to 20 years.
75. **d** When performed by experienced individuals, laparoscopy is neither time consuming nor inaccurate.
76. **d** In chimpanzees, gestation lasts 216-260 days.
77. **a**
78. **d** Basenjis are one of the few breeds that truly cycle once per year. The Tibetan Mastiff (rarely seen as a pet) is another.
79. **c** Items a, b and e will probably induce ovulation. Item d will pharmacologically overcome estrogen-expressed signs of heat. Item c will prolong the signs of heat.
80. **c** Parabasal and uncornified epithelial cells are synonymous. Their numbers decrease as estrogen levels increase. PMNs disappear and RBC numbers are highly variable.
81. **e** Estrogen is produced by the ovulatory follicle during estrus.
82. **e** This is the only indisputable sign of estrus.
83. **d** This is a neverending management problem.

84. **a** Mares normally cycle during periods of longer day length, which, in the Northern Hemisphere, is in the spring (March-July).
85. **c** In estrus, the mare has a flaccid uterus and flaccid cervix because of the influence of estrogen.
86. **b** A second ejaculate, collected 1 hour after the first, should have the same volume and half as many spermatozoa. If this is not the case, one of the ejaculates is not representative.
87. **e** Though the other factors listed may influence the time of onset of puberty, exposure of gilts of the proper age to a mature boar is the most consistent factor influencing the onset of puberty.
88. **d**
89. **d**
90. **a** The left ovary is more well developed than the right ovary.

Notes

Notes

Section 31

Surgical Nursing

T. Colville, R.L. Leighton

Recommended Reading

Bojrab MJ: *Current Techniques in Small Animal Surgery.* 3rd ed. Lea & Febiger, Philadelphia, 1990.
Gourley IM and Vasseur PB: *General Small Animal Surgery.* Lippincott, Philadelphia, 1985.
Harvey CE *et al: Small Animal Surgery.* Lippincott, Philadelphia, 1990.
Jennings PB: *The Practice of Large Animal Surgery.* Saunders, Philadelphia, 1984.
Knecht CD *et al: Fundamental Techniques in Veterinary Surgery.* Saunders, Philadelphia, 1987.
McCurnin DM *et al: Clinical Textbook for Veterinary Technicians.* 2nd ed. Saunders, Philadelphia, 1990.
Newton CD and Nunamaker DM: *Textbook of Small Animal Orthopaedics.* Lippincott, Philadelphia, 1985.
Slatter DH: *Textbook of Small Animal Surgery.* Saunders, Philadelphia, 1985.
Swaim SA and Henderson RA: *Small Animal Wound Management.* Lea & Febiger, Philadelphia, 1990.
Tracy DL *et al: Small Animal Surgical Nursing.* Mosby, St. Louis, 1983.

Practice answer sheet is on page 405.

Questions

1. *Which surgical instrument is primarily used to hold organs and tissues out of the way to facilitate exposure of the operative field?*

   a. elevator
   b. forceps
   c. retractor
   d. rongeur
   e. hemostat

2. *Which orthopedic instrument has sharp, opposing, cup-shaped jaws used to shape bone by "chewing" out small pieces?*

   a. chisel
   b. curette
   c. osteotome
   d. rongeur
   e. trephine

Correct answers are on pages

3. *Which of the following is the correct surgical term for declawing?*

   a. celiotomy
   b. cystotomy
   c. onychectomy
   d. hysterectomy
   e. colpotomy

4. *The type of needle most appropriate for suturing internal organs, such as gastrointestinal structures, is the:*

   a. blunt
   b. cutting
   c. reverse cutting
   d. tapered
   e. trocar

5. *Which type of needle is most commonly used for suturing in general surgery?*

   a. straight
   b. 3/8 circle
   c. 1/2 circle
   d. 5/8 circle
   e. 1/2 curved

6. *Which of the following surgical procedures is* ***not*** *considered an elective procedure?*

   a. correction of a proptosed eye
   b. dew claw removal in a field trial dog
   c. mastectomy to remove a benign tumor
   d. ovariohysterectomy in a healthy 6-month-old cat
   e. tail docking in 3-day-old Boxer puppies

7. *Healing of a properly sutured surgical wound is most appropriately termed:*

   a. first-intention healing
   b. granulation
   c. secondary union
   d. second-intention healing
   e. wound contraction

8. *Which of the following has the* ***poorest*** *potential for healing and return to normal function after damage and effective surgical repair?*

   a. bone
   b. intestine
   c. liver
   d. nervous tissue
   e. uterus

9. *Which surgical term describes removal of necrotic tissue from a wound?*

   a. debride
   b. exudate
   c. incise
   d. retract
   e. suture

10. *Which of the following best describes the location of an incision extending from the xiphoid process to the umbilicus of an animal?*

   a. dorsal midline
   b. flank
   c. paracostal
   d. paramedian
   e. ventral midline

For Questions 11 through 13, select the correct answer from the 5 choices below.

   a. autoclave
   b. boiling
   c. dry heat
   d. ethylene oxide gas
   e. liquid chemical disinfectant

11. *Most appropriate for sterilization of an electric drill to be used in an orthopedic surgical procedure.*

12. *Most appropriate for sterilization of a needle holder to be used in a surgical procedure.*

13. *Most appropriate for sterilization of dissecting scissors to be used in a surgical procedure.*

14. Which of the following describes the minimal exposure time and temperature for autoclaving of a surgical pack?

a. 121 C for 15 minutes
b. 121 F for 15 minutes
c. 250 F for 5 minutes
d. 250 C for 20 minutes
e. 250 F for 20 minutes

15. Which of the following is the most effective and immediate indicator that the conditions for sterilization have been met in an autoclaved surgery pack?

a. appearance of the instruments
b. autoclave tape
c. chemical indicator
d. culture results
e. melting pellet

16. What is the proper term for entrance of microorganisms to an incision during a surgical procedure?

a. contamination
b. debridement
c. dehiscence
d. infection
e. septicemia

*17. Which of the following items does **not** have to be sterile during a surgical procedure involving aseptic technique?*

a. drapes
b. gloves
c. gown
d. mask
e. suture material

18. Which of the following is the agent for sterilization by autoclaving?

a. chemical disinfectant solution
b. dry heat
c. ethylene oxide gas
d. ionizing radiation
e. steam

19. Which size of electrical clipper blade is most commonly used for clipping the hair from a surgical site?

a. # 10
b. # 20
c. # 30
d. # 40
e. # 50

*20. Which suture size is the **smallest** in diameter?*

a. 0
b. 0000
c. 2-0
d. # 2
e. 3/0

*21. Which suture material shows the **least** conduction of fluid by capillary action?*

a. braided cotton
b. braided polyglycolic acid
c. braided silk
d. monofilament nylon
e. chromic catgut

*22. All of the following are nonabsorbable suture materials **except**:*

a. cotton
b. nylon
c. silk
d. stainless-steel wire
e. chromic catgut

23. Which type of surgical gut is absorbed most rapidly from tissues after surgery?

a. extra chromic
b. heavy chromic
c. medium chromic
d. mild chromic
e. plain gut

Correct answers are on pages

24. *Which of the following is* ***not*** *an effective form of surgical hemostasis?*

a. crushing
b. curettage
c. electrocoagulation
d. ligation
e. pressure

25. *Which of the following is* ***not*** *a likely cause of dehiscence of an abdominal incision?*

a. chronic vomiting
b. excessive physical activity
c. stormy recovery from anesthesia
d. surgical wound infection
e. suture material larger than needed

26. *Concerning aseptic surgical technique, which statement is* ***least*** *accurate?*

a. A sterile item touched by a nonsterile item becomes nonsterile.
b. If the sterility of an item is in doubt, consider it sterile.
c. Nonscrubbed personnel can touch only nonsterile items.
d. Only sterile items can contact exposed patient tissue.
e. Only sterile items can contact other sterile items.

27. *Which of the following is an everting suture pattern that should only be used to close skin incisions?*

a. Cushing
b. Lembert
c. Parker-Kerr
d. simple interrupted
e. vertical mattress

28. *Which of the following is an inverting suture pattern used mainly to suture hollow internal organs?*

a. horizontal mattress
b. Lembert
c. pursestring
d. simple interrupted or continuous
e. vertical mattress

29. *Which of the following is most effective in minimizing the scarring from skin sutures and achieving good wound healing?*

a. leaving sutures permanently in place
b. removing the sutures 2 days after insertion
c. removing the sutures 7 days after insertion
d. using large-diameter suture material
e. using suture material that produces significant inflammation

30. *Which of the following does* ***not*** *enhance healing of an open wound?*

a. debridement
b. exuberant granulation tissue
c. granulation tissue
d. wound contraction
e. wound flushing

31. *Which of the following is* ***not*** *a characteristic of first-intention wound healing?*

a. minimal contamination
b. minimal tissue damage
c. minimal role of wound contraction
d. wound edges are not approximated
e. wound edges are sutured

32. *Which incision is most appropriate for exploratory surgery in a dog's abdomen, in which the precise location of the problem is* ***not*** *known?*

a. dorsal midline
b. flank
c. paracostal
d. paramedian
e. ventral midline

33. *Which of the following is* ***not*** *an early sign of wound dehiscence during the first 24 hours after abdominal surgery?*

a. body temperature elevation of 1 - 2 F

b. change in texture of the wound edges
c. serosanguineous discharge from the incision
d. swollen incision
e. very warm incision

34. *The main goal of aseptic surgical technique is to prevent contamination of the:*

a. operative personnel
b. sterile fields
c. sterile zones
d. surgical instruments
e. surgical wound

35. *Which factor related to infection of a surgical wound is most significantly affected by aseptic technique?*

a. number of microorganisms entering the wound
b. pathogenicity of microorganisms entering the wound
c. species of microorganisms entering the wound
d. route of exposure to infectious microorganisms
e. susceptibility of the patient

36. *The effectiveness of a bactericidal surgical scrub of one's hands and arms depends on the:*

a. combination of contact time and scrubbing action
b. length of time the soap is in contact with the skin
c. pH of the skin surface
d. scrubbing action of the brush
e. temperature of the water

37. *Which of the following, when used alone as a surgical scrub soap, forms a bacteriostatic film over the skin?*

a. chlorhexidine
b. chlorpheniramine
c. hexadimethrine
d. hexachlorophene
e. povidone-iodine

38. *Which of the following does **not** normally have to be sterilized as part of good aseptic surgical technique?*

a. cap
b. drapes
c. gloves
d. gown
e. scrub brush

39. *Liquid chemical sterilization is used primarily for:*

a. electrical equipment
b. hemostatic forceps
c. instruments with sharp edges
d. orthopedic equipment
e. surgical drapes

40. *The time necessary to achieve disinfection of surgical instruments with liquid chemicals can be shortened by:*

a. agitating the solution
b. cooling the solution
c. using a lower concentration than recommended
d. using a higher concentration than recommended
e. warming the solution

41. *Which surgical wire size is the **smallest** in diameter?*

a. 40 gauge
b. 10 gauge
c. 26 gauge
d. 32 gauge
e. 20 gauge

42. *Which surgical drape material prevents passage of bacteria through the drape to the patient's skin by capillary action when the top surface of the drape becomes wet?*

a. cloth
b. fenestrated paper
c. muslin
d. paper
e. plastic

Correct answers are on pages

43. *Which suture size is **smaller** in diameter than 3-0?*

a. 2-0
b. #1
c. #3
d. #4
e. 4-0

44. *Which suture material is absorbable?*

a. cotton
b. nylon
c. polypropylene
d. silk
e. chromic catgut

45. *Which surgical instrument should **not** be routinely steam sterilized?*

a. Backhaus towel clamp
b. Halsted mosquito forceps
c. Mayo-Hegar needle holder
d. Metzenbaum scissors
e. Bard-Parker scalpel handle

46. *Castration of a healthy 6-month-old cat is an example of:*

a. cosmetic surgery
b. elective surgery
c. emergency surgery
d. exploratory surgery
e. first-intention surgery

47. *Which solution causes the **least** tissue damage and is most appropriate for wound flushing?*

a. hydrogen peroxide
b. isotonic saline
c. povidone-iodine scrub
d. povidone-iodine solution
e. tap water

48. *Which incision provides the best overall exposure of the abdominal cavity?*

a. dorsal midline
b. flank
c. paracostal
d. paramedian
e. ventral midline

49. *What is the most appropriate suture pattern to close an incision in an animal's stomach?*

a. horizontal mattress
b. Lembert
c. pursestring
d. simple interrupted
e. vertical mattress

50. *Which operating room personnel should try to face away from sterile fields during a surgical procedure?*

a. all personnel
b. nonscrubbed personnel only
c. scrubbed personnel only
d. both nonscrubbed and scrubbed personnel
e. neither nonscrubbed nor scrubbed personnel

51. *What is the significance of dehiscence of the muscle, subcutaneous tissue and skin layers in a ventral midline surgical wound?*

a. acute emergency
b. cosmetic problem only
c. minor significance
d. no significance
e. serious but not an acute emergency

52. *Why is a recent surgical wound usually slightly warmer than the surrounding normal tissues?*

a. contamination
b. debridement
c. infection
d. inflammation
e. septicemia

53. When does a sutured surgical wound begin to gain significant strength from production of collagen strands, so that the wound edges are beginning to be held together by tissue as well as sutures?

a. 6-8 hours
b. 4-6 days
c. 12-14 days
d. 24-26 days
e. 28-30 days

54. Wound contraction is produced by:

a. movement of only the dermis
b. movement of only the epidermis
c. movement of all layers of the skin
d. reproduction of epidermal cells
e. reproduction of all skin cells

55. As a part of effective aseptic technique, surgical gowns:

a. are commonly made of cloth or paper
b. are put on by touching only the outside
c. are routinely sterilized by ethylene oxide gas
d. do not need to be sterile, only clean
e. protect against contamination from the waist down

56. Which suture size is larger in diameter than size #2?

a. 0
b. #1
c. 2-0
d. #3
e. 3-0

57. Which suture material is synthetic?

a. chromic catgut
b. cotton
c. nylon
d. plain catgut
e. silk

*58. Which of the following is **not** a typical sign of hemorrhagic shock in a postsurgical patient?*

a. deep, slow breathing
b. pale mucous membranes
c. slow capillary refill
d. tachycardia
e. weakness

59. What is the most appropriate suture pattern to use in closing an incision of the urinary bladder?

a. Cushing
b. horizontal mattress
c. simple continuous
d. simple interrupted
e. vertical mattress

60. Suture material used to close a surgical wound represents what kind of irritant to body tissues?

a. chemical
b. infectious
c. photic
d. physical
e. thermal

61. What is the usual significance of a small seroma deep to (beneath) the skin suture line after aseptic surgery?

a. acute emergency
b. cosmetic problem only
c. minor significance
d. no significance
e. serious but not an acute emergency

*62. Which suture pattern is **neither** an inverting **nor** an everting pattern?*

a. Cushing
b. horizontal mattress
c. Lembert
d. simple interrupted or continuous
e. vertical mattress

Correct answers are on pages

63. *What is the healing potential of a fractured bone that is properly aligned and kept immobile?*

a. excellent
b. good
c. fair
d. poor
e. very poor

64. *Which of the following indicates the best blood supply to the edges of a wound in unpigmented skin?*

a. black wound edges
b. bluish-purple wound edges
c. gray wound edges
d. pink wound edges
e. white wound edges

65. *Which abdominal incision is most appropriate for cesarean section on a standing heifer?*

a. dorsal midline
b. flank
c. paracostal
d. paramedian
e. ventral midline

66. *What portion of a surgical gown is considered sterile during surgery?*

a. entire outside of the gown
b. front and sides of the gown, from the neck to the bottom, including the arms
c. front of the gown, from the neck to the bottom, including the arms
d. front and sides of the gown, from the neck to the waist
e. front of the gown, from the waist up, including the arms

67. *Which bacterial form is most easily destroyed by common sterilization methods?*

a. spores of aerobes
b. hyphated form
c. dormant form
d. spores of anaerobes
e. vegetative form

68. *The first phase of the wound healing process is the:*

a. epithelial phase
b. fibroblast phase
c. inflammatory phase
d. maturation phase
e. scarring phase

69. *In the first 24 hours of primary union wound healing, most of the resistance to opening of the sutured wound is provided by:*

a. collagen strands
b. fibrin strands
c. fibroblasts
d. granulation tissue
e. sutures

70. *Assuming no complications, how long after surgery should skin sutures generally be removed?*

a. 2-3 days
b. 4-5 days
c. 7-10 days
d. 15-17 days
e. 18-21 days

71. *What is the correct surgical term for incision of the urinary bladder?*

a. cystectomy
b. cystopexy
c. cystoscopy
d. cystostomy
e. cystotomy

72. *What is the correct surgical term for removal of the kidney?*

a. nephrectomy

b. nephropexy
c. nephroscopy
d. nephrostomy
e. nephrotomy

73. *What is the correct surgical term for suturing the stomach to the body wall to fix the stomach in place?*

a. gastrectomy
b. gastropexy
c. gastroscopy
d. gastrostomy
e. gastrotomy

74. *What is the correct surgical term for creation of a permanent artificial opening in the esophagus?*

a. esophagectomy
b. esophagopexy
c. esophagoscopy
d. esophagostomy
e. esophagotomy

75. *With which type of abdominal incision can the abdominal wall be most effectively closed using a single layer of sutures?*

a. high flank
b. low flank
c. paracostal
d. paramedian
e. ventral midline

76. *Scrubbed surgical personnel become contaminated if they touch:*

a. objects in sterile fields
b. objects outside the sterile zone
c. properly sterilized surgical instruments
d. sterile objects
e. freshly exposed tissues of the patient

77. *Nonscrubbed surgical personnel may properly touch anything that is:*

a. contaminated
b. inside the patient
c. inside the sterile zone
d. part of a sterile field
e. sterile

78. *How should scrubbed personnel pass each other when moving about in the operating room?*

a. any way that is convenient
b. back to back
c. back to front
d. front to back
e. front to front

79. *When not otherwise occupied, scrubbed surgical personnel should stand with their:*

a. arms folded across the chest
b. hands held apart and above shoulder level
c. hands clapsed between waist and shoulder level
d. hands held down and to each side
e. hands on the surgery table

80. *During surgery, when is it permissible for nonscrubbed surgical personnel to pass between scrubbed personnel and the patient?*

a. at any convenient time
b. never
c. when opening suture material
d. when adjusting the anesthesia machine
e. when adjusting the intravenous drip

81. *When aseptically opening a sterile surgical pack on an instrument stand, it is **not** proper for nonscrubbed surgical personnel to touch the:*

a. autoclave tape
b. contents of the pack
c. corners of the wrap
d. instrument stand
e. outside of the wrap

Correct answers are on pages

82. *Which of the following characteristics applies to ethylene oxide gas?*

a. flammable
b. exposure is not considered a health hazard
c. noncombustible
d. nontoxic to tissues
e. safe to breathe

83. *Which type of needle is most appropriate for suturing muscle?*

a. blunt
b. cutting
c. reverse cutting
d. tapered
e. trocar

84. *Which type of needle is most appropriate for suturing a ligament?*

a. blunt
b. cutting
c. reverse cutting
d. tapered
e. trocar

85. *Which type of needle is most appropriate for suturing the uterus?*

a. blunt
b. cutting
c. reverse cutting
d. tapered
e. trocar

86. *Surgical removal of a ruptured spleen is an example of:*

a. cosmetic surgery
b. elective surgery
c. emergency surgery
d. exploratory surgery
e. first-intention surgery

87. *Removal of a large skin tumor has left a large skin defect to be closed. Which suture pattern is* ***least*** *likely to cause skin tearing when large wounds are closed under tension?*

a. Cushing
b. horizontal mattress
c. Lembert
d. pursestring
e. simple interrupted

88. *Surgical removal of a cancerous eye from a Hereford cow is an example of:*

a. cosmetic surgery
b. elective surgery
c. emergency surgery
d. exploratory surgery
e. first-intention surgery

89. *Which of the following is* ***not*** *a likely contributor to dehiscence of an abdominal surgical incision?*

a. chronic vomiting
b. internal suture ends cut too short
c. infection
d. skin sutures left in place too long
e. suture material of too-small diameter

90. *Which type of dressing, when removed, provides the* ***least*** *traumatic and* ***least*** *irritating means of debriding a wound with extensive tissue damage?*

a. dry gauze
b. dry nonadhesive pad
c. gauze dressing with an oily antiseptic
d. gauze dressing with a water-soluble antiseptic
e. wet saline dressing

91. *Most of the clinical signs seen in animals in shock related to excessive blood loss are attributable to:*

a. acidosis
b. alkalosis
c. cell death

d. redistribution of blood flow
e. tissue hyperoxia

92. Which of the following is a noncapillary suture material suitable for skin closure?

a. braided cotton
b. braided polyglycolic acid
c. braided silk
d. monofilament stainless steel
e. monofilament cotton

93. The main goal of surgery to remove a pus-filled uterus (pyometra) is to:

a. prevent subsequent pregnancy
b. alter the behavior of the animal
c. make a diagnosis
d. restore the animal to a normal reproductive state
e. restore health despite loss of normal reproductive function

94. With what kind of knot should sutures be routinely tied?

a. bowline
b. granny knot
c. square knot
d. slip knot
e. half hitch

*95. Concerning the principles of cryosurgery, which statement is **least** accurate?*

a. Frozen tissues should be thawed slowly.
b. Little aftercare is required.
c. Multiple freeze-thaw cycles should be applied.
d. Tissues should be frozen to -25 C.
e. Tissues should be frozen rapidly.

96. When does the strength of a sutured surgical skin wound return to its original preoperative strength?

a. 7-10 days
b. 21-28 days
c. 60 days
d. 2-3 years
e. never

97. In second-intention healing, which of the following must be present before wound contraction or epithelial regeneration can occur?

a. collagen fibers
b. exudative tissue
c. fibrin clot
d. granulation tissue
e. scar tissue

*98. When putting on sterile gloves for aseptic surgery, which of the following is **not** permitted?*

a. touching one gloved thumb with the other gloved thumb
b. touching the outside of the glove with scrubbed fingers
c. touching the outside of the gown cuff with the inside of the glove cuff
d. touching the outside of one glove with the outside of the other glove
e. touching the inside of the glove cuff with scrubbed fingers

99. How should packs be placed in an autoclave for sterilization?

a. diagonally
b. horizontally
c. tightly packed
d. unwrapped
e. vertically

100. The use of extreme cold to destroy unwanted tissue is termed:

a. cosmetic surgery
b. cryosurgery
c. elective surgery
d. orthopedic surgery
e. prophylactic surgery

Correct answers are on pages

101. Which of the following suture materials is badly damaged by steam sterilization (autoclaving)?

a. polyglycolic acid
b. polyester
c. nylon
d. polypropylene
e. silk

*102. The likelihood of postoperative wound infection is **decreased** by use of:*

a. monofilament sutures
b. the fewest possible number of large-diameter sutures
c. a multilayered surgical closure
d. adequate postoperative drains
e. the fewest possible number of fine-diameter sutures

103. An autoclaved instrument pack protected by double-wrapped muslin and stored on an open shelf will remain sterile for:

a. 10 weeks
b. 8 weeks
c. 3 weeks
d. 12 weeks
e. 2 weeks

*104. Though hexachlorophene is a very effective antiseptic, a serious **disadvantage** is that it:*

a. is easily inactivated
b. is highly allergenic
c. is unstable and rapidly loses its effectiveness
d. is absorbed through the skin and is neurotoxic
e. tends to sear tissues, trapping pockets of bacteria

105. Concerning use of antibiotics for prophylaxis of wound infections, which statement is most accurate?

a. Antibiotics should be given IV at induction of anesthesia and continued for 12-24 hours after surgery.
b. Antibiotics should be given 24 hours before surgery and then discontinued after surgery is completed.
c. Antibiotics should be given for 24 hours before surgery and for 5 days after surgery.
d. Antibiotics should be given per os just before surgery and for 12-24 hours after surgery.
e. Antibiotics should be given IV 12 hours before anesthesia and discontinued after complete recovery from anesthesia.

*106. Concerning polypropylene (Prolene) suture material, which statement is **least** accurate?*

a. It is inert and retains strength after implantation.
b. It is degraded by hydrolysis and is absorbed by 180 days after implantation.
c. It is frequently used in vascular surgery.
d. Its slippery quality may make knot tying and handling difficult.
e. It has relatively low tensile strength but excellent knot security.

*107. Which suture material is **not** appropriate for tendon repair?*

a. chromic catgut
b. polyglycolic acid
c. polyglactin
d. polypropylene
e. nylon

*108. Concerning stainless-steel suture material, which statement is **least** accurate?*

a. It is biologically inert.
b. It has the greatest tensile strength of all suture materials.
c. It should not be used in tissues that heal slowly.
d. It offers excellent knot security and causes no inflammation.
e. It tends to cut through tissues.

109. The gripping surface of Rochester-Carmalt forceps has:

a. longitudinal grooves, with cross grooves at the tip
b. longitudinal grooves along its entire length
c. longitudinal grooves, with a large tooth at the tip
d. transverse grooves along its entire length
e. transverse grooves, with a large tooth at the tip

110. The gripping surface of Kelly forceps has:

a. transverse grooves along its entire length
b. transverse grooves only near the tip
c. transverse grooves, with a tooth at the tip
d. longitudinal grooves, with cross grooves at the tip
e. longitudinal grooves along its entire length

111. Allis forceps are best used for grasping:

a. calculi
b. skin
c. bone
d. lung
e. fascia and subcutaneous tissues

112. When scrubbing one's hands before surgery, the recommended contact time with an antiseptic is:

a. 1 1/2-2 minutes
b. 6-8 minutes
c. 10-12 minutes
d. 3-5 minutes
e. 9 minutes

113. A nosocomial infection is one arising from the patient's:

a. bloodstream
b. environment
c. intestinal tract
d. skin
e. respiratory system

114. Which suture material is subject to rapid loss of strength when exposed to urine?

a. nylon
b. polyglycolic acid
c. silk
d. chromic catgut
e. polydioxanone

115. Concerning dry-to-dry wound dressings, which statement is most accurate?

a. They are applied dry and covered with a nonabsorptive intermediate layer and a nonporous outer bandage.
b. Their excellent absorptive capacity causes necrotic tissue and foreign material to adhere to them.
c. They should be left in place for 5 days and removed only after the exudative phase of healing.
d. They should be soaked in 0.05% chlorhexidine before application to the wound.
e. A major advantage is that they cause no pain on removal.

Answers

1. **c** The instrument is named for its function of retracting organs and tissues out of the way.
2. **d** None of the other instruments listed has opposing jaws.
3. **c** Declawing involves removal (-ectomy) of the nails or claws (onych-).
4. **d** A tapered-point needle easily passes through soft organs, making a tunnel through which the suture material is drawn.
5. **c** The half-circle needle offers the best compromise of shape, allowing use in both shallow and deep incisions.

6. **a** A proptosed eye must be returned to the eye socket quickly so as to prevent permanent damage to the eye.

7. **a** The basic requirements for healing by first intention are minimal tissue damage and apposition of the edges of the wound, usually with sutures.

8. **d** The basic functional unit of the nervous system, the neuron, is incapable of reproduction, so damage to the nervous system is often repaired by scar tissue. The other organs and tissues listed have excellent healing potential.

9. **a** Debridement of a wound facilitates healing by minimizing the amount of inflammation necessary before filling of the defect can begin.

10. **e** The xiphoid process and umbilicus are both on the animal's ventral midline.

11. **d** An electric drill would be damaged or inadequately sterilized by any of the other methods.

12. **a** Steam sterilization in an autoclave is most commonly used for instruments and equipment not damaged by moisture or heat.

13. **e** The sharp edges of scissors are dulled by steam in an autoclave. Boiling and dry heat are not sufficiently effective. The expense and hazards of ethylene oxide are not warranted.

14. **a** The minimal standard for sterilization of surgical instruments in an autoclave is 121 C (250 F) for at least 15 minutes.

15. **c** Chemical autoclave indicators are the only type listed that can give immediate information on all 3 basic criteria for autoclave sterilization (presence of steam at the proper combination of exposure time and temperature).

16. **a** Microorganisms in a wound during surgery are considered contaminants until, or unless, they multiply and cause damage.

17. **d** A surgical mask does not come in contact with anything sterile during a surgical procedure, so it need only be clean.

18. **e** An autoclave sterilizes by exposing packs to steam under pressure.

19. **d** A #40 clipper blade is a "surgical" blade. It clips the hair off at the skin surface.

20. **b** Numbered suture sizes (*eg*, #2) decrease in size as the number gets smaller, down to size 0. From that point on the sizes get smaller as the number of 0s (or the number in front of the 0) increases.

21. **d** All of the other suture materials listed are either braided or twisted and have the potential for considerable capillary action.

22. **e** Surgical gut is absorbed by the body.

23. **e** Treatment with chromic acid delays absorption of surgical gut by the body.

24. **b** Curettage involves the scraping of a tissue or cavity.

25. **e** Use of overly large suture material would not cause a wound to dehisce. It would actually provide greater holding power than smaller suture material.

26. **b** Contaminated items appear identical to sterile items. If there is any doubt about the sterility of an item, it must be considered contaminated.

27. **e** All of the other patterns are inverting or appositional.

28. **b** The other patterns are inverting (mattress patterns), appositional (simple pattern) or used only to close off an orifice (pursestring).

29. **c** All of the other choices promote increased scarring or early disruption of the wound.

30. **b** Exuberant granulation tissue (proud flesh) acts to block wound healing and epithelial regeneration. The other choices would likely enhance wound healing.

31. **d** One of the most important characteristics of wound healing by first intention is approximation of the wound edges.

32. **e** The ventral midline approach to the abdomen gives the most extensive access to the abdominal cavity.

33. **a** Slight elevation of body temperature for 1-2 days is normal after major surgery. The other choices are all early indicators of wound dehiscence.

34. **e** Prevention of surgical wound contamination is the whole purpose of aseptic technique in the operating room.

35. **a** This is the only choice that can be influenced by aseptic technique. The others are inherent to the patient, the surgical procedure being performed, or the microorganisms in the environment.

36. **a** The antimicrobial effect of a surgical scrub depends on sufficient exposure of the skin to the soap, as well as the scrubbing action that loosens dead skin and debris, and works the soap down into the cracks and crevices of the skin.

37. **d** Hexachlorophene forms a bacteriostatic film on the skin if used exclusively to wash the hands and arms. Other soaps remove the protective film.

38. **a** The surgical cap does not come in contact with tissues of the patient directly or indirectly, so it need only be clean, not sterile.

39. **c** Liquid chemical sterilization does not dull sharp edges.

40. **e** Warming the solution accelerates the chemical reactions necessary to kill microorganisms.

41. **a** The relative size of the wire, as measured by gauge, is inversely proportional to the gauge number. For example, 40-gauge wire is smaller than 32-gauge wire.

42. **e** Cloth and paper drapes are subject to capillary action. Plastic drapes are not.

43. **e** From largest to smallest, these sizes are ranked as follows: #4, #3, #1, 2-0 and 4-0. 3-0 is midway in size between 2-0 and 4-0.

44. **e** All of the other suture materials listed are nonabsorbable.

45. **d** Steam dulls the sharp edges of scissors.

46. **b** Elective surgery is done by choice, so it can be performed when conditions are most appropriate.

47. **b** The other listed solutions are irritating to the tissues or are not isotonic with the patient's tissue fluids.

48. **e** The ventral midline approach provides the most extensive access to the abdominal cavity.

49. **b** Incisions in viscera are best closed with inverting suture patterns. The other listed patterns are everting, appositional or inappropriate for wound closure.

50. **e** All personnel in the operating room should face toward sterile fields so they are aware of their relationship to them.

51. **a** Dehiscence of all layers of the body wall exposes abdominal viscera. Repair must be immediate to prevent serious damage to abdominal structures.

52. **d** Inflammation results from any insult to the body, whether intentional (surgical) or unintentional (traumatic, infectious). Increased blood supply to an inflamed area produces the increased warmth of the area. Good surgical technique minimizes inflammation but does not eliminate it.

53. **b** It takes 4-6 days for production of collagen strands in a wound to reach a significant level. Until that time, the wound is held together by sutures.

54. **c** Wound contraction represents movement of the entire thickness of the skin toward the center of the wound.

55. **a** All of the other choices are incorrect.

56. **d** All of the other choices are smaller.

57. **c** All of the other choices are from natural sources.

58. **a** A patient in shock would show rapid, shallow breathing in an effort to oxygenate the blood as rapidly as possible.

59. **a** The Cushing pattern is the only one listed that is an inverting pattern appropriate for closure of a hollow organ.

60. **d** Suture material acts as a physical irritant until it is absorbed, removed, or encapsulated with scar tissue.

61. **b** Unless very large or ruptured, postoperative seromas are unsightly but of little other importance to the animal's health.

62. **d** The simple pattern is an appositional pattern. It brings the incision edges together without inverting or everting them.

63. **a** Bone has excellent healing capacities, provided the fracture fragments are properly aligned and movement is kept to a minimum.

64. **b** Bluish-purple wound edges indicate that blood vessels in and under the skin are congested with blood.

65. **b** None of the other approaches is appropriate for a standing animal.

66. **e** This is the only portion of a surgical gown that is considered sterile during surgery.

67. **e** The vegetative bacterial form is the actively feeding, growing, reproducing form. It is most easily destroyed by common sterilization and disinfection methods.

68. **c** Inflammation is the first step in wound healing. It "cleans up" the damage so the defect can be repaired by the balance of the healing process.

69. **e** Other than sutures, a surgical wound has no appreciable strength until significant numbers of collagen fibers are produced at about 4-6 days.

70. **c** Before 7 days, the wound may not have enough strength to resist separation. After 10 days, inflammatory reaction to the suture material may cause significant scarring.

71. **e** The suffix -otomy means to make an incision into something.

72. **a** The suffix -ectomy means to surgically remove something.

73. **b** The suffix -pexy means to fix something in place.

74. **d** The suffix -ostomy means to create an artificial opening in an organ or tissue.

75. **e** The linea alba, on the ventral midline of the abdominal muscle wall, is the tendinous attachment of the ventral abdominal muscles. One layer of sutures in this area effectively closes the whole thickness of the abdominal wall, after which the skin is closed.

76. **b** Anything outside the sterile zone in an operating room is considered contaminated.

77. **a** Nonscrubbed personnel should only touch things that are not sterile.

78. **b** Passing back to back prevents accidental contamination of the front, sterile portions of their gown.

79. **c** The hands of scrubbed personnel should always be held between waist level and shoulder level to help prevent inadvertent contamination. Clasping the hands, when not otherwise occupied, helps prevent fatigue from compromising the position of the hands and arms.

80. **b** Nonscrubbed personnel should never violate the sterile zone in which scrubbed personnel are working.

81. **b** The sterility of the pack contents would be destroyed if touched by a nonscrubbed person.

82. **a** Ethylene oxide gas is very flammable.

83. **d** A tapered-point needle easily passes through muscle, making a tunnel through which the suture material is drawn.

84. **c** A reverse-cutting needle cuts a tunnel through the tough tissue of a ligament that is less likely to tear through than the tunnel created by a standard (inside-curve) cutting needle. The other needle points would not easily pass through this tough tissue.

85. **d** A tapered-point needle easily passes through muscle, making a tunnel through which the suture material is drawn.

86. **c** Splenic rupture is a potentially life-threatening condition. If surgery is indicated, it must be performed immediately.

87. **b** Mattress suture patterns spread the tension created by each suture over a broad area and are less likely to tear out due to tension on the suture line.

88. **b** While important, a tumor that is not immediately life threatening can be removed when conditions are most favorable.

89. **d** Leaving skin sutures in place too long increases scarring but does not directly contribute to breakdown of the surgical wound.

90. **e** Wet saline dressings are useful to help debride wounds with extensive tissue damage. They absorb and remove inflammatory products from the wound.

91. **d** Redistribution of blood flow results in the pale mucous membranes, poor capillary refill and cold extremities seen in shock.

92. **d** The other suture materials listed are braided or twisted and can conduct fluid and microorganisms by capillary action from the surface of the skin to the deeper layers.

93. **e** Removal of the uterus may restore health, but it also precludes future breeding.

94. **c** A square knot is conveniently tied and provides a very secure knot.

95. **b** The principal action of cryosurgery is destruction of unwanted tissue by freezing. This leaves dead tissue that must be liquefied and removed by inflammation. Such areas must be monitored closely and kept clean, and frequently require bandaging.

96. **e** The strength of the scar that results from healing of a surgical skin wound never reaches that of the normal skin around it.

97. **d** After dead and damaged tisuse has been removed from a wound by inflammation, a bed

of granulation tissue, consisting primarily of collagen fibers and capillaries, must form on the floor of the wound so that the processes that reduce the size of the wound can begin.

98. **b** If the outside of the glove is touched by anything that is not sterile, including freshly scrubbed fingers, it becomes contaminated and must not be used for surgery.

99. **e** Packs placed vertically in the autoclave receive the best circulation of steam around their contents.

100. **b** The prefix cryo- means cold.

101. **a**

102. **e**

103. **c**

104. **d**

105. **a**

106. **b**

107. **a**

108. **c**

109. **a**

110. **b**

111. **e**

112. **d**

113. **b**

114. **b**

115. **b**

Notes

Notes

Section 32

Terminology

P.W. Pratt

Recommended Reading

Blood DC and Studdert VP: *Bailliere's Comprehensive Veterinary Dictionary.* Saunders, Philadelphia, 1989.

Cochran PE: *Guide to Veterinary Medical Terminology.* American Veterinary Publications, Goleta, CA, 1991.

Prendergast A: *Medical Terminology: A Text/Workbook.* 2nd ed. Addison-Wesley Publishing, Menlo Park, CA, 1983

Wroble EM: *Terminology for the Health Professions.* Lippincott, Philadelphia, 1982.

Practice answer sheet is on page 407.

Questions

For Questions 1 through 5, select the correct answer from the 5 choices below:

a. dys –
b. poly –
c. micro –
d. hydro –
e. cryo –

1. *Prefix meaning very small.*

2. *Prefix relating to use of ultra-cold liquids.*

3. *Prefix relating to water.*

4. *Prefix meaning impaired or difficult.*

5. *Prefix meaning too much, in excess, many, or multiple.*

For Questions 6 through 10, select the correct answer from the 5 choices below:

a. – phagia
b. – emia
c. – ectomy
d. – uria
e. – itis

6. *Suffix meaning inflammation of.*

7. *Suffix meaning excision or surgical removal of.*

8. *Suffix relating to ingestion or swallowing.*

9. *Suffix relating to urine or urination.*

10. *Suffix relating to blood or blood cells.*

Correct answers are on pages 338-339.

For Questions 11 through 15, select the correct answer from the 5 choices below:

a. – tomy
b. – stomy
c. – rrhaphy
d. – pexy
e. – plasty

11. *Suffix meaning to surgically repair by joining in a seam or by suturing together.*

12. *Suffix meaning to shape or surgically form.*

13. *Suffix meaning to surgically create a new opening in a hollow organ, connecting it to the outside of the body or to another hollow organ.*

14. *Suffix meaning to incise or cut into.*

15. *Suffix relating to surgical fixation by suturing.*

For Questions 16 through 20, select the correct answer from the 5 choices below:

a. – algia
b. – cele
c. – ectasia
d. – iasis
e. – pathy

16. *Suffix relating to pain.*

17. *Suffix relating to infestation or infection.*

18. *Suffix relating to dilation, expansion or distention.*

19. *Suffix relating to a disorder or disease condition.*

20. *Suffix relating to a swelling, especially one with a cavity or associated with a hernia.*

For Questions 21 through 25, select the correct answer from the 5 choices below:

a. an –
b. brady –
c. contra –
d. hypo –
e. pyo –

21. *Prefix meaning against or opposed.*

22. *Prefix meaning insufficient or abnormally low.*

23. *Prefix meaning without or not having.*

24. *Prefix meaning abnormally slow.*

25. *Prefix relating to pus.*

For Questions 26 through 30, select the correct answer from the 5 choices below:

a. salpingo –
b. phlebo –
c. orchi –
d. hystero –
e. episio –

26. *Combining form relating to the uterus.*

27. *Combining form relating to veins.*

28. *Combining form relating to the vulva.*

29. *Combining form relating to the oviducts.*

30. *Combining form relating to the testes.*

For Questions 31 through 35, select the correct answer from the 5 choices below:

a. costo –
b. adipo –
c. myringo –
d. gnatho –
e. chordo –

31. Combining form relating to fat.

32. Combining form relating to the jaw.

33. Combining form relating to the spinal cord.

34. Combining form relating to the ribs.

35. Combining form relating to the eardrum.

For Questions 36 through 40, select the correct answer from the 5 choices below:

a. histo –
b. syndesmo –
c. spondylo –
d. pilo –
e. onycho –

36. Combining form relating to the claw or hoof.

37. Combining form relating to hair.

38. Combining form relating to ligaments or connective tissue.

39. Combining form relating to tissue.

40. Combining form relating to the vertebrae or spinal column.

For Questions 41 through 45, select the correct answer from the 5 choices below:

a. sclero –
b. megalo –
c. ankylo –
d. crypto –
e. litho –

41. Prefix meaning bent, looped or fused.

42. Prefix relating to a stone or calculus.

43. Prefix relating to hardening.

44. Prefix meaning hidden, concealed or a depression on a surface.

45. Prefix meaning abnormally large.

For Questions 46 through 50, select the correct answer from the 5 choices below:

a. – paresis
b. – lysis
c. – plasia
d. – plegia
e. – rrhexis

46. Suffix relating to paralysis.

47. Suffix relating to destruction of.

48. Suffix meaning rupture.

49. Suffix relating to weakness or partial paralysis.

50. Suffix relating to development or cell numbers.

Correct answers are on pages 338-339.

For Questions 51 through 55, select the correct answer from the 5 choices below:

a. mesial
b. axial
c. supine
d. sagittal
e. oblique

51. *In dorsal recumbency.*

52. *On a plane parallel to the median plane.*

53. *Contact surface of a tooth, closest to the midline of the dental arcade.*

54. *Pertaining to or situated near a longitudinal line about which a body or structure would rotate.*

55. *On a plane not parallel to 1 of the 3 major directional axes.*

For Questions 56 through 60, select the correct answer from the 5 choices below:

a. amb –
b. ecto –
c. para –
d. meta –
e. infra –

56. *Prefix meaning outer or on the outside.*

57. *Prefix meaning beneath or below.*

58. *Prefix meaning both or on both sides.*

59. *Prefix meaning beside, beyond, accessory to, or apart from.*

60. *Prefix meaning change, exchange or transformation.*

For Questions 61 through 65, select the correct answer from the 5 choices below:

a. *Streptobacillus*
b. *Staphylococcus*
c. *Bacillus*
d. *Streptococcus*
e. *Diplococcus*

61. *Spherical bacterium found in pairs.*

62. *Rod-shaped bacterium found singly or in chains that are not twisted.*

63. *Spherical bacterium found grouped in clusters or bunches.*

64. *Rod-shaped bacterium found grouped in twisted chains.*

65. *Spherical bacterium found grouped in chains.*

For Questions 66 through 70, select the correct answer from the 5 choices below:

a. chloro –
b. leuko –
c. cyano –
d. melano –
e. xantho –

66. *Prefix relating to the color blue.*

67. *Prefix relating to the color yellow.*

68. *Prefix relating to the color green.*

69. *Prefix relating to the color white.*

70. *Prefix relating to the color black.*

For Questions 71 through 75, select the correct answer from the 5 choices below:

a. picornavirus
b. rotavirus
c. papovavirus
d. oncornavirus
e. coronavirus

71. *Virus resembling a wheel.*

72. *RNA virus that causes neoplasia.*

73. *Small RNA virus.*

74. *Virus that causes papillomas, poliomas and vacuolization.*

75. *Virus resembling a crown.*

For Questions 76 through 80, select the correct answer from the 5 choices below:

a. intra –
b. syn –
c. toco –
d. amblyo –
e. aniso –

76. *Prefix meaning together, union or in association with.*

77. *Prefix meaning within or inside.*

78. *Prefix meaning unequal or dissimilar.*

79. *Prefix meaning dull, dim or not clear.*

80. *Prefix relating to birth.*

For Questions 81 through 85, select the correct answer from the 5 choices below:

a. prn
b. qd
c. qh
d. od
e. qid

81. *In prescriptions and medical records, the abbreviation meaning every day.*

82. *In prescriptions and medical records, the abbreviation meaning 4 times a day.*

83. *In prescriptions and medical records, the abbreviation meaning right eye.*

84. *In prescriptions and medical records, the abbreviation meaning every hour.*

85. *In prescriptions and medical records, the abbreviation meaning as needed.*

For Questions 86 through 90, select the correct answer from the 5 choices below:

a. $\leq$
b. μ
c. $\propto$
d. γ
e. $>$

86. *Symbol meaning gamma.*

87. *Symbol meaning less than or equal to.*

88. *Symbol meaning micron.*

89. *Symbol meaning greater than.*

90. *Symbol meaning proportional to.*

Correct answers are on pages 338-339.

For Questions 91 through 95, select the correct answer from the 5 choices below:

a. dacryo –
b. kerato –
c. oligo –
d. dactylo –
e. xero –

91. *Combining form meaning dry.*

92. *Combining form relating to the digits or toes.*

93. *Combining form relating to tears or the lacrimal gland.*

94. *Combining form meaning few or scanty.*

95. *Combining form relating to horny tissue or the cornea.*

For Questions 96 through 100, select the correct answer from the 5 choices below:

a. lavage
b. phytobezoar
c. scoliosis
d. petechia
e. morbidity

96. *A concretion or solid mass of vegetable matter found in the stomach or intestine.*

97. *Lateral deviation of the spine.*

98. *A pinpoint, circular hemorrhage on the skin or on a serosal surface.*

99. *To irrigate or flush out an organ or cavity.*

100. *The proportion of sick animals to healthy animals in a population.*

Answers

1. **c**
2. **e**
3. **d**
4. **a**
5. **b**
6. **e**
7. **c**
8. **a**
9. **d**
10. **b**
11. **c**
12. **e**
13. **b**
14. **a**
15. **d**
16. **a**
17. **d**
18. **c**
19. **e**
20. **b**
21. **c**
22. **d**
23. **a**
24. **b**
25. **e**
26. **d**
27. **b**
28. **e**
29. **a**
30. **c**

31. **b**
32. **d**
33. **e**
34. **a**
35. **c**
36. **e**
37. **d**
38. **b**
39. **a**
40. **c**
41. **c**
42. **e**
43. **a**
44. **d**
45. **b**
46. **d**
47. **b**
48. **e**
49. **a**
50. **c**
51. **c**
52. **d**
53. **a**
54. **b**
55. **e**
56. **b**
57. **e**
58. **a**
59. **c**
60. **d**
61. **e**
62. **c**
63. **b**
64. **a**
65. **d**
66. **c**
67. **e**
68. **a**
69. **b**
70. **d**
71. **b**
72. **d**
73. **a**
74. **c**
75. **e**
76. **b**
77. **a**
78. **e**
79. **d**
80. **c**
81. **b**
82. **e**
83. **d**
84. **c**
85. **a**
86. **d**
87. **a**
88. **b**
89. **e**
90. **c**
91. **e**
92. **d**
93. **a**
94. **c**
95. **b**
96. **b**
97. **c**
98. **d**
99. **a**
100. **e**

Notes

Section 33

Toxicology

G.D. Osweiler

Recommended Reading

Beasley VR *et al: A Systems Affected Approach to Small Animal Toxicology.* Univ Illinois, Coll Vet Med, Urbana, IL, 1990.

Beasley VR: Toxicology of selected pesticides, drugs and chemicals. *Vet Clin No Am* (Small Anim Pract) 20:283-563, 1990.

Blood DC and Radostits OM: *Veterinary Medicine.* Balliere Tindall, Philadelphia, 1989.

Fraser: *Merck Veterinary Manual.* 7th ed. Merck, Rahway, NJ, 1991.

Hatch RC, in Booth NH and McDonald LE: *Veterinary Pharmacology and Therapeutics.* 6th ed. Iowa State Univ, Ames, 1991.

Howard JL: *Current Veterinary Therapy: Food Animal Practice 3.* Saunders, Philadelphia, 1992.

Kirk RW: *Current Veterinary Therapy X: Small Animal Practice.* Saunders, Philadelphia, 1989.

Morgan RB: *Handbook of Small Animal Practice.* 2nd ed. Churchill Livingstone, New York, 1992.

Osweiler GD *et al: Clinical and Diagnostic Veterinary Toxicology.* 3rd ed. Kendall-Hunt, Dubuque, IA, 1985.

Practice answer sheet is on page 409.

Questions

1. *A concentration of 0.01% is equivalent to how many parts per million (ppm)?*
   a. 1 ppm
   b. 10 ppm
   c. 100 ppm
   d. 1,000 ppm
   e. 10,000 ppm

2. *Which category of insecticidal compounds presents a problem of persistent residues in fatty tissues of animals?*
   a. carbamates
   b. organochlorines
   c. organophosphates
   d. pyrethrins
   e. juvenile hormones

3. *If acute organophosphate insecticide poisoning is suspected, an appropriate sample from a live animal for initial diagnostic testing is:*
   a. serum
   b. whole blood
   c. urine
   d. stomach contents
   e. fat biopsy

Correct answers are on page 343.

For Questions 4 through 8, select the correct answer from the 5 choices below.

a. anticoagulant rodenticides
b. strychnine
c. cholecalciferol
d. bromethalin
e. sodium fluoroacetate

4. *No longer legal to use because of high toxicity to dogs and probability of secondary or relay toxicosis.*

5. *Can cause acute tetanic seizures, with marked hyperesthesia, hyperreflexia and death from respiratory muscle failure.*

6. *Can cause acute to chronic neurologic signs by altering central nervous system fluid balance, leading to cerebral edema.*

7. *Clinical signs may be delayed for 1-2 days after exposure, regardless of dosage.*

8. *Can cause acute renal damage, hypercalcemia and tissue mineralization.*

For Questions 9 through 13, select the correct answer from the 5 choices below.

a. acetaminophen
b. aspirin
c. ibuprofen
d. caffeine
e. amphetamine

9. *Central nervous system stimulant used for appetite suppression and mood elevation.*

10. *1 or 2 350-mg tablets can cause methemoglobinemia, facial edema and hepatic damage.*

11. *Chronic use or excessive short-term use causes gastric ulcers, vomiting, depression, anorexia and toxic hepatitis. More toxic to cats than to dogs.*

12. *Can cause acute central nervous system stimulation, with hyperreflexia, tonic seizures, tachycardia, polypnea and hyperthermia.*

13. *Acute toxicosis causes oliguria, renal papillary necrosis and uremia. Chronic overuse may cause gastric ulcers in dogs.*

For Questions 14 through 18, select the correct answer from the 5 choices below.

a. Japanese yew
b. red maple
c. redroot pigweed
d. white snakeroot
e. *Crotalaria*

14. *Ornamental evergreen shrub with an acute cardiotoxic principle that causes sudden death in horses and cattle.*

15. *Nitrate-accumulating plant common in gardens, crop fields and feedlots. Causes acute toxic tubular nephrosis with perirenal edema and ascites in swine and cattle.*

16. *Causes acute hemolytic anemia in horses.*

17. *Causes tremors and myocardial damage in grazing horses. Passed in the milk of lactating animals.*

18. *Its seeds contaminate small grains. Causes acute to chronic liver and pulmonary damage, especially in swine and poultry.*

19. *Bone is the site of long-term storage of:*

a. arsenic
b. copper
c. iron
d. lead
e. mercury

20. Overheated Teflon-coated frying pans release vapors that are especially toxic to:

a. cats
b. dogs
c. gerbils
d. parakeets
e. reptiles

Answers

1. **c** Convert % to ppm by moving the decimal point 4 places to the right.
2. **b** Chlorinated hydrocarbon insecticides are highly lipophilic.
3. **b** Cholinesterase activity is most concentrated in red blood cells.
4. **e** Fluoroacetate is more toxic to dogs than to rodents.
5. **b** Signs are due to suppression of inhibitory interneurons in the spinal reflex arc.
6. **d** Bromethalin affects Na-K ATPase, leading to loss of cellular fluid control.
7. **a** Clinical signs do not appear until coagulation factors are depleted.
8. **c** Acute tissue damage is followed by mineralization when vitamin D rodenticides are consumed.
9. **e** Amphetamines are commonly used in people. At high dosages, nervous signs predominate.
10. **a** These effects are especially predominant in cats.
11. **b** Aspirin should be used at the recommended dosages in animals, especially in cats.
12. **d** Methylxanthine alkaloids (caffeine, theobromine) are hazardous to dogs.
13. **c** Large doses of nonsteroidal antiinflammatory drugs may induce toxicosis after several days' exposure.
14. **a** Japanese yew is a common cause of toxicosis in horses and cattle, and is also toxic to dogs.
15. **c** The toxic principle causing nephrosis has not been defined, but lesions are similar to those seen in oak (acorn) toxicosis.
16. **b** It causes early oxidant damage and Heinz body formation in red blood cells.
17. **d** This plant is hazardous both to adult animals and to nursing foals or calves.
18. **e** It contains high concentrations of pyrrolizidine alkaloids, which cause liver damage.
19. **d** Lead is stored in an inactive form, except in growing animals, in which metaphyses may be affected.
20. **d** Teflon fumes sensitize the budgerigar's heart to epinephrine and endogenous catecholamines.

Notes

Practice Answer Sheet

Section 1

Anatomy

Fill in a circled letter to indicate your answer choice.

1. ⓐ ⓑ ⓒ ⓓ ⓔ	25. ⓐ ⓑ ⓒ ⓓ ⓔ	49. ⓐ ⓑ ⓒ ⓓ ⓔ	73. ⓐ ⓑ ⓒ ⓓ ⓔ
2. ⓐ ⓑ ⓒ ⓓ ⓔ	26. ⓐ ⓑ ⓒ ⓓ ⓔ	50. ⓐ ⓑ ⓒ ⓓ ⓔ	74. ⓐ ⓑ ⓒ ⓓ ⓔ
3. ⓐ ⓑ ⓒ ⓓ ⓔ	27. ⓐ ⓑ ⓒ ⓓ ⓔ	51. ⓐ ⓑ ⓒ ⓓ ⓔ	75. ⓐ ⓑ ⓒ ⓓ ⓔ
4. ⓐ ⓑ ⓒ ⓓ ⓔ	28. ⓐ ⓑ ⓒ ⓓ ⓔ	52. ⓐ ⓑ ⓒ ⓓ ⓔ	76. ⓐ ⓑ ⓒ ⓓ ⓔ
5. ⓐ ⓑ ⓒ ⓓ ⓔ	29. ⓐ ⓑ ⓒ ⓓ ⓔ	53. ⓐ ⓑ ⓒ ⓓ ⓔ	77. ⓐ ⓑ ⓒ ⓓ ⓔ
6. ⓐ ⓑ ⓒ ⓓ ⓔ	30. ⓐ ⓑ ⓒ ⓓ ⓔ	54. ⓐ ⓑ ⓒ ⓓ ⓔ	78. ⓐ ⓑ ⓒ ⓓ ⓔ
7. ⓐ ⓑ ⓒ ⓓ ⓔ	31. ⓐ ⓑ ⓒ ⓓ ⓔ	55. ⓐ ⓑ ⓒ ⓓ ⓔ	79. ⓐ ⓑ ⓒ ⓓ ⓔ
8. ⓐ ⓑ ⓒ ⓓ ⓔ	32. ⓐ ⓑ ⓒ ⓓ ⓔ	56. ⓐ ⓑ ⓒ ⓓ ⓔ	80. ⓐ ⓑ ⓒ ⓓ ⓔ
9. ⓐ ⓑ ⓒ ⓓ ⓔ	33. ⓐ ⓑ ⓒ ⓓ ⓔ	57. ⓐ ⓑ ⓒ ⓓ ⓔ	81. ⓐ ⓑ ⓒ ⓓ ⓔ
10. ⓐ ⓑ ⓒ ⓓ ⓔ	34. ⓐ ⓑ ⓒ ⓓ ⓔ	58. ⓐ ⓑ ⓒ ⓓ ⓔ	82. ⓐ ⓑ ⓒ ⓓ ⓔ
11. ⓐ ⓑ ⓒ ⓓ ⓔ	35. ⓐ ⓑ ⓒ ⓓ ⓔ	59. ⓐ ⓑ ⓒ ⓓ ⓔ	83. ⓐ ⓑ ⓒ ⓓ ⓔ
12. ⓐ ⓑ ⓒ ⓓ ⓔ	36. ⓐ ⓑ ⓒ ⓓ ⓔ	60. ⓐ ⓑ ⓒ ⓓ ⓔ	84. ⓐ ⓑ ⓒ ⓓ ⓔ
13. ⓐ ⓑ ⓒ ⓓ ⓔ	37. ⓐ ⓑ ⓒ ⓓ ⓔ	61. ⓐ ⓑ ⓒ ⓓ ⓔ	85. ⓐ ⓑ ⓒ ⓓ ⓔ
14. ⓐ ⓑ ⓒ ⓓ ⓔ	38. ⓐ ⓑ ⓒ ⓓ ⓔ	62. ⓐ ⓑ ⓒ ⓓ ⓔ	86. ⓐ ⓑ ⓒ ⓓ ⓔ
15. ⓐ ⓑ ⓒ ⓓ ⓔ	39. ⓐ ⓑ ⓒ ⓓ ⓔ	63. ⓐ ⓑ ⓒ ⓓ ⓔ	87. ⓐ ⓑ ⓒ ⓓ ⓔ
16. ⓐ ⓑ ⓒ ⓓ ⓔ	40. ⓐ ⓑ ⓒ ⓓ ⓔ	64. ⓐ ⓑ ⓒ ⓓ ⓔ	88. ⓐ ⓑ ⓒ ⓓ ⓔ
17. ⓐ ⓑ ⓒ ⓓ ⓔ	41. ⓐ ⓑ ⓒ ⓓ ⓔ	65. ⓐ ⓑ ⓒ ⓓ ⓔ	89. ⓐ ⓑ ⓒ ⓓ ⓔ
18. ⓐ ⓑ ⓒ ⓓ ⓔ	42. ⓐ ⓑ ⓒ ⓓ ⓔ	66. ⓐ ⓑ ⓒ ⓓ ⓔ	90. ⓐ ⓑ ⓒ ⓓ ⓔ
19. ⓐ ⓑ ⓒ ⓓ ⓔ	43. ⓐ ⓑ ⓒ ⓓ ⓔ	67. ⓐ ⓑ ⓒ ⓓ ⓔ	
20. ⓐ ⓑ ⓒ ⓓ ⓔ	44. ⓐ ⓑ ⓒ ⓓ ⓔ	68. ⓐ ⓑ ⓒ ⓓ ⓔ	
21. ⓐ ⓑ ⓒ ⓓ ⓔ	45. ⓐ ⓑ ⓒ ⓓ ⓔ	69. ⓐ ⓑ ⓒ ⓓ ⓔ	
22. ⓐ ⓑ ⓒ ⓓ ⓔ	46. ⓐ ⓑ ⓒ ⓓ ⓔ	70. ⓐ ⓑ ⓒ ⓓ ⓔ	
23. ⓐ ⓑ ⓒ ⓓ ⓔ	47. ⓐ ⓑ ⓒ ⓓ ⓔ	71. ⓐ ⓑ ⓒ ⓓ ⓔ	
24. ⓐ ⓑ ⓒ ⓓ ⓔ	48. ⓐ ⓑ ⓒ ⓓ ⓔ	72. ⓐ ⓑ ⓒ ⓓ ⓔ	

This page intentionally left blank.

Practice Answer Sheet

Section 5

Care of Cage/Aviary Birds

Fill in a circled letter to indicate your answer choice.

1. ⓐ ⓑ ⓒ ⓓ ⓔ	17. ⓐ ⓑ ⓒ ⓓ ⓔ	33. ⓐ ⓑ ⓒ ⓓ ⓔ	49. ⓐ ⓑ ⓒ ⓓ ⓔ
2. ⓐ ⓑ ⓒ ⓓ ⓔ	18. ⓐ ⓑ ⓒ ⓓ ⓔ	34. ⓐ ⓑ ⓒ ⓓ ⓔ	50. ⓐ ⓑ ⓒ ⓓ ⓔ
3. ⓐ ⓑ ⓒ ⓓ ⓔ	19. ⓐ ⓑ ⓒ ⓓ ⓔ	35. ⓐ ⓑ ⓒ ⓓ ⓔ	51. ⓐ ⓑ ⓒ ⓓ ⓔ
4. ⓐ ⓑ ⓒ ⓓ ⓔ	20. ⓐ ⓑ ⓒ ⓓ ⓔ	36. ⓐ ⓑ ⓒ ⓓ ⓔ	52. ⓐ ⓑ ⓒ ⓓ ⓔ
5. ⓐ ⓑ ⓒ ⓓ ⓔ	21. ⓐ ⓑ ⓒ ⓓ ⓔ	37. ⓐ ⓑ ⓒ ⓓ ⓔ	53. ⓐ ⓑ ⓒ ⓓ ⓔ
6. ⓐ ⓑ ⓒ ⓓ ⓔ	22. ⓐ ⓑ ⓒ ⓓ ⓔ	38. ⓐ ⓑ ⓒ ⓓ ⓔ	54. ⓐ ⓑ ⓒ ⓓ ⓔ
7. ⓐ ⓑ ⓒ ⓓ ⓔ	23. ⓐ ⓑ ⓒ ⓓ ⓔ	39. ⓐ ⓑ ⓒ ⓓ ⓔ	55. ⓐ ⓑ ⓒ ⓓ ⓔ
8. ⓐ ⓑ ⓒ ⓓ ⓔ	24. ⓐ ⓑ ⓒ ⓓ ⓔ	40. ⓐ ⓑ ⓒ ⓓ ⓔ	56. ⓐ ⓑ ⓒ ⓓ ⓔ
9. ⓐ ⓑ ⓒ ⓓ ⓔ	25. ⓐ ⓑ ⓒ ⓓ ⓔ	41. ⓐ ⓑ ⓒ ⓓ ⓔ	57. ⓐ ⓑ ⓒ ⓓ ⓔ
10. ⓐ ⓑ ⓒ ⓓ ⓔ	26. ⓐ ⓑ ⓒ ⓓ ⓔ	42. ⓐ ⓑ ⓒ ⓓ ⓔ	58. ⓐ ⓑ ⓒ ⓓ ⓔ
11. ⓐ ⓑ ⓒ ⓓ ⓔ	27. ⓐ ⓑ ⓒ ⓓ ⓔ	43. ⓐ ⓑ ⓒ ⓓ ⓔ	59. ⓐ ⓑ ⓒ ⓓ ⓔ
12. ⓐ ⓑ ⓒ ⓓ ⓔ	28. ⓐ ⓑ ⓒ ⓓ ⓔ	44. ⓐ ⓑ ⓒ ⓓ ⓔ	60. ⓐ ⓑ ⓒ ⓓ ⓔ
13. ⓐ ⓑ ⓒ ⓓ ⓔ	29. ⓐ ⓑ ⓒ ⓓ ⓔ	45. ⓐ ⓑ ⓒ ⓓ ⓔ	
14. ⓐ ⓑ ⓒ ⓓ ⓔ	30. ⓐ ⓑ ⓒ ⓓ ⓔ	46. ⓐ ⓑ ⓒ ⓓ ⓔ	
15. ⓐ ⓑ ⓒ ⓓ ⓔ	31. ⓐ ⓑ ⓒ ⓓ ⓔ	47. ⓐ ⓑ ⓒ ⓓ ⓔ	
16. ⓐ ⓑ ⓒ ⓓ ⓔ	32. ⓐ ⓑ ⓒ ⓓ ⓔ	48. ⓐ ⓑ ⓒ ⓓ ⓔ	

This page intentionally left blank.

Practice Answer Sheet

Section 6

Care of Food Animals

Fill in a circled letter to indicate your answer choice.

1. ⓐ ⓑ ⓒ ⓓ ⓔ
2. ⓐ ⓑ ⓒ ⓓ ⓔ
3. ⓐ ⓑ ⓒ ⓓ ⓔ
4. ⓐ ⓑ ⓒ ⓓ ⓔ
5. ⓐ ⓑ ⓒ ⓓ ⓔ
6. ⓐ ⓑ ⓒ ⓓ ⓔ
7. ⓐ ⓑ ⓒ ⓓ ⓔ
8. ⓐ ⓑ ⓒ ⓓ ⓔ
9. ⓐ ⓑ ⓒ ⓓ ⓔ
10. ⓐ ⓑ ⓒ ⓓ ⓔ
11. ⓐ ⓑ ⓒ ⓓ ⓔ
12. ⓐ ⓑ ⓒ ⓓ ⓔ
13. ⓐ ⓑ ⓒ ⓓ ⓔ
14. ⓐ ⓑ ⓒ ⓓ ⓔ
15. ⓐ ⓑ ⓒ ⓓ ⓔ
16. ⓐ ⓑ ⓒ ⓓ ⓔ
17. ⓐ ⓑ ⓒ ⓓ ⓔ
18. ⓐ ⓑ ⓒ ⓓ ⓔ
19. ⓐ ⓑ ⓒ ⓓ ⓔ
20. ⓐ ⓑ ⓒ ⓓ ⓔ
21. ⓐ ⓑ ⓒ ⓓ ⓔ
22. ⓐ ⓑ ⓒ ⓓ ⓔ
23. ⓐ ⓑ ⓒ ⓓ ⓔ
24. ⓐ ⓑ ⓒ ⓓ ⓔ
25. ⓐ ⓑ ⓒ ⓓ ⓔ
26. ⓐ ⓑ ⓒ ⓓ ⓔ
27. ⓐ ⓑ ⓒ ⓓ ⓔ
28. ⓐ ⓑ ⓒ ⓓ ⓔ
29. ⓐ ⓑ ⓒ ⓓ ⓔ
30. ⓐ ⓑ ⓒ ⓓ ⓔ
31. ⓐ ⓑ ⓒ ⓓ ⓔ
32. ⓐ ⓑ ⓒ ⓓ ⓔ
33. ⓐ ⓑ ⓒ ⓓ ⓔ
34. ⓐ ⓑ ⓒ ⓓ ⓔ
35. ⓐ ⓑ ⓒ ⓓ ⓔ
36. ⓐ ⓑ ⓒ ⓓ ⓔ
37. ⓐ ⓑ ⓒ ⓓ ⓔ
38. ⓐ ⓑ ⓒ ⓓ ⓔ
39. ⓐ ⓑ ⓒ ⓓ ⓔ
40. ⓐ ⓑ ⓒ ⓓ ⓔ
41. ⓐ ⓑ ⓒ ⓓ ⓔ
42. ⓐ ⓑ ⓒ ⓓ ⓔ
43. ⓐ ⓑ ⓒ ⓓ ⓔ
44. ⓐ ⓑ ⓒ ⓓ ⓔ
45. ⓐ ⓑ ⓒ ⓓ ⓔ
46. ⓐ ⓑ ⓒ ⓓ ⓔ
47. ⓐ ⓑ ⓒ ⓓ ⓔ
48. ⓐ ⓑ ⓒ ⓓ ⓔ
49. ⓐ ⓑ ⓒ ⓓ ⓔ
50. ⓐ ⓑ ⓒ ⓓ ⓔ
51. ⓐ ⓑ ⓒ ⓓ ⓔ
52. ⓐ ⓑ ⓒ ⓓ ⓔ
53. ⓐ ⓑ ⓒ ⓓ ⓔ
54. ⓐ ⓑ ⓒ ⓓ ⓔ
55. ⓐ ⓑ ⓒ ⓓ ⓔ
56. ⓐ ⓑ ⓒ ⓓ ⓔ
57. ⓐ ⓑ ⓒ ⓓ ⓔ
58. ⓐ ⓑ ⓒ ⓓ ⓔ
59. ⓐ ⓑ ⓒ ⓓ ⓔ
60. ⓐ ⓑ ⓒ ⓓ ⓔ
61. ⓐ ⓑ ⓒ ⓓ ⓔ
62. ⓐ ⓑ ⓒ ⓓ ⓔ
63. ⓐ ⓑ ⓒ ⓓ ⓔ
64. ⓐ ⓑ ⓒ ⓓ ⓔ
65. ⓐ ⓑ ⓒ ⓓ ⓔ
66. ⓐ ⓑ ⓒ ⓓ ⓔ
67. ⓐ ⓑ ⓒ ⓓ ⓔ
68. ⓐ ⓑ ⓒ ⓓ ⓔ
69. ⓐ ⓑ ⓒ ⓓ ⓔ
70. ⓐ ⓑ ⓒ ⓓ ⓔ
71. ⓐ ⓑ ⓒ ⓓ ⓔ
72. ⓐ ⓑ ⓒ ⓓ ⓔ
73. ⓐ ⓑ ⓒ ⓓ ⓔ
74. ⓐ ⓑ ⓒ ⓓ ⓔ
75. ⓐ ⓑ ⓒ ⓓ ⓔ
76. ⓐ ⓑ ⓒ ⓓ ⓔ
77. ⓐ ⓑ ⓒ ⓓ ⓔ
78. ⓐ ⓑ ⓒ ⓓ ⓔ
79. ⓐ ⓑ ⓒ ⓓ ⓔ
80. ⓐ ⓑ ⓒ ⓓ ⓔ
81. ⓐ ⓑ ⓒ ⓓ ⓔ
82. ⓐ ⓑ ⓒ ⓓ ⓔ
83. ⓐ ⓑ ⓒ ⓓ ⓔ
84. ⓐ ⓑ ⓒ ⓓ ⓔ
85. ⓐ ⓑ ⓒ ⓓ ⓔ
86. ⓐ ⓑ ⓒ ⓓ ⓔ
87. ⓐ ⓑ ⓒ ⓓ ⓔ
88. ⓐ ⓑ ⓒ ⓓ ⓔ
89. ⓐ ⓑ ⓒ ⓓ ⓔ
90. ⓐ ⓑ ⓒ ⓓ ⓔ
91. ⓐ ⓑ ⓒ ⓓ ⓔ
92. ⓐ ⓑ ⓒ ⓓ ⓔ
93. ⓐ ⓑ ⓒ ⓓ ⓔ
94. ⓐ ⓑ ⓒ ⓓ ⓔ
95. ⓐ ⓑ ⓒ ⓓ ⓔ
96. ⓐ ⓑ ⓒ ⓓ ⓔ
97. ⓐ ⓑ ⓒ ⓓ ⓔ
98. ⓐ ⓑ ⓒ ⓓ ⓔ
99. ⓐ ⓑ ⓒ ⓓ ⓔ
100. ⓐ ⓑ ⓒ ⓓ ⓔ
101. ⓐ ⓑ ⓒ ⓓ ⓔ
102. ⓐ ⓑ ⓒ ⓓ ⓔ
103. ⓐ ⓑ ⓒ ⓓ ⓔ
104. ⓐ ⓑ ⓒ ⓓ ⓔ
105. ⓐ ⓑ ⓒ ⓓ ⓔ
106. ⓐ ⓑ ⓒ ⓓ ⓔ
107. ⓐ ⓑ ⓒ ⓓ ⓔ
108. ⓐ ⓑ ⓒ ⓓ ⓔ
109. ⓐ ⓑ ⓒ ⓓ ⓔ
110. ⓐ ⓑ ⓒ ⓓ ⓔ
111. ⓐ ⓑ ⓒ ⓓ ⓔ
112. ⓐ ⓑ ⓒ ⓓ ⓔ
113. ⓐ ⓑ ⓒ ⓓ ⓔ
114. ⓐ ⓑ ⓒ ⓓ ⓔ
115. ⓐ ⓑ ⓒ ⓓ ⓔ
116. ⓐ ⓑ ⓒ ⓓ ⓔ
117. ⓐ ⓑ ⓒ ⓓ ⓔ
118. ⓐ ⓑ ⓒ ⓓ ⓔ
119. ⓐ ⓑ ⓒ ⓓ ⓔ
120. ⓐ ⓑ ⓒ ⓓ ⓔ
121. ⓐ ⓑ ⓒ ⓓ ⓔ
122. ⓐ ⓑ ⓒ ⓓ ⓔ
123. ⓐ ⓑ ⓒ ⓓ ⓔ
124. ⓐ ⓑ ⓒ ⓓ ⓔ
125. ⓐ ⓑ ⓒ ⓓ ⓔ
126. ⓐ ⓑ ⓒ ⓓ ⓔ
127. ⓐ ⓑ ⓒ ⓓ ⓔ
128. ⓐ ⓑ ⓒ ⓓ ⓔ
129. ⓐ ⓑ ⓒ ⓓ ⓔ
130. ⓐ ⓑ ⓒ ⓓ ⓔ
131. ⓐ ⓑ ⓒ ⓓ ⓔ
132. ⓐ ⓑ ⓒ ⓓ ⓔ
133. ⓐ ⓑ ⓒ ⓓ ⓔ
134. ⓐ ⓑ ⓒ ⓓ ⓔ
135. ⓐ ⓑ ⓒ ⓓ ⓔ
136. ⓐ ⓑ ⓒ ⓓ ⓔ
137. ⓐ ⓑ ⓒ ⓓ ⓔ
138. ⓐ ⓑ ⓒ ⓓ ⓔ
139. ⓐ ⓑ ⓒ ⓓ ⓔ
140. ⓐ ⓑ ⓒ ⓓ ⓔ
141. ⓐ ⓑ ⓒ ⓓ ⓔ
142. ⓐ ⓑ ⓒ ⓓ ⓔ
143. ⓐ ⓑ ⓒ ⓓ ⓔ
144. ⓐ ⓑ ⓒ ⓓ ⓔ
145. ⓐ ⓑ ⓒ ⓓ ⓔ
146. ⓐ ⓑ ⓒ ⓓ ⓔ
147. ⓐ ⓑ ⓒ ⓓ ⓔ

This page intentionally left blank.

Practice Answer Sheet

Section 7

Care of Horses

Fill in a circled letter to indicate your answer choice.

1. (a) (b) (c) (d) (e)
2. (a) (b) (c) (d) (e)
3. (a) (b) (c) (d) (e)
4. (a) (b) (c) (d) (e)
5. (a) (b) (c) (d) (e)
6. (a) (b) (c) (d) (e)
7. (a) (b) (c) (d) (e)
8. (a) (b) (c) (d) (e)
9. (a) (b) (c) (d) (e)
10. (a) (b) (c) (d) (e)
11. (a) (b) (c) (d) (e)
12. (a) (b) (c) (d) (e)
13. (a) (b) (c) (d) (e)
14. (a) (b) (c) (d) (e)
15. (a) (b) (c) (d) (e)
16. (a) (b) (c) (d) (e)
17. (a) (b) (c) (d) (e)
18. (a) (b) (c) (d) (e)
19. (a) (b) (c) (d) (e)
20. (a) (b) (c) (d) (e)
21. (a) (b) (c) (d) (e)
22. (a) (b) (c) (d) (e)
23. (a) (b) (c) (d) (e)
24. (a) (b) (c) (d) (e)
25. (a) (b) (c) (d) (e)
26. (a) (b) (c) (d) (e)
27. (a) (b) (c) (d) (e)
28. (a) (b) (c) (d) (e)
29. (a) (b) (c) (d) (e)
30. (a) (b) (c) (d) (e)
31. (a) (b) (c) (d) (e)
32. (a) (b) (c) (d) (e)
33. (a) (b) (c) (d) (e)
34. (a) (b) (c) (d) (e)
35. (a) (b) (c) (d) (e)
36. (a) (b) (c) (d) (e)
37. (a) (b) (c) (d) (e)
38. (a) (b) (c) (d) (e)
39. (a) (b) (c) (d) (e)
40. (a) (b) (c) (d) (e)
41. (a) (b) (c) (d) (e)
42. (a) (b) (c) (d) (e)
43. (a) (b) (c) (d) (e)
44. (a) (b) (c) (d) (e)
45. (a) (b) (c) (d) (e)
46. (a) (b) (c) (d) (e)
47. (a) (b) (c) (d) (e)
48. (a) (b) (c) (d) (e)
49. (a) (b) (c) (d) (e)
50. (a) (b) (c) (d) (e)
51. (a) (b) (c) (d) (e)
52. (a) (b) (c) (d) (e)
53. (a) (b) (c) (d) (e)
54. (a) (b) (c) (d) (e)
55. (a) (b) (c) (d) (e)
56. (a) (b) (c) (d) (e)
57. (a) (b) (c) (d) (e)
58. (a) (b) (c) (d) (e)
59. (a) (b) (c) (d) (e)
60. (a) (b) (c) (d) (e)
61. (a) (b) (c) (d) (e)
62. (a) (b) (c) (d) (e)
63. (a) (b) (c) (d) (e)
64. (a) (b) (c) (d) (e)
65. (a) (b) (c) (d) (e)
66. (a) (b) (c) (d) (e)
67. (a) (b) (c) (d) (e)
68. (a) (b) (c) (d) (e)
69. (a) (b) (c) (d) (e)
70. (a) (b) (c) (d) (e)
71. (a) (b) (c) (d) (e)
72. (a) (b) (c) (d) (e)
73. (a) (b) (c) (d) (e)
74. (a) (b) (c) (d) (e)
75. (a) (b) (c) (d) (e)
76. (a) (b) (c) (d) (e)
77. (a) (b) (c) (d) (e)
78. (a) (b) (c) (d) (e)
79. (a) (b) (c) (d) (e)
80. (a) (b) (c) (d) (e)
81. (a) (b) (c) (d) (e)
82. (a) (b) (c) (d) (e)
83. (a) (b) (c) (d) (e)
84. (a) (b) (c) (d) (e)
85. (a) (b) (c) (d) (e)
86. (a) (b) (c) (d) (e)
87. (a) (b) (c) (d) (e)
88. (a) (b) (c) (d) (e)
89. (a) (b) (c) (d) (e)
90. (a) (b) (c) (d) (e)
91. (a) (b) (c) (d) (e)
92. (a) (b) (c) (d) (e)
93. (a) (b) (c) (d) (e)
94. (a) (b) (c) (d) (e)
95. (a) (b) (c) (d) (e)
96. (a) (b) (c) (d) (e)
97. (a) (b) (c) (d) (e)
98. (a) (b) (c) (d) (e)
99. (a) (b) (c) (d) (e)
100. (a) (b) (c) (d) (e)
101. (a) (b) (c) (d) (e)
102. (a) (b) (c) (d) (e)
103. (a) (b) (c) (d) (e)
104. (a) (b) (c) (d) (e)
105. (a) (b) (c) (d) (e)
106. (a) (b) (c) (d) (e)
107. (a) (b) (c) (d) (e)
108. (a) (b) (c) (d) (e)
109. (a) (b) (c) (d) (e)
110. (a) (b) (c) (d) (e)
111. (a) (b) (c) (d) (e)
112. (a) (b) (c) (d) (e)
113. (a) (b) (c) (d) (e)
114. (a) (b) (c) (d) (e)
115. (a) (b) (c) (d) (e)
116. (a) (b) (c) (d) (e)
117. (a) (b) (c) (d) (e)
118. (a) (b) (c) (d) (e)
119. (a) (b) (c) (d) (e)
120. (a) (b) (c) (d) (e)
121. (a) (b) (c) (d) (e)
122. (a) (b) (c) (d) (e)
123. (a) (b) (c) (d) (e)
124. (a) (b) (c) (d) (e)
125. (a) (b) (c) (d) (e)
126. (a) (b) (c) (d) (e)
127. (a) (b) (c) (d) (e)
128. (a) (b) (c) (d) (e)

This page intentionally left blank.

Section 8

Care of Laboratory Animals

Fill in a circled letter to indicate your answer choice.

1. ⓐ ⓑ ⓒ ⓓ ⓔ	11. ⓐ ⓑ ⓒ ⓓ ⓔ	21. ⓐ ⓑ ⓒ ⓓ ⓔ	31. ⓐ ⓑ ⓒ ⓓ ⓔ
2. ⓐ ⓑ ⓒ ⓓ ⓔ	12. ⓐ ⓑ ⓒ ⓓ ⓔ	22. ⓐ ⓑ ⓒ ⓓ ⓔ	32. ⓐ ⓑ ⓒ ⓓ ⓔ
3. ⓐ ⓑ ⓒ ⓓ ⓔ	13. ⓐ ⓑ ⓒ ⓓ ⓔ	23. ⓐ ⓑ ⓒ ⓓ ⓔ	33. ⓐ ⓑ ⓒ ⓓ ⓔ
4. ⓐ ⓑ ⓒ ⓓ ⓔ	14. ⓐ ⓑ ⓒ ⓓ ⓔ	24. ⓐ ⓑ ⓒ ⓓ ⓔ	34. ⓐ ⓑ ⓒ ⓓ ⓔ
5. ⓐ ⓑ ⓒ ⓓ ⓔ	15. ⓐ ⓑ ⓒ ⓓ ⓔ	25. ⓐ ⓑ ⓒ ⓓ ⓔ	35. ⓐ ⓑ ⓒ ⓓ ⓔ
6. ⓐ ⓑ ⓒ ⓓ ⓔ	16. ⓐ ⓑ ⓒ ⓓ ⓔ	26. ⓐ ⓑ ⓒ ⓓ ⓔ	36. ⓐ ⓑ ⓒ ⓓ ⓔ
7. ⓐ ⓑ ⓒ ⓓ ⓔ	17. ⓐ ⓑ ⓒ ⓓ ⓔ	27. ⓐ ⓑ ⓒ ⓓ ⓔ	37. ⓐ ⓑ ⓒ ⓓ ⓔ
8. ⓐ ⓑ ⓒ ⓓ ⓔ	18. ⓐ ⓑ ⓒ ⓓ ⓔ	28. ⓐ ⓑ ⓒ ⓓ ⓔ	38. ⓐ ⓑ ⓒ ⓓ ⓔ
9. ⓐ ⓑ ⓒ ⓓ ⓔ	19. ⓐ ⓑ ⓒ ⓓ ⓔ	29. ⓐ ⓑ ⓒ ⓓ ⓔ	39. ⓐ ⓑ ⓒ ⓓ ⓔ
10. ⓐ ⓑ ⓒ ⓓ ⓔ	20. ⓐ ⓑ ⓒ ⓓ ⓔ	30. ⓐ ⓑ ⓒ ⓓ ⓔ	40. ⓐ ⓑ ⓒ ⓓ ⓔ

This page intentionally left blank.

Practice Answer Sheet

Section 9

Care of Marine Mammals

Fill in a circled letter to indicate your answer choice.

1. ⓐ ⓑ ⓒ ⓓ ⓔ	5. ⓐ ⓑ ⓒ ⓓ ⓔ	9. ⓐ ⓑ ⓒ ⓓ ⓔ
2. ⓐ ⓑ ⓒ ⓓ ⓔ	6. ⓐ ⓑ ⓒ ⓓ ⓔ	10. ⓐ ⓑ ⓒ ⓓ ⓔ
3. ⓐ ⓑ ⓒ ⓓ ⓔ	7. ⓐ ⓑ ⓒ ⓓ ⓔ	
4. ⓐ ⓑ ⓒ ⓓ ⓔ	8. ⓐ ⓑ ⓒ ⓓ ⓔ	

This page intentionally left blank.

Practice Answer Sheet

Section 10

Care of Poultry and Wild Fowl

Fill in a circled letter to indicate your answer choice.

1. ⓐ ⓑ ⓒ ⓓ ⓔ
2. ⓐ ⓑ ⓒ ⓓ ⓔ
3. ⓐ ⓑ ⓒ ⓓ ⓔ
4. ⓐ ⓑ ⓒ ⓓ ⓔ
5. ⓐ ⓑ ⓒ ⓓ ⓔ
6. ⓐ ⓑ ⓒ ⓓ ⓔ
7. ⓐ ⓑ ⓒ ⓓ ⓔ
8. ⓐ ⓑ ⓒ ⓓ ⓔ
9. ⓐ ⓑ ⓒ ⓓ ⓔ
10. ⓐ ⓑ ⓒ ⓓ ⓔ
11. ⓐ ⓑ ⓒ ⓓ ⓔ
12. ⓐ ⓑ ⓒ ⓓ ⓔ
13. ⓐ ⓑ ⓒ ⓓ ⓔ
14. ⓐ ⓑ ⓒ ⓓ ⓔ
15. ⓐ ⓑ ⓒ ⓓ ⓔ

This page intentionally left blank.

Section 11

Care of Small Animals

Fill in a circled letter to indicate your answer choice.

1. (a) (b) (c) (d) (e)
2. (a) (b) (c) (d) (e)
3. (a) (b) (c) (d) (e)
4. (a) (b) (c) (d) (e)
5. (a) (b) (c) (d) (e)
6. (a) (b) (c) (d) (e)
7. (a) (b) (c) (d) (e)
8. (a) (b) (c) (d) (e)
9. (a) (b) (c) (d) (e) (f)
10. (a) (b) (c) (d) (e) (f)
11. (a) (b) (c) (d) (e) (f)
12. (a) (b) (c) (d) (e) (f)
13. (a) (b) (c) (d) (e) (f)
14. (a) (b) (c) (d) (e) (f)
15. (a) (b) (c) (d) (e)
16. (a) (b) (c) (d) (e)
17. (a) (b) (c) (d) (e)
18. (a) (b) (c) (d) (e)
19. (a) (b) (c) (d) (e)
20. (a) (b) (c) (d) (e)
21. (a) (b) (c) (d) (e)
22. (a) (b) (c) (d) (e)
23. (a) (b) (c) (d) (e)
24. (a) (b) (c) (d) (e)
25. (a) (b) (c) (d) (e)
26. (a) (b) (c) (d) (e)
27. (a) (b) (c) (d) (e)
28. (a) (b) (c) (d) (e)
29. (a) (b) (c) (d) (e)
30. (a) (b) (c) (d) (e)
31. (a) (b) (c) (d) (e)
32. (a) (b) (c) (d) (e)
33. (a) (b) (c) (d) (e)
34. (a) (b) (c) (d) (e)
35. (a) (b) (c) (d) (e)
36. (a) (b) (c) (d) (e)
37. (a) (b) (c) (d) (e)
38. (a) (b) (c) (d) (e)
39. (a) (b) (c) (d) (e)
40. (a) (b) (c) (d) (e)
41. (a) (b) (c) (d) (e)
42. (a) (b) (c) (d) (e)
43. (a) (b) (c) (d) (e)
44. (a) (b) (c) (d) (e)
45. (a) (b) (c) (d) (e) (f)
46. (a) (b) (c) (d) (e) (f)
47. (a) (b) (c) (d) (e) (f)
48. (a) (b) (c) (d) (e) (f)
49. (a) (b) (c) (d) (e) (f)
50. (a) (b) (c) (d) (e) (f)
51. (a) (b) (c) (d) (e)
52. (a) (b) (c) (d) (e)
53. (a) (b) (c) (d) (e)
54. (a) (b) (c) (d) (e)
55. (a) (b) (c) (d) (e)
56. (a) (b) (c) (d) (e)
57. (a) (b) (c) (d) (e)
58. (a) (b) (c) (d) (e)
59. (a) (b) (c) (d) (e)
60. (a) (b) (c) (d) (e)
61. (a) (b) (c) (d) (e)
62. (a) (b) (c) (d) (e)
63. (a) (b) (c) (d) (e)
64. (a) (b) (c) (d) (e)
65. (a) (b) (c) (d) (e)
66. (a) (b) (c) (d) (e)
67. (a) (b) (c) (d) (e)
68. (a) (b) (c) (d) (e)
69. (a) (b) (c) (d) (e)
70. (a) (b) (c) (d) (e)
71. (a) (b) (c) (d) (e)
72. (a) (b) (c) (d) (e)
73. (a) (b) (c) (d) (e)
74. (a) (b) (c) (d) (e)
75. (a) (b) (c) (d) (e)
76. (a) (b) (c) (d) (e)
77. (a) (b) (c) (d) (e)
78. (a) (b) (c) (d) (e)
79. (a) (b) (c) (d) (e)
80. (a) (b) (c) (d) (e)
81. (a) (b) (c) (d) (e)
82. (a) (b) (c) (d) (e)
83. (a) (b) (c) (d) (e)
84. (a) (b) (c) (d) (e)
85. (a) (b) (c) (d) (e)
86. (a) (b) (c) (d) (e)
87. (a) (b) (c) (d) (e)
88. (a) (b) (c) (d) (e)
89. (a) (b) (c) (d) (e)
90. (a) (b) (c) (d) (e)
91. (a) (b) (c) (d) (e)
92. (a) (b) (c) (d) (e)
93. (a) (b) (c) (d) (e)
94. (a) (b) (c) (d) (e)
95. (a) (b) (c) (d) (e)
96. (a) (b) (c) (d) (e)
97. (a) (b) (c) (d) (e)
98. (a) (b) (c) (d) (e)
99. (a) (b) (c) (d) (e)
100. (a) (b) (c) (d) (e)
101. (a) (b) (c) (d) (e)
102. (a) (b) (c) (d) (e)
103. (a) (b) (c) (d) (e)
104. (a) (b) (c) (d) (e)
105. (a) (b) (c) (d) (e)
106. (a) (b) (c) (d) (e)
107. (a) (b) (c) (d) (e)
108. (a) (b) (c) (d) (e)
109. (a) (b) (c) (d) (e)
110. (a) (b) (c) (d) (e)
111. (a) (b) (c) (d) (e)
112. (a) (b) (c) (d) (e)
113. (a) (b) (c) (d) (e)
114. (a) (b) (c) (d) (e)
115. (a) (b) (c) (d) (e)
116. (a) (b) (c) (d) (e)
117. (a) (b) (c) (d) (e)
118. (a) (b) (c) (d) (e)
119. (a) (b) (c) (d) (e)
120. (a) (b) (c) (d) (e)
121. (a) (b) (c) (d) (e)
122. (a) (b) (c) (d) (e)
123. (a) (b) (c) (d) (e)
124. (a) (b) (c) (d) (e)
125. (a) (b) (c) (d) (e)

This page intentionally left blank.

Practice Answer Sheet

Section 12

Care of Zoo and Exotic Animals

Fill in a circled letter to indicate your answer choice.

1. ⓐ ⓑ ⓒ ⓓ ⓔ	17. ⓐ ⓑ ⓒ ⓓ ⓔ	33. ⓐ ⓑ ⓒ ⓓ ⓔ	49. ⓐ ⓑ ⓒ ⓓ ⓔ
2. ⓐ ⓑ ⓒ ⓓ ⓔ	18. ⓐ ⓑ ⓒ ⓓ ⓔ	34. ⓐ ⓑ ⓒ ⓓ ⓔ	50. ⓐ ⓑ ⓒ ⓓ ⓔ
3. ⓐ ⓑ ⓒ ⓓ ⓔ	19. ⓐ ⓑ ⓒ ⓓ ⓔ	35. ⓐ ⓑ ⓒ ⓓ ⓔ	51. ⓐ ⓑ ⓒ ⓓ ⓔ
4. ⓐ ⓑ ⓒ ⓓ ⓔ	20. ⓐ ⓑ ⓒ ⓓ ⓔ	36. ⓐ ⓑ ⓒ ⓓ ⓔ	52. ⓐ ⓑ ⓒ ⓓ ⓔ
5. ⓐ ⓑ ⓒ ⓓ ⓔ	21. ⓐ ⓑ ⓒ ⓓ ⓔ	37. ⓐ ⓑ ⓒ ⓓ ⓔ	53. ⓐ ⓑ ⓒ ⓓ ⓔ
6. ⓐ ⓑ ⓒ ⓓ ⓔ	22. ⓐ ⓑ ⓒ ⓓ ⓔ	38. ⓐ ⓑ ⓒ ⓓ ⓔ	54. ⓐ ⓑ ⓒ ⓓ ⓔ
7. ⓐ ⓑ ⓒ ⓓ ⓔ	23. ⓐ ⓑ ⓒ ⓓ ⓔ	39. ⓐ ⓑ ⓒ ⓓ ⓔ	55. ⓐ ⓑ ⓒ ⓓ ⓔ
8. ⓐ ⓑ ⓒ ⓓ ⓔ	24. ⓐ ⓑ ⓒ ⓓ ⓔ	40. ⓐ ⓑ ⓒ ⓓ ⓔ	56. ⓐ ⓑ ⓒ ⓓ ⓔ
9. ⓐ ⓑ ⓒ ⓓ ⓔ	25. ⓐ ⓑ ⓒ ⓓ ⓔ	41. ⓐ ⓑ ⓒ ⓓ ⓔ	57. ⓐ ⓑ ⓒ ⓓ ⓔ
10. ⓐ ⓑ ⓒ ⓓ ⓔ	26. ⓐ ⓑ ⓒ ⓓ ⓔ	42. ⓐ ⓑ ⓒ ⓓ ⓔ	58. ⓐ ⓑ ⓒ ⓓ ⓔ
11. ⓐ ⓑ ⓒ ⓓ ⓔ	27. ⓐ ⓑ ⓒ ⓓ ⓔ	43. ⓐ ⓑ ⓒ ⓓ ⓔ	59. ⓐ ⓑ ⓒ ⓓ ⓔ
12. ⓐ ⓑ ⓒ ⓓ ⓔ	28. ⓐ ⓑ ⓒ ⓓ ⓔ	44. ⓐ ⓑ ⓒ ⓓ ⓔ	60. ⓐ ⓑ ⓒ ⓓ ⓔ
13. ⓐ ⓑ ⓒ ⓓ ⓔ	29. ⓐ ⓑ ⓒ ⓓ ⓔ	45. ⓐ ⓑ ⓒ ⓓ ⓔ	61. ⓐ ⓑ ⓒ ⓓ ⓔ
14. ⓐ ⓑ ⓒ ⓓ ⓔ	30. ⓐ ⓑ ⓒ ⓓ ⓔ	46. ⓐ ⓑ ⓒ ⓓ ⓔ	62. ⓐ ⓑ ⓒ ⓓ ⓔ
15. ⓐ ⓑ ⓒ ⓓ ⓔ	31. ⓐ ⓑ ⓒ ⓓ ⓔ	47. ⓐ ⓑ ⓒ ⓓ ⓔ	63. ⓐ ⓑ ⓒ ⓓ ⓔ
16. ⓐ ⓑ ⓒ ⓓ ⓔ	32. ⓐ ⓑ ⓒ ⓓ ⓔ	48. ⓐ ⓑ ⓒ ⓓ ⓔ	

This page intentionally left blank.

Section 13

Clinic Administration and Client Relations

Fill in a circled letter to indicate your answer choice.

1. (a) (b) (c) (d) (e)
2. (a) (b) (c) (d) (e)
3. (a) (b) (c) (d) (e)
4. (a) (b) (c) (d) (e)
5. (a) (b) (c) (d) (e)
6. (a) (b) (c) (d) (e)
7. (a) (b) (c) (d) (e)
8. (a) (b) (c) (d) (e)
9. (a) (b) (c) (d) (e)
10. (a) (b) (c) (d) (e)
11. (a) (b) (c) (d) (e)
12. (a) (b) (c) (d) (e)
13. (a) (b) (c) (d) (e)
14. (a) (b) (c) (d) (e)
15. (a) (b) (c) (d) (e)
16. (a) (b) (c) (d) (e)
17. (a) (b) (c) (d) (e)
18. (a) (b) (c) (d) (e)
19. (a) (b) (c) (d) (e)
20. (a) (b) (c) (d) (e)
21. (a) (b) (c) (d) (e)
22. (a) (b) (c) (d) (e)
23. (a) (b) (c) (d) (e)
24. (a) (b) (c) (d) (e)
25. (a) (b) (c) (d) (e)
26. (a) (b) (c) (d) (e)
27. (a) (b) (c) (d) (e)
28. (a) (b) (c) (d) (e)
29. (a) (b) (c) (d) (e)
30. (a) (b) (c) (d) (e)
31. (a) (b) (c) (d) (e)
32. (a) (b) (c) (d) (e)
33. (a) (b) (c) (d) (e)
34. (a) (b) (c) (d) (e)
35. (a) (b) (c) (d) (e)
36. (a) (b) (c) (d)
37. (a) (b) (c) (d)
38. (a) (b) (c) (d)
39. (a) (b) (c) (d)
40. (a) (b) (c) (d)
41. (a) (b) (c) (d)
42. (a) (b) (c) (d)
43. (a) (b) (c) (d)
44. (a) (b) (c) (d) (e)
45. (a) (b) (c) (d) (e)
46. (a) (b) (c) (d) (e)
47. (a) (b) (c) (d) (e)
48. (a) (b) (c) (d) (e)
49. (a) (b) (c) (d) (e)
50. (a) (b) (c) (d) (e)
51. (a) (b) (c) (d) (e)
52. (a) (b) (c) (d) (e)
53. (a) (b) (c) (d) (e)
54. (a) (b) (c) (d) (e)
55. (a) (b) (c) (d) (e)
56. (a) (b) (c) (d) (e)
57. (a) (b) (c) (d) (e)
58. (a) (b) (c) (d) (e)
59. (a) (b) (c) (d) (e)
60. (a) (b) (c) (d) (e)
61. (a) (b) (c) (d) (e)
62. (a) (b) (c) (d) (e)
63. (a) (b) (c) (d) (e)
64. (a) (b) (c) (d) (e)
65. (a) (b) (c) (d) (e)

This page intentionally left blank.

Practice Answer Sheet

Section 14

Dentistry

Fill in a circled letter to indicate your answer choice.

1. ⓐ ⓑ ⓒ ⓓ ⓔ	23. ⓐ ⓑ ⓒ ⓓ ⓔ	45. ⓐ ⓑ ⓒ ⓓ ⓔ	67. ⓐ ⓑ ⓒ ⓓ ⓔ
2. ⓐ ⓑ ⓒ ⓓ ⓔ	24. ⓐ ⓑ ⓒ ⓓ ⓔ	46. ⓐ ⓑ ⓒ ⓓ ⓔ	68. ⓐ ⓑ ⓒ ⓓ ⓔ
3. ⓐ ⓑ ⓒ ⓓ ⓔ	25. ⓐ ⓑ ⓒ ⓓ ⓔ	47. ⓐ ⓑ ⓒ ⓓ ⓔ	69. ⓐ ⓑ ⓒ ⓓ ⓔ
4. ⓐ ⓑ ⓒ ⓓ ⓔ	26. ⓐ ⓑ ⓒ ⓓ ⓔ	48. ⓐ ⓑ ⓒ ⓓ ⓔ	70. ⓐ ⓑ ⓒ ⓓ ⓔ
5. ⓐ ⓑ ⓒ ⓓ ⓔ	27. ⓐ ⓑ ⓒ ⓓ ⓔ	49. ⓐ ⓑ ⓒ ⓓ ⓔ	71. ⓐ ⓑ ⓒ ⓓ ⓔ
6. ⓐ ⓑ ⓒ ⓓ ⓔ	28. ⓐ ⓑ ⓒ ⓓ ⓔ	50. ⓐ ⓑ ⓒ ⓓ ⓔ	72. ⓐ ⓑ ⓒ ⓓ ⓔ
7. ⓐ ⓑ ⓒ ⓓ ⓔ	29. ⓐ ⓑ ⓒ ⓓ ⓔ	51. ⓐ ⓑ ⓒ ⓓ ⓔ	73. ⓐ ⓑ ⓒ ⓓ ⓔ
8. ⓐ ⓑ ⓒ ⓓ ⓔ	30. ⓐ ⓑ ⓒ ⓓ ⓔ	52. ⓐ ⓑ ⓒ ⓓ ⓔ	74. ⓐ ⓑ ⓒ ⓓ ⓔ
9. ⓐ ⓑ ⓒ ⓓ ⓔ	31. ⓐ ⓑ ⓒ ⓓ ⓔ	53. ⓐ ⓑ ⓒ ⓓ ⓔ	75. ⓐ ⓑ ⓒ ⓓ ⓔ
10. ⓐ ⓑ ⓒ ⓓ ⓔ	32. ⓐ ⓑ ⓒ ⓓ ⓔ	54. ⓐ ⓑ ⓒ ⓓ ⓔ	76. ⓐ ⓑ ⓒ ⓓ ⓔ
11. ⓐ ⓑ ⓒ ⓓ ⓔ	33. ⓐ ⓑ ⓒ ⓓ ⓔ	55. ⓐ ⓑ ⓒ ⓓ ⓔ	77. ⓐ ⓑ ⓒ ⓓ
12. ⓐ ⓑ ⓒ ⓓ ⓔ	34. ⓐ ⓑ ⓒ ⓓ ⓔ	56. ⓐ ⓑ ⓒ ⓓ ⓔ	78. ⓐ ⓑ ⓒ ⓓ
13. ⓐ ⓑ ⓒ ⓓ ⓔ	35. ⓐ ⓑ ⓒ ⓓ ⓔ	57. ⓐ ⓑ ⓒ ⓓ ⓔ	79. ⓐ ⓑ ⓒ ⓓ
14. ⓐ ⓑ ⓒ ⓓ ⓔ	36. ⓐ ⓑ ⓒ ⓓ ⓔ	58. ⓐ ⓑ ⓒ ⓓ ⓔ	80. ⓐ ⓑ ⓒ ⓓ
15. ⓐ ⓑ ⓒ ⓓ ⓔ	37. ⓐ ⓑ ⓒ ⓓ ⓔ	59. ⓐ ⓑ ⓒ ⓓ ⓔ	81. ⓐ ⓑ ⓒ ⓓ ⓔ
16. ⓐ ⓑ ⓒ ⓓ ⓔ	38. ⓐ ⓑ ⓒ ⓓ ⓔ	60. ⓐ ⓑ ⓒ ⓓ ⓔ	82. ⓐ ⓑ ⓒ ⓓ ⓔ
17. ⓐ ⓑ ⓒ ⓓ ⓔ	39. ⓐ ⓑ ⓒ ⓓ ⓔ	61. ⓐ ⓑ ⓒ ⓓ ⓔ	83. ⓐ ⓑ ⓒ ⓓ ⓔ
18. ⓐ ⓑ ⓒ ⓓ ⓔ	40. ⓐ ⓑ ⓒ ⓓ ⓔ	62. ⓐ ⓑ ⓒ ⓓ ⓔ	
19. ⓐ ⓑ ⓒ ⓓ ⓔ	41. ⓐ ⓑ ⓒ ⓓ ⓔ	63. ⓐ ⓑ ⓒ ⓓ ⓔ	
20. ⓐ ⓑ ⓒ ⓓ ⓔ	42. ⓐ ⓑ ⓒ ⓓ ⓔ	64. ⓐ ⓑ ⓒ ⓓ ⓔ	
21. ⓐ ⓑ ⓒ ⓓ ⓔ	43. ⓐ ⓑ ⓒ ⓓ ⓔ	65. ⓐ ⓑ ⓒ ⓓ ⓔ	
22. ⓐ ⓑ ⓒ ⓓ ⓔ	44. ⓐ ⓑ ⓒ ⓓ ⓔ	66. ⓐ ⓑ ⓒ ⓓ ⓔ	

This page intentionally left blank.

Practice Answer Sheet

Section 15

Diagnostic Imaging and Recordings

Fill in a circled letter to indicate your answer choice.

1. ⓐ ⓑ ⓒ ⓓ ⓔ
2. ⓐ ⓑ ⓒ ⓓ ⓔ
3. ⓐ ⓑ ⓒ ⓓ ⓔ
4. ⓐ ⓑ ⓒ ⓓ ⓔ
5. ⓐ ⓑ ⓒ ⓓ ⓔ
6. ⓐ ⓑ ⓒ ⓓ ⓔ
7. ⓐ ⓑ ⓒ ⓓ ⓔ
8. ⓐ ⓑ ⓒ ⓓ ⓔ
9. ⓐ ⓑ ⓒ ⓓ ⓔ
10. ⓐ ⓑ ⓒ ⓓ ⓔ
11. ⓐ ⓑ ⓒ ⓓ ⓔ
12. ⓐ ⓑ ⓒ ⓓ ⓔ
13. ⓐ ⓑ ⓒ ⓓ ⓔ
14. ⓐ ⓑ ⓒ ⓓ ⓔ
15. ⓐ ⓑ ⓒ ⓓ ⓔ
16. ⓐ ⓑ ⓒ ⓓ ⓔ
17. ⓐ ⓑ ⓒ ⓓ ⓔ
18. ⓐ ⓑ ⓒ ⓓ ⓔ
19. ⓐ ⓑ ⓒ ⓓ ⓔ ⓕ ⓖ
20. ⓐ ⓑ ⓒ ⓓ ⓔ ⓕ ⓖ
21. ⓐ ⓑ ⓒ ⓓ ⓔ ⓕ ⓖ
22. ⓐ ⓑ ⓒ ⓓ ⓔ ⓕ ⓖ
23. ⓐ ⓑ ⓒ ⓓ ⓔ ⓕ ⓖ
24. ⓐ ⓑ ⓒ ⓓ ⓔ ⓕ ⓖ
25. ⓐ ⓑ ⓒ ⓓ ⓔ ⓕ ⓖ
26. ⓐ ⓑ ⓒ ⓓ ⓔ
27. ⓐ ⓑ ⓒ ⓓ ⓔ
28. ⓐ ⓑ ⓒ ⓓ ⓔ
29. ⓐ ⓑ ⓒ ⓓ ⓔ ⓕ ⓖ ⓗ ⓘ ⓙ ⓚ
30. ⓐ ⓑ ⓒ ⓓ ⓔ ⓕ ⓖ ⓗ ⓘ ⓙ ⓚ
31. ⓐ ⓑ ⓒ ⓓ ⓔ ⓕ ⓖ ⓗ ⓘ ⓙ ⓚ
32. ⓐ ⓑ ⓒ ⓓ ⓔ ⓕ ⓖ ⓗ ⓘ ⓙ ⓚ
33. ⓐ ⓑ ⓒ ⓓ ⓔ ⓕ ⓖ ⓗ ⓘ ⓙ ⓚ
34. ⓐ ⓑ ⓒ ⓓ ⓔ ⓕ ⓖ ⓗ ⓘ ⓙ ⓚ
35. ⓐ ⓑ ⓒ ⓓ ⓔ ⓕ ⓖ ⓗ ⓘ ⓙ ⓚ
36. ⓐ ⓑ ⓒ ⓓ ⓔ ⓕ ⓖ ⓗ ⓘ ⓙ ⓚ
37. ⓐ ⓑ ⓒ ⓓ ⓔ ⓕ ⓖ ⓗ ⓘ ⓙ ⓚ
38. ⓐ ⓑ ⓒ ⓓ ⓔ ⓕ ⓖ ⓗ ⓘ ⓙ ⓚ
39. ⓐ ⓑ ⓒ ⓓ ⓔ ⓕ ⓖ ⓗ ⓘ ⓙ ⓚ
40. ⓐ ⓑ ⓒ ⓓ ⓔ
41. ⓐ ⓑ ⓒ ⓓ ⓔ
42. ⓐ ⓑ ⓒ ⓓ ⓔ
43. ⓐ ⓑ ⓒ ⓓ ⓔ
44. ⓐ ⓑ ⓒ ⓓ ⓔ
45. ⓐ ⓑ ⓒ ⓓ ⓔ
46. ⓐ ⓑ ⓒ ⓓ ⓔ
47. ⓐ ⓑ ⓒ ⓓ ⓔ
48. ⓐ ⓑ ⓒ ⓓ ⓔ
49. ⓐ ⓑ ⓒ ⓓ ⓔ
50. ⓐ ⓑ ⓒ ⓓ ⓔ
51. ⓐ ⓑ ⓒ ⓓ ⓔ
52. ⓐ ⓑ ⓒ ⓓ ⓔ
53. ⓐ ⓑ ⓒ ⓓ ⓔ
54. ⓐ ⓑ ⓒ ⓓ ⓔ
55. ⓐ ⓑ ⓒ ⓓ ⓔ
56. ⓐ ⓑ ⓒ ⓓ ⓔ
57. ⓐ ⓑ ⓒ ⓓ ⓔ
58. ⓐ ⓑ ⓒ ⓓ ⓔ
59. ⓐ ⓑ ⓒ ⓓ ⓔ
60. ⓐ ⓑ ⓒ ⓓ ⓔ
61. ⓐ ⓑ ⓒ ⓓ ⓔ
62. ⓐ ⓑ ⓒ ⓓ ⓔ
63. ⓐ ⓑ ⓒ ⓓ ⓔ
64. ⓐ ⓑ ⓒ ⓓ ⓔ
65. ⓐ ⓑ ⓒ ⓓ ⓔ
66. ⓐ ⓑ ⓒ ⓓ ⓔ
67. ⓐ ⓑ ⓒ
68. ⓐ ⓑ ⓒ
69. ⓐ ⓑ ⓒ
70. ⓐ ⓑ ⓒ ⓓ ⓔ
71. ⓐ ⓑ ⓒ ⓓ ⓔ
72. ⓐ ⓑ ⓒ ⓓ ⓔ
73. ⓐ ⓑ ⓒ ⓓ ⓔ
74. ⓐ ⓑ ⓒ ⓓ ⓔ
75. ⓐ ⓑ ⓒ ⓓ ⓔ
76. ⓐ ⓑ ⓒ ⓓ ⓔ
77. ⓐ ⓑ ⓒ ⓓ ⓔ
78. ⓐ ⓑ ⓒ ⓓ ⓔ
79. ⓐ ⓑ ⓒ ⓓ ⓔ
80. ⓐ ⓑ ⓒ ⓓ ⓔ
81. ⓐ ⓑ ⓒ ⓓ ⓔ
82. ⓐ ⓑ ⓒ ⓓ ⓔ
83. ⓐ ⓑ ⓒ ⓓ ⓔ
84. ⓐ ⓑ ⓒ ⓓ ⓔ

This page intentionally left blank.

Section 16

Epidemiology and Public Health

Fill in a circled letter to indicate your answer choice.

1. ⓐ ⓑ ⓒ ⓓ ⓔ	15. ⓐ ⓑ ⓒ ⓓ ⓔ	29. ⓐ ⓑ ⓒ ⓓ ⓔ	43. ⓐ ⓑ ⓒ ⓓ ⓔ
2. ⓐ ⓑ ⓒ ⓓ ⓔ	16. ⓐ ⓑ ⓒ ⓓ ⓔ	30. ⓐ ⓑ ⓒ ⓓ ⓔ	44. ⓐ ⓑ ⓒ ⓓ ⓔ
3. ⓐ ⓑ ⓒ ⓓ ⓔ	17. ⓐ ⓑ ⓒ ⓓ ⓔ	31. ⓐ ⓑ ⓒ ⓓ ⓔ	45. ⓐ ⓑ ⓒ ⓓ ⓔ
4. ⓐ ⓑ ⓒ ⓓ ⓔ	18. ⓐ ⓑ ⓒ ⓓ ⓔ	32. ⓐ ⓑ ⓒ ⓓ ⓔ	46. ⓐ ⓑ ⓒ ⓓ ⓔ
5. ⓐ ⓑ ⓒ ⓓ ⓔ	19. ⓐ ⓑ ⓒ ⓓ ⓔ	33. ⓐ ⓑ ⓒ ⓓ ⓔ	47. ⓐ ⓑ ⓒ ⓓ ⓔ
6. ⓐ ⓑ ⓒ ⓓ ⓔ	20. ⓐ ⓑ ⓒ ⓓ ⓔ	34. ⓐ ⓑ ⓒ ⓓ ⓔ	48. ⓐ ⓑ ⓒ ⓓ ⓔ
7. ⓐ ⓑ ⓒ ⓓ ⓔ	21. ⓐ ⓑ ⓒ ⓓ ⓔ	35. ⓐ ⓑ ⓒ ⓓ ⓔ	49. ⓐ ⓑ ⓒ ⓓ ⓔ
8. ⓐ ⓑ ⓒ ⓓ ⓔ	22. ⓐ ⓑ ⓒ ⓓ ⓔ	36. ⓐ ⓑ ⓒ ⓓ ⓔ	50. ⓐ ⓑ ⓒ ⓓ ⓔ
9. ⓐ ⓑ ⓒ ⓓ ⓔ	23. ⓐ ⓑ ⓒ ⓓ ⓔ	37. ⓐ ⓑ ⓒ ⓓ ⓔ	
10. ⓐ ⓑ ⓒ ⓓ ⓔ	24. ⓐ ⓑ ⓒ ⓓ ⓔ	38. ⓐ ⓑ ⓒ ⓓ ⓔ	
11. ⓐ ⓑ ⓒ ⓓ ⓔ	25. ⓐ ⓑ ⓒ ⓓ ⓔ	39. ⓐ ⓑ ⓒ ⓓ ⓔ	
12. ⓐ ⓑ ⓒ ⓓ ⓔ	26. ⓐ ⓑ ⓒ ⓓ ⓔ	40. ⓐ ⓑ ⓒ ⓓ ⓔ	
13. ⓐ ⓑ ⓒ ⓓ ⓔ	27. ⓐ ⓑ ⓒ ⓓ ⓔ	41. ⓐ ⓑ ⓒ ⓓ ⓔ	
14. ⓐ ⓑ ⓒ ⓓ ⓔ	28. ⓐ ⓑ ⓒ ⓓ ⓔ	42. ⓐ ⓑ ⓒ ⓓ ⓔ	

This page intentionally left blank.

Section 17

Ethics, Law and Animal Welfare

Fill in a circled letter to indicate your answer choice.

1. ⓐ ⓑ ⓒ ⓓ ⓔ	9. ⓐ ⓑ ⓒ ⓓ ⓔ	17. ⓐ ⓑ ⓒ ⓓ ⓔ	25. ⓐ ⓑ ⓒ ⓓ ⓔ
2. ⓐ ⓑ ⓒ ⓓ ⓔ	10. ⓐ ⓑ ⓒ ⓓ ⓔ	18. ⓐ ⓑ ⓒ ⓓ ⓔ	
3. ⓐ ⓑ ⓒ ⓓ ⓔ	11. ⓐ ⓑ ⓒ ⓓ ⓔ	19. ⓐ ⓑ ⓒ ⓓ ⓔ	
4. ⓐ ⓑ ⓒ ⓓ ⓔ	12. ⓐ ⓑ ⓒ ⓓ ⓔ	20. ⓐ ⓑ ⓒ ⓓ ⓔ	
5. ⓐ ⓑ ⓒ ⓓ ⓔ	13. ⓐ ⓑ ⓒ ⓓ ⓔ	21. ⓐ ⓑ ⓒ ⓓ ⓔ	
6. ⓐ ⓑ ⓒ ⓓ ⓔ	14. ⓐ ⓑ ⓒ ⓓ ⓔ	22. ⓐ ⓑ ⓒ ⓓ ⓔ	
7. ⓐ ⓑ ⓒ ⓓ ⓔ	15. ⓐ ⓑ ⓒ ⓓ ⓔ	23. ⓐ ⓑ ⓒ ⓓ ⓔ	
8. ⓐ ⓑ ⓒ ⓓ ⓔ	16. ⓐ ⓑ ⓒ ⓓ ⓔ	24. ⓐ ⓑ ⓒ ⓓ ⓔ	

This page intentionally left blank.

Practice Answer Sheet

Section 18

Hematology and Cytology

Fill in a circled letter to indicate your answer choice.

1. ⓐ ⓑ ⓒ ⓓ ⓔ	25. ⓐ ⓑ ⓒ ⓓ ⓔ	49. ⓐ ⓑ ⓒ ⓓ ⓔ	73. ⓐ ⓑ ⓒ ⓓ ⓔ
2. ⓐ ⓑ ⓒ ⓓ ⓔ	26. ⓐ ⓑ ⓒ ⓓ ⓔ	50. ⓐ ⓑ ⓒ ⓓ ⓔ	74. ⓐ ⓑ ⓒ ⓓ ⓔ
3. ⓐ ⓑ ⓒ ⓓ ⓔ	27. ⓐ ⓑ ⓒ ⓓ ⓔ	51. ⓐ ⓑ ⓒ ⓓ ⓔ	75. ⓐ ⓑ ⓒ ⓓ ⓔ
4. ⓐ ⓑ ⓒ ⓓ ⓔ	28. ⓐ ⓑ ⓒ ⓓ ⓔ	52. ⓐ ⓑ ⓒ ⓓ ⓔ	76. ⓐ ⓑ ⓒ ⓓ ⓔ
5. ⓐ ⓑ ⓒ ⓓ ⓔ	29. ⓐ ⓑ ⓒ ⓓ ⓔ	53. ⓐ ⓑ ⓒ ⓓ ⓔ	77. ⓐ ⓑ ⓒ ⓓ ⓔ
6. ⓐ ⓑ ⓒ ⓓ ⓔ	30. ⓐ ⓑ ⓒ ⓓ ⓔ	54. ⓐ ⓑ ⓒ ⓓ ⓔ	78. ⓐ ⓑ ⓒ ⓓ ⓔ
7. ⓐ ⓑ ⓒ ⓓ ⓔ	31. ⓐ ⓑ ⓒ ⓓ ⓔ	55. ⓐ ⓑ ⓒ ⓓ ⓔ	79. ⓐ ⓑ ⓒ ⓓ ⓔ
8. ⓐ ⓑ ⓒ ⓓ ⓔ	32. ⓐ ⓑ ⓒ ⓓ ⓔ	56. ⓐ ⓑ ⓒ ⓓ ⓔ	80. ⓐ ⓑ ⓒ ⓓ ⓔ
9. ⓐ ⓑ ⓒ ⓓ ⓔ	33. ⓐ ⓑ ⓒ ⓓ ⓔ	57. ⓐ ⓑ ⓒ ⓓ ⓔ	81. ⓐ ⓑ ⓒ ⓓ ⓔ
10. ⓐ ⓑ ⓒ ⓓ ⓔ	34. ⓐ ⓑ ⓒ ⓓ ⓔ	58. ⓐ ⓑ ⓒ ⓓ ⓔ	82. ⓐ ⓑ ⓒ ⓓ ⓔ
11. ⓐ ⓑ ⓒ ⓓ ⓔ	35. ⓐ ⓑ ⓒ ⓓ ⓔ	59. ⓐ ⓑ ⓒ ⓓ ⓔ	83. ⓐ ⓑ ⓒ ⓓ ⓔ
12. ⓐ ⓑ ⓒ ⓓ ⓔ	36. ⓐ ⓑ ⓒ ⓓ ⓔ	60. ⓐ ⓑ ⓒ ⓓ ⓔ	84. ⓐ ⓑ ⓒ ⓓ ⓔ
13. ⓐ ⓑ ⓒ ⓓ ⓔ	37. ⓐ ⓑ ⓒ ⓓ ⓔ	61. ⓐ ⓑ ⓒ ⓓ ⓔ	85. ⓐ ⓑ ⓒ ⓓ ⓔ
14. ⓐ ⓑ ⓒ ⓓ ⓔ	38. ⓐ ⓑ ⓒ ⓓ ⓔ	62. ⓐ ⓑ ⓒ ⓓ ⓔ	86. ⓐ ⓑ ⓒ ⓓ ⓔ
15. ⓐ ⓑ ⓒ ⓓ ⓔ	39. ⓐ ⓑ ⓒ ⓓ ⓔ	63. ⓐ ⓑ ⓒ ⓓ ⓔ	87. ⓐ ⓑ ⓒ ⓓ ⓔ
16. ⓐ ⓑ ⓒ ⓓ ⓔ	40. ⓐ ⓑ ⓒ ⓓ ⓔ	64. ⓐ ⓑ ⓒ ⓓ ⓔ	88. ⓐ ⓑ ⓒ ⓓ ⓔ
17. ⓐ ⓑ ⓒ ⓓ ⓔ	41. ⓐ ⓑ ⓒ ⓓ ⓔ	65. ⓐ ⓑ ⓒ ⓓ ⓔ	89. ⓐ ⓑ ⓒ ⓓ ⓔ
18. ⓐ ⓑ ⓒ ⓓ ⓔ	42. ⓐ ⓑ ⓒ ⓓ ⓔ	66. ⓐ ⓑ ⓒ ⓓ ⓔ	90. ⓐ ⓑ ⓒ ⓓ ⓔ
19. ⓐ ⓑ ⓒ ⓓ ⓔ	43. ⓐ ⓑ ⓒ ⓓ ⓔ	67. ⓐ ⓑ ⓒ ⓓ ⓔ	
20. ⓐ ⓑ ⓒ ⓓ ⓔ	44. ⓐ ⓑ ⓒ ⓓ ⓔ	68. ⓐ ⓑ ⓒ ⓓ ⓔ	
21. ⓐ ⓑ ⓒ ⓓ ⓔ	45. ⓐ ⓑ ⓒ ⓓ ⓔ	69. ⓐ ⓑ ⓒ ⓓ ⓔ	
22. ⓐ ⓑ ⓒ ⓓ ⓔ	46. ⓐ ⓑ ⓒ ⓓ ⓔ	70. ⓐ ⓑ ⓒ ⓓ ⓔ	
23. ⓐ ⓑ ⓒ ⓓ ⓔ	47. ⓐ ⓑ ⓒ ⓓ ⓔ	71. ⓐ ⓑ ⓒ ⓓ ⓔ	
24. ⓐ ⓑ ⓒ ⓓ ⓔ	48. ⓐ ⓑ ⓒ ⓓ ⓔ	72. ⓐ ⓑ ⓒ ⓓ ⓔ	

This page intentionally left blank.

Practice Answer Sheet

Section 19

Immunology

Fill in a circled letter to indicate your answer choice.

1. ⓐ ⓑ ⓒ ⓓ ⓔ	5. ⓐ ⓑ ⓒ ⓓ ⓔ	9. ⓐ ⓑ ⓒ ⓓ ⓔ	13. ⓐ ⓑ ⓒ ⓓ ⓔ
2. ⓐ ⓑ ⓒ ⓓ ⓔ	6. ⓐ ⓑ ⓒ ⓓ ⓔ	10. ⓐ ⓑ ⓒ ⓓ ⓔ	14. ⓐ ⓑ ⓒ ⓓ ⓔ
3. ⓐ ⓑ ⓒ ⓓ ⓔ	7. ⓐ ⓑ ⓒ ⓓ ⓔ	11. ⓐ ⓑ ⓒ ⓓ ⓔ	15. ⓐ ⓑ ⓒ ⓓ ⓔ
4. ⓐ ⓑ ⓒ ⓓ ⓔ	8. ⓐ ⓑ ⓒ ⓓ ⓔ	12. ⓐ ⓑ ⓒ ⓓ ⓔ	

This page intentionally left blank.

Section 20

Laboratory Procedures

Fill in a circled letter to indicate your answer choice.

1. a b c d e
2. a b c d e
3. a b c d e
4. a b c d e
5. a b c d e
6. a b c d e
7. a b c d e
8. a b c d e
9. a b c d e
10. a b c d e
11. a b c d e
12. a b c d e
13. a b c d e
14. a b c d e
15. a b c d e
16. a b c d e
17. a b c d e
18. a b c d e
19. a b c d e
20. a b c d e
21. a b c d e
22. a b c d e
23. a b c d e
24. a b c d e
25. a b c d e
26. a b c d e
27. a b c d e
28. a b c d e
29. a b c d e
30. a b c d e
31. a b c d e
32. a b c d e
33. a b c d e
34. a b c d e
35. a b c d e
36. a b c d e
37. a b c d e
38. a b c d e
39. a b c d e
40. a b c d e
41. a b c d e
42. a b c d e
43. a b c d e
44. a b c d e
45. a b c d e
46. a b c d e
47. a b c d e
48. a b c d e
49. a b c d e
50. a b c d e
51. a b c d e
52. a b c d e
53. a b c d e
54. a b c d e
55. a b c d e
56. a b c d e
57. a b c d e
58. a b c d e
59. a b c d e
60. a b c d e
61. a b c d e
62. a b c d e
63. a b c d e
64. a b c d e
65. a b c d e
66. a b c d e
67. a b c d e
68. a b c d e
69. a b c d e
70. a b c d e
71. a b c d e
72. a b c d e
73. a b c d e
74. a b c d e
75. a b c d e
76. a b c d e
77. a b c d e
78. a b c d e
79. a b c d e
80. a b c d e
81. a b c d e
82. a b c d e
83. a b c d e
84. a b c d e
85. a b c d e
86. a b c d e
87. a b c d e
88. a b c d e
89. a b c d e
90. a b c d e
91. a b c d e
92. a b c d e
93. a b c d e
94. a b c d e
95. a b c d e
96. a b c d e
97. a b c d e
98. a b c d e
99. a b c d e
100. a b c d e
101. a b c d e
102. a b c d e
103. a b c d e
104. a b c d e
105. a b c d e
106. a b c d e
107. a b c d e
108. a b c d e
109. a b c d e
110. a b c d e
111. a b c d e
112. a b c d e
113. a b c d e
114. a b c d e
115. a b c d e

This page intentionally left blank.

Practice Answer Sheet

Section 21

Microbiology

Fill in a circled letter to indicate your answer choice.

1. (a) (b) (c) (d) (e)
2. (a) (b) (c) (d) (e)
3. (a) (b) (c) (d) (e)
4. (a) (b) (c) (d) (e)
5. (a) (b) (c) (d) (e)
6. (a) (b) (c) (d) (e)
7. (a) (b) (c) (d) (e)
8. (a) (b) (c) (d) (e)
9. (a) (b) (c) (d) (e)
10. (a) (b) (c) (d) (e)
11. (a) (b) (c) (d) (e)
12. (a) (b) (c) (d) (e)
13. (a) (b) (c) (d) (e)
14. (a) (b) (c) (d) (e)
15. (a) (b) (c) (d) (e)
16. (a) (b) (c) (d) (e)
17. (a) (b) (c) (d) (e)
18. (a) (b) (c) (d) (e)
19. (a) (b) (c) (d) (e)
20. (a) (b) (c) (d) (e)
21. (a) (b) (c) (d) (e)
22. (a) (b) (c) (d) (e)
23. (a) (b) (c) (d) (e)
24. (a) (b) (c) (d) (e)
25. (a) (b) (c) (d) (e)
26. (a) (b) (c) (d) (e)
27. (a) (b) (c) (d) (e)
28. (a) (b) (c) (d) (e)
29. (a) (b) (c) (d) (e)
30. (a) (b) (c) (d) (e)
31. (a) (b) (c) (d) (e)
32. (a) (b) (c) (d) (e)
33. (a) (b) (c) (d) (e)
34. (a) (b) (c) (d) (e)
35. (a) (b) (c) (d) (e)
36. (a) (b) (c) (d) (e)
37. (a) (b) (c) (d) (e)
38. (a) (b) (c) (d) (e)
39. (a) (b) (c) (d) (e)
40. (a) (b) (c) (d) (e)
41. (a) (b) (c) (d) (e)
42. (a) (b) (c) (d) (e)
43. (a) (b) (c) (d) (e)
44. (a) (b) (c) (d) (e)
45. (a) (b) (c) (d) (e)
46. (a) (b) (c) (d) (e)
47. (a) (b) (c) (d) (e)
48. (a) (b) (c) (d) (e)
49. (a) (b) (c) (d) (e)
50. (a) (b) (c) (d) (e)
51. (a) (b) (c) (d) (e)
52. (a) (b) (c) (d) (e)
53. (a) (b) (c) (d) (e)
54. (a) (b) (c) (d) (e)
55. (a) (b) (c) (d) (e)
56. (a) (b) (c) (d) (e)
57. (a) (b) (c) (d) (e)
58. (a) (b) (c) (d) (e)
59. (a) (b) (c) (d) (e)
60. (a) (b) (c) (d) (e)
61. (a) (b) (c) (d) (e)
62. (a) (b) (c) (d) (e)
63. (a) (b) (c) (d) (e)
64. (a) (b) (c) (d) (e)
65. (a) (b) (c) (d) (e)
66. (a) (b) (c) (d) (e)
67. (a) (b) (c) (d) (e)
68. (a) (b) (c) (d) (e)
69. (a) (b) (c) (d) (e)
70. (a) (b) (c) (d) (e)
71. (a) (b) (c) (d) (e)
72. (a) (b) (c) (d) (e)
73. (a) (b) (c) (d) (e)
74. (a) (b) (c) (d) (e)
75. (a) (b) (c) (d) (e)
76. (a) (b) (c) (d) (e)
77. (a) (b) (c) (d) (e)
78. (a) (b) (c) (d) (e)
79. (a) (b) (c) (d) (e)
80. (a) (b) (c) (d) (e)
81. (a) (b) (c) (d) (e)
82. (a) (b) (c) (d) (e)
83. (a) (b) (c) (d) (e)
84. (a) (b) (c) (d) (e)
85. (a) (b) (c) (d) (e)
86. (a) (b) (c) (d) (e)
87. (a) (b) (c) (d) (e)
88. (a) (b) (c) (d) (e)
89. (a) (b) (c) (d) (e)
90. (a) (b) (c) (d) (e)
91. (a) (b) (c) (d) (e)
92. (a) (b) (c) (d) (e)
93. (a) (b) (c) (d) (e)
94. (a) (b) (c) (d) (e)
95. (a) (b) (c) (d) (e)
96. (a) (b) (c) (d) (e)
97. (a) (b) (c) (d) (e)
98. (a) (b) (c) (d) (e)
99. (a) (b) (c) (d) (e)
100. (a) (b) (c) (d) (e)

This page intentionally left blank.

Practice Answer Sheet

Section 22

Necropsy

Fill in a circled letter to indicate your answer choice.

1. ⓐ ⓑ ⓒ ⓓ ⓔ
2. ⓐ ⓑ ⓒ ⓓ ⓔ
3. ⓐ ⓑ ⓒ ⓓ ⓔ
4. ⓐ ⓑ ⓒ ⓓ ⓔ
5. ⓐ ⓑ ⓒ ⓓ ⓔ
6. ⓐ ⓑ ⓒ ⓓ ⓔ
7. ⓐ ⓑ ⓒ ⓓ ⓔ
8. ⓐ ⓑ ⓒ ⓓ ⓔ
9. ⓐ ⓑ ⓒ ⓓ ⓔ
10. ⓐ ⓑ ⓒ ⓓ ⓔ
11. ⓐ ⓑ ⓒ ⓓ ⓔ
12. ⓐ ⓑ ⓒ ⓓ ⓔ
13. ⓐ ⓑ ⓒ ⓓ ⓔ
14. ⓐ ⓑ ⓒ ⓓ ⓔ
15. ⓐ ⓑ ⓒ ⓓ ⓔ
16. ⓐ ⓑ ⓒ ⓓ ⓔ
17. ⓐ ⓑ ⓒ ⓓ ⓔ
18. ⓐ ⓑ ⓒ ⓓ ⓔ
19. ⓐ ⓑ ⓒ ⓓ ⓔ
20. ⓐ ⓑ ⓒ ⓓ ⓔ
21. ⓐ ⓑ ⓒ ⓓ ⓔ
22. ⓐ ⓑ ⓒ ⓓ ⓔ
23. ⓐ ⓑ ⓒ ⓓ ⓔ
24. ⓐ ⓑ ⓒ ⓓ ⓔ
25. ⓐ ⓑ ⓒ ⓓ ⓔ

This page intentionally left blank.

Practice Answer Sheet

Section 23

Nutrition

Fill in a circled letter to indicate your answer choice.

1. ⓐ ⓑ ⓒ ⓓ ⓔ
2. ⓐ ⓑ ⓒ ⓓ ⓔ
3. ⓐ ⓑ ⓒ ⓓ ⓔ
4. ⓐ ⓑ ⓒ ⓓ ⓔ
5. ⓐ ⓑ ⓒ ⓓ ⓔ
6. ⓐ ⓑ ⓒ ⓓ ⓔ
7. ⓐ ⓑ ⓒ ⓓ ⓔ
8. ⓐ ⓑ ⓒ ⓓ ⓔ
9. ⓐ ⓑ ⓒ ⓓ ⓔ
10. ⓐ ⓑ ⓒ ⓓ ⓔ
11. ⓐ ⓑ ⓒ ⓓ ⓔ
12. ⓐ ⓑ ⓒ ⓓ ⓔ
13. ⓐ ⓑ ⓒ ⓓ ⓔ
14. ⓐ ⓑ ⓒ ⓓ ⓔ
15. ⓐ ⓑ ⓒ ⓓ ⓔ
16. ⓐ ⓑ ⓒ ⓓ ⓔ
17. ⓐ ⓑ ⓒ ⓓ ⓔ
18. ⓐ ⓑ ⓒ ⓓ ⓔ
19. ⓐ ⓑ ⓒ ⓓ ⓔ
20. ⓐ ⓑ ⓒ ⓓ ⓔ
21. ⓐ ⓑ ⓒ ⓓ ⓔ
22. ⓐ ⓑ ⓒ ⓓ ⓔ
23. ⓐ ⓑ ⓒ ⓓ ⓔ
24. ⓐ ⓑ ⓒ ⓓ ⓔ ⓕ ⓖ ⓗ
25. ⓐ ⓑ ⓒ ⓓ ⓔ ⓕ ⓖ ⓗ
26. ⓐ ⓑ ⓒ ⓓ ⓔ ⓕ ⓖ ⓗ
27. ⓐ ⓑ ⓒ ⓓ ⓔ ⓕ ⓖ ⓗ
28. ⓐ ⓑ ⓒ ⓓ ⓔ ⓕ ⓖ ⓗ
29. ⓐ ⓑ ⓒ ⓓ ⓔ ⓕ ⓖ ⓗ
30. ⓐ ⓑ ⓒ ⓓ ⓔ ⓕ ⓖ ⓗ
31. ⓐ ⓑ ⓒ ⓓ ⓔ ⓕ ⓖ ⓗ
32. ⓐ ⓑ ⓒ ⓓ ⓔ
33. ⓐ ⓑ ⓒ ⓓ ⓔ
34. ⓐ ⓑ ⓒ ⓓ ⓔ
35. ⓐ ⓑ ⓒ ⓓ ⓔ
36. ⓐ ⓑ ⓒ ⓓ ⓔ
37. ⓐ ⓑ ⓒ ⓓ ⓔ
38. ⓐ ⓑ ⓒ ⓓ ⓔ
39. ⓐ ⓑ ⓒ ⓓ ⓔ
40. ⓐ ⓑ ⓒ ⓓ ⓔ
41. ⓐ ⓑ ⓒ ⓓ ⓔ
42. ⓐ ⓑ ⓒ ⓓ ⓔ ⓕ ⓖ ⓗ ⓘ
43. ⓐ ⓑ ⓒ ⓓ ⓔ ⓕ ⓖ ⓗ ⓘ
44. ⓐ ⓑ ⓒ ⓓ ⓔ ⓕ ⓖ ⓗ ⓘ
45. ⓐ ⓑ ⓒ ⓓ ⓔ ⓕ ⓖ ⓗ ⓘ
46. ⓐ ⓑ ⓒ ⓓ ⓔ ⓕ ⓖ ⓗ ⓘ
47. ⓐ ⓑ ⓒ ⓓ ⓔ ⓕ ⓖ ⓗ ⓘ
48. ⓐ ⓑ ⓒ ⓓ ⓔ ⓕ ⓖ ⓗ ⓘ
49. ⓐ ⓑ ⓒ ⓓ ⓔ ⓕ ⓖ ⓗ ⓘ
50. ⓐ ⓑ ⓒ ⓓ ⓔ ⓕ ⓖ ⓗ ⓘ

This page intentionally left blank.

Practice Answer Sheet

Section 24

Parasitology

Fill in a circled letter to indicate your answer choice.

1. ⓐ ⓑ ⓒ ⓓ ⓔ	25. ⓐ ⓑ ⓒ ⓓ ⓔ	49. ⓐ ⓑ ⓒ ⓓ ⓔ	73. ⓐ ⓑ ⓒ ⓓ ⓔ
2. ⓐ ⓑ ⓒ ⓓ ⓔ	26. ⓐ ⓑ ⓒ ⓓ ⓔ	50. ⓐ ⓑ ⓒ ⓓ ⓔ	74. ⓐ ⓑ ⓒ ⓓ ⓔ
3. ⓐ ⓑ ⓒ ⓓ ⓔ	27. ⓐ ⓑ ⓒ ⓓ ⓔ	51. ⓐ ⓑ ⓒ ⓓ ⓔ	75. ⓐ ⓑ ⓒ ⓓ ⓔ
4. ⓐ ⓑ ⓒ ⓓ ⓔ	28. ⓐ ⓑ ⓒ ⓓ ⓔ	52. ⓐ ⓑ ⓒ ⓓ ⓔ	76. ⓐ ⓑ ⓒ ⓓ ⓔ
5. ⓐ ⓑ ⓒ ⓓ ⓔ	29. ⓐ ⓑ ⓒ ⓓ ⓔ	53. ⓐ ⓑ ⓒ ⓓ ⓔ	77. ⓐ ⓑ ⓒ ⓓ ⓔ
6. ⓐ ⓑ ⓒ ⓓ ⓔ	30. ⓐ ⓑ ⓒ ⓓ ⓔ	54. ⓐ ⓑ ⓒ ⓓ ⓔ	78. ⓐ ⓑ ⓒ ⓓ ⓔ
7. ⓐ ⓑ ⓒ ⓓ ⓔ	31. ⓐ ⓑ ⓒ ⓓ ⓔ	55. ⓐ ⓑ ⓒ ⓓ ⓔ	79. ⓐ ⓑ ⓒ ⓓ ⓔ
8. ⓐ ⓑ ⓒ ⓓ ⓔ	32. ⓐ ⓑ ⓒ ⓓ ⓔ	56. ⓐ ⓑ ⓒ ⓓ ⓔ	80. ⓐ ⓑ ⓒ ⓓ ⓔ
9. ⓐ ⓑ ⓒ ⓓ ⓔ	33. ⓐ ⓑ ⓒ ⓓ ⓔ	57. ⓐ ⓑ ⓒ ⓓ ⓔ	81. ⓐ ⓑ ⓒ ⓓ ⓔ
10. ⓐ ⓑ ⓒ ⓓ ⓔ	34. ⓐ ⓑ ⓒ ⓓ ⓔ	58. ⓐ ⓑ ⓒ ⓓ ⓔ	82. ⓐ ⓑ ⓒ ⓓ ⓔ
11. ⓐ ⓑ ⓒ ⓓ ⓔ	35. ⓐ ⓑ ⓒ ⓓ ⓔ	59. ⓐ ⓑ ⓒ ⓓ ⓔ	83. ⓐ ⓑ ⓒ ⓓ ⓔ
12. ⓐ ⓑ ⓒ ⓓ ⓔ	36. ⓐ ⓑ ⓒ ⓓ ⓔ	60. ⓐ ⓑ ⓒ ⓓ ⓔ	84. ⓐ ⓑ ⓒ ⓓ ⓔ
13. ⓐ ⓑ ⓒ ⓓ ⓔ	37. ⓐ ⓑ ⓒ ⓓ ⓔ	61. ⓐ ⓑ ⓒ ⓓ ⓔ	85. ⓐ ⓑ ⓒ ⓓ ⓔ
14. ⓐ ⓑ ⓒ ⓓ ⓔ	38. ⓐ ⓑ ⓒ ⓓ ⓔ	62. ⓐ ⓑ ⓒ ⓓ ⓔ	86. ⓐ ⓑ ⓒ ⓓ ⓔ
15. ⓐ ⓑ ⓒ ⓓ ⓔ	39. ⓐ ⓑ ⓒ ⓓ ⓔ	63. ⓐ ⓑ ⓒ ⓓ ⓔ	87. ⓐ ⓑ ⓒ ⓓ ⓔ
16. ⓐ ⓑ ⓒ ⓓ ⓔ	40. ⓐ ⓑ ⓒ ⓓ ⓔ	64. ⓐ ⓑ ⓒ ⓓ ⓔ	88. ⓐ ⓑ ⓒ ⓓ ⓔ
17. ⓐ ⓑ ⓒ ⓓ ⓔ	41. ⓐ ⓑ ⓒ ⓓ ⓔ	65. ⓐ ⓑ ⓒ ⓓ ⓔ	89. ⓐ ⓑ ⓒ ⓓ ⓔ
18. ⓐ ⓑ ⓒ ⓓ ⓔ	42. ⓐ ⓑ ⓒ ⓓ ⓔ	66. ⓐ ⓑ ⓒ ⓓ ⓔ	90. ⓐ ⓑ ⓒ ⓓ ⓔ
19. ⓐ ⓑ ⓒ ⓓ ⓔ	43. ⓐ ⓑ ⓒ ⓓ ⓔ	67. ⓐ ⓑ ⓒ ⓓ ⓔ	
20. ⓐ ⓑ ⓒ ⓓ ⓔ	44. ⓐ ⓑ ⓒ ⓓ ⓔ	68. ⓐ ⓑ ⓒ ⓓ ⓔ	
21. ⓐ ⓑ ⓒ ⓓ ⓔ	45. ⓐ ⓑ ⓒ ⓓ ⓔ	69. ⓐ ⓑ ⓒ ⓓ ⓔ	
22. ⓐ ⓑ ⓒ ⓓ ⓔ	46. ⓐ ⓑ ⓒ ⓓ ⓔ	70. ⓐ ⓑ ⓒ ⓓ ⓔ	
23. ⓐ ⓑ ⓒ ⓓ ⓔ	47. ⓐ ⓑ ⓒ ⓓ ⓔ	71. ⓐ ⓑ ⓒ ⓓ ⓔ	
24. ⓐ ⓑ ⓒ ⓓ ⓔ	48. ⓐ ⓑ ⓒ ⓓ ⓔ	72. ⓐ ⓑ ⓒ ⓓ ⓔ	

This page intentionally left blank.

Practice Answer Sheet

Section 25

Pharmacology and Pharmacy Procedures

Fill in a circled letter to indicate your answer choice.

1. (a) (b) (c) (d) (e)
2. (a) (b) (c) (d) (e)
3. (a) (b) (c) (d) (e)
4. (a) (b) (c) (d) (e)
5. (a) (b) (c) (d) (e)
6. (a) (b) (c) (d) (e)
7. (a) (b) (c) (d) (e)
8. (a) (b) (c) (d) (e)
9. (a) (b) (c) (d) (e)
10. (a) (b) (c) (d) (e)
11. (a) (b) (c) (d) (e)
12. (a) (b) (c) (d) (e)
13. (a) (b) (c) (d) (e)
14. (a) (b) (c) (d) (e)
15. (a) (b) (c) (d) (e)
16. (a) (b) (c) (d) (e)
17. (a) (b) (c) (d) (e)
18. (a) (b) (c) (d) (e)
19. (a) (b) (c) (d) (e)
20. (a) (b) (c) (d) (e)
21. (a) (b) (c) (d) (e)
22. (a) (b) (c) (d) (e)
23. (a) (b) (c) (d) (e)
24. (a) (b) (c) (d) (e)
25. (a) (b) (c) (d) (e)
26. (a) (b) (c) (d) (e)
27. (a) (b) (c) (d) (e)
28. (a) (b) (c) (d) (e)
29. (a) (b) (c) (d) (e)
30. (a) (b) (c) (d) (e)
31. (a) (b) (c) (d) (e)
32. (a) (b) (c) (d) (e)
33. (a) (b) (c) (d) (e)
34. (a) (b) (c) (d) (e)
35. (a) (b) (c) (d) (e)
36. (a) (b) (c) (d) (e)
37. (a) (b) (c) (d) (e)
38. (a) (b) (c) (d) (e)
39. (a) (b) (c) (d) (e)
40. (a) (b) (c) (d) (e)
41. (a) (b) (c) (d) (e)
42. (a) (b) (c) (d) (e)
43. (a) (b) (c) (d) (e)
44. (a) (b) (c) (d) (e)
45. (a) (b) (c) (d) (e)
46. (a) (b) (c) (d) (e)
47. (a) (b) (c) (d) (e)
48. (a) (b) (c) (d) (e)
49. (a) (b) (c) (d) (e)
50. (a) (b) (c) (d) (e)
51. (a) (b) (c) (d) (e)
52. (a) (b) (c) (d) (e)
53. (a) (b) (c) (d) (e)
54. (a) (b) (c) (d) (e)
55. (a) (b) (c) (d) (e)
56. (a) (b) (c) (d) (e)
57. (a) (b) (c) (d) (e)
58. (a) (b) (c) (d) (e)
59. (a) (b) (c) (d) (e)
60. (a) (b) (c) (d) (e)
61. (a) (b) (c) (d) (e)
62. (a) (b) (c) (d) (e)
63. (a) (b) (c) (d) (e)
64. (a) (b) (c) (d) (e)
65. (a) (b) (c) (d) (e)
66. (a) (b) (c) (d) (e)
67. (a) (b) (c) (d) (e)
68. (a) (b) (c) (d) (e)
69. (a) (b) (c) (d) (e)
70. (a) (b) (c) (d) (e)
71. (a) (b) (c) (d) (e)
72. (a) (b) (c) (d) (e)
73. (a) (b) (c) (d) (e)
74. (a) (b) (c) (d) (e)
75. (a) (b) (c) (d) (e)
76. (a) (b) (c) (d) (e)
77. (a) (b) (c) (d) (e)
78. (a) (b) (c) (d) (e)
79. (a) (b) (c) (d) (e)
80. (a) (b) (c) (d) (e)
81. (a) (b) (c) (d) (e)
82. (a) (b) (c) (d) (e)
83. (a) (b) (c) (d) (e)
84. (a) (b) (c) (d) (e)
85. (a) (b) (c) (d) (e)
86. (a) (b) (c) (d) (e)
87. (a) (b) (c) (d) (e)
88. (a) (b) (c) (d) (e)
89. (a) (b) (c) (d) (e)
90. (a) (b) (c) (d) (e)

This page intentionally left blank.

Practice Answer Sheet

Section 26

Physical Restraint

Fill in a circled letter to indicate your answer choice.

1. ⓐ ⓑ ⓒ ⓓ ⓔ	9. ⓐ ⓑ ⓒ ⓓ ⓔ	17. ⓐ ⓑ ⓒ ⓓ ⓔ	25. ⓐ ⓑ ⓒ ⓓ ⓔ
2. ⓐ ⓑ ⓒ ⓓ ⓔ	10. ⓐ ⓑ ⓒ ⓓ ⓔ	18. ⓐ ⓑ ⓒ ⓓ ⓔ	
3. ⓐ ⓑ ⓒ ⓓ ⓔ	11. ⓐ ⓑ ⓒ ⓓ ⓔ	19. ⓐ ⓑ ⓒ ⓓ ⓔ	
4. ⓐ ⓑ ⓒ ⓓ ⓔ	12. ⓐ ⓑ ⓒ ⓓ ⓔ	20. ⓐ ⓑ ⓒ ⓓ ⓔ	
5. ⓐ ⓑ ⓒ ⓓ ⓔ	13. ⓐ ⓑ ⓒ ⓓ ⓔ	21. ⓐ ⓑ ⓒ ⓓ ⓔ	
6. ⓐ ⓑ ⓒ ⓓ ⓔ	14. ⓐ ⓑ ⓒ ⓓ ⓔ	22. ⓐ ⓑ ⓒ ⓓ ⓔ	
7. ⓐ ⓑ ⓒ ⓓ ⓔ	15. ⓐ ⓑ ⓒ ⓓ ⓔ	23. ⓐ ⓑ ⓒ ⓓ ⓔ	
8. ⓐ ⓑ ⓒ ⓓ ⓔ	16. ⓐ ⓑ ⓒ ⓓ ⓔ	24. ⓐ ⓑ ⓒ ⓓ ⓔ	

This page intentionally left blank.

Practice Answer Sheet

Section 27

Physiology

Fill in a circled letter to indicate your answer choice.

1. ⓐ ⓑ ⓒ ⓓ ⓔ	17. ⓐ ⓑ ⓒ ⓓ ⓔ	33. ⓐ ⓑ ⓒ ⓓ ⓔ	49. ⓐ ⓑ ⓒ ⓓ ⓔ
2. ⓐ ⓑ ⓒ ⓓ ⓔ	18. ⓐ ⓑ ⓒ ⓓ ⓔ	34. ⓐ ⓑ ⓒ ⓓ ⓔ	50. ⓐ ⓑ ⓒ ⓓ ⓔ
3. ⓐ ⓑ ⓒ ⓓ ⓔ	19. ⓐ ⓑ ⓒ ⓓ ⓔ	35. ⓐ ⓑ ⓒ ⓓ ⓔ	51. ⓐ ⓑ ⓒ ⓓ ⓔ
4. ⓐ ⓑ ⓒ ⓓ ⓔ	20. ⓐ ⓑ ⓒ ⓓ ⓔ	36. ⓐ ⓑ ⓒ ⓓ ⓔ	52. ⓐ ⓑ ⓒ ⓓ ⓔ
5. ⓐ ⓑ ⓒ ⓓ ⓔ	21. ⓐ ⓑ ⓒ ⓓ ⓔ	37. ⓐ ⓑ ⓒ ⓓ ⓔ	53. ⓐ ⓑ ⓒ ⓓ ⓔ
6. ⓐ ⓑ ⓒ ⓓ ⓔ	22. ⓐ ⓑ ⓒ ⓓ ⓔ	38. ⓐ ⓑ ⓒ ⓓ ⓔ	54. ⓐ ⓑ ⓒ ⓓ ⓔ
7. ⓐ ⓑ ⓒ ⓓ ⓔ	23. ⓐ ⓑ ⓒ ⓓ ⓔ	39. ⓐ ⓑ ⓒ ⓓ ⓔ	55. ⓐ ⓑ ⓒ ⓓ ⓔ
8. ⓐ ⓑ ⓒ ⓓ ⓔ	24. ⓐ ⓑ ⓒ ⓓ ⓔ	40. ⓐ ⓑ ⓒ ⓓ ⓔ	56. ⓐ ⓑ ⓒ ⓓ ⓔ
9. ⓐ ⓑ ⓒ ⓓ ⓔ	25. ⓐ ⓑ ⓒ ⓓ ⓔ	41. ⓐ ⓑ ⓒ ⓓ ⓔ	57. ⓐ ⓑ ⓒ ⓓ ⓔ
10. ⓐ ⓑ ⓒ ⓓ ⓔ	26. ⓐ ⓑ ⓒ ⓓ ⓔ	42. ⓐ ⓑ ⓒ ⓓ ⓔ	58. ⓐ ⓑ ⓒ ⓓ ⓔ
11. ⓐ ⓑ ⓒ ⓓ ⓔ	27. ⓐ ⓑ ⓒ ⓓ ⓔ	43. ⓐ ⓑ ⓒ ⓓ ⓔ	59. ⓐ ⓑ ⓒ ⓓ ⓔ
12. ⓐ ⓑ ⓒ ⓓ ⓔ	28. ⓐ ⓑ ⓒ ⓓ ⓔ	44. ⓐ ⓑ ⓒ ⓓ ⓔ	60. ⓐ ⓑ ⓒ ⓓ ⓔ
13. ⓐ ⓑ ⓒ ⓓ ⓔ	29. ⓐ ⓑ ⓒ ⓓ ⓔ	45. ⓐ ⓑ ⓒ ⓓ ⓔ	
14. ⓐ ⓑ ⓒ ⓓ ⓔ	30. ⓐ ⓑ ⓒ ⓓ ⓔ	46. ⓐ ⓑ ⓒ ⓓ ⓔ	
15. ⓐ ⓑ ⓒ ⓓ ⓔ	31. ⓐ ⓑ ⓒ ⓓ ⓔ	47. ⓐ ⓑ ⓒ ⓓ ⓔ	
16. ⓐ ⓑ ⓒ ⓓ ⓔ	32. ⓐ ⓑ ⓒ ⓓ ⓔ	48. ⓐ ⓑ ⓒ ⓓ ⓔ	

This page intentionally left blank.

Practice Answer Sheet

Section 28

Preventive Medicine

Fill in a circled letter to indicate your answer choice.

1. ⓐ ⓑ ⓒ ⓓ ⓔ	13. ⓐ ⓑ ⓒ ⓓ ⓔ	25. ⓐ ⓑ ⓒ ⓓ ⓔ	37. ⓐ ⓑ ⓒ ⓓ ⓔ
2. ⓐ ⓑ ⓒ ⓓ ⓔ	14. ⓐ ⓑ ⓒ ⓓ ⓔ	26. ⓐ ⓑ ⓒ ⓓ ⓔ	38. ⓐ ⓑ ⓒ ⓓ ⓔ
3. ⓐ ⓑ ⓒ ⓓ ⓔ	15. ⓐ ⓑ ⓒ ⓓ ⓔ	27. ⓐ ⓑ ⓒ ⓓ ⓔ	39. ⓐ ⓑ ⓒ ⓓ ⓔ
4. ⓐ ⓑ ⓒ ⓓ ⓔ	16. ⓐ ⓑ ⓒ ⓓ ⓔ	28. ⓐ ⓑ ⓒ ⓓ ⓔ	40. ⓐ ⓑ ⓒ ⓓ ⓔ
5. ⓐ ⓑ ⓒ ⓓ ⓔ	17. ⓐ ⓑ ⓒ ⓓ ⓔ	29. ⓐ ⓑ ⓒ ⓓ ⓔ	41. ⓐ ⓑ ⓒ ⓓ ⓔ
6. ⓐ ⓑ ⓒ ⓓ ⓔ	18. ⓐ ⓑ ⓒ ⓓ ⓔ	30. ⓐ ⓑ ⓒ ⓓ ⓔ	42. ⓐ ⓑ ⓒ ⓓ ⓔ
7. ⓐ ⓑ ⓒ ⓓ ⓔ	19. ⓐ ⓑ ⓒ ⓓ ⓔ	31. ⓐ ⓑ ⓒ ⓓ ⓔ	43. ⓐ ⓑ ⓒ ⓓ ⓔ
8. ⓐ ⓑ ⓒ ⓓ ⓔ	20. ⓐ ⓑ ⓒ ⓓ ⓔ	32. ⓐ ⓑ ⓒ ⓓ ⓔ	44. ⓐ ⓑ ⓒ ⓓ ⓔ
9. ⓐ ⓑ ⓒ ⓓ ⓔ	21. ⓐ ⓑ ⓒ ⓓ ⓔ	33. ⓐ ⓑ ⓒ ⓓ ⓔ	45. ⓐ ⓑ ⓒ ⓓ ⓔ
10. ⓐ ⓑ ⓒ ⓓ ⓔ	22. ⓐ ⓑ ⓒ ⓓ ⓔ	34. ⓐ ⓑ ⓒ ⓓ ⓔ	46. ⓐ ⓑ ⓒ ⓓ ⓔ
11. ⓐ ⓑ ⓒ ⓓ ⓔ	23. ⓐ ⓑ ⓒ ⓓ ⓔ	35. ⓐ ⓑ ⓒ ⓓ ⓔ	
12. ⓐ ⓑ ⓒ ⓓ ⓔ	24. ⓐ ⓑ ⓒ ⓓ ⓔ	36. ⓐ ⓑ ⓒ ⓓ ⓔ	

This page intentionally left blank.

Practice Answer Sheet

Section 29

Principles of Disease

Fill in a circled letter to indicate your answer choice.

1. ⓐ ⓑ ⓒ ⓓ ⓔ	15. ⓐ ⓑ ⓒ ⓓ ⓔ	29. ⓐ ⓑ ⓒ ⓓ ⓔ	43. ⓐ ⓑ ⓒ ⓓ ⓔ
2. ⓐ ⓑ ⓒ ⓓ ⓔ	16. ⓐ ⓑ ⓒ ⓓ ⓔ	30. ⓐ ⓑ ⓒ ⓓ ⓔ	44. ⓐ ⓑ ⓒ ⓓ ⓔ
3. ⓐ ⓑ ⓒ ⓓ ⓔ	17. ⓐ ⓑ ⓒ ⓓ ⓔ	31. ⓐ ⓑ ⓒ ⓓ ⓔ	45. ⓐ ⓑ ⓒ ⓓ ⓔ
4. ⓐ ⓑ ⓒ ⓓ ⓔ	18. ⓐ ⓑ ⓒ ⓓ ⓔ	32. ⓐ ⓑ ⓒ ⓓ ⓔ	46. ⓐ ⓑ ⓒ ⓓ ⓔ
5. ⓐ ⓑ ⓒ ⓓ ⓔ	19. ⓐ ⓑ ⓒ ⓓ ⓔ	33. ⓐ ⓑ ⓒ ⓓ ⓔ	47. ⓐ ⓑ ⓒ ⓓ ⓔ
6. ⓐ ⓑ ⓒ ⓓ ⓔ	20. ⓐ ⓑ ⓒ ⓓ ⓔ	34. ⓐ ⓑ ⓒ ⓓ ⓔ	48. ⓐ ⓑ ⓒ ⓓ ⓔ
7. ⓐ ⓑ ⓒ ⓓ ⓔ	21. ⓐ ⓑ ⓒ ⓓ ⓔ	35. ⓐ ⓑ ⓒ ⓓ ⓔ	49. ⓐ ⓑ ⓒ ⓓ ⓔ
8. ⓐ ⓑ ⓒ ⓓ ⓔ	22. ⓐ ⓑ ⓒ ⓓ ⓔ	36. ⓐ ⓑ ⓒ ⓓ ⓔ	50. ⓐ ⓑ ⓒ ⓓ ⓔ
9. ⓐ ⓑ ⓒ ⓓ ⓔ	23. ⓐ ⓑ ⓒ ⓓ ⓔ	37. ⓐ ⓑ ⓒ ⓓ ⓔ	
10. ⓐ ⓑ ⓒ ⓓ ⓔ	24. ⓐ ⓑ ⓒ ⓓ ⓔ	38. ⓐ ⓑ ⓒ ⓓ ⓔ	
11. ⓐ ⓑ ⓒ ⓓ ⓔ	25. ⓐ ⓑ ⓒ ⓓ ⓔ	39. ⓐ ⓑ ⓒ ⓓ ⓔ	
12. ⓐ ⓑ ⓒ ⓓ ⓔ	26. ⓐ ⓑ ⓒ ⓓ ⓔ	40. ⓐ ⓑ ⓒ ⓓ ⓔ	
13. ⓐ ⓑ ⓒ ⓓ ⓔ	27. ⓐ ⓑ ⓒ ⓓ ⓔ	41. ⓐ ⓑ ⓒ ⓓ ⓔ	
14. ⓐ ⓑ ⓒ ⓓ ⓔ	28. ⓐ ⓑ ⓒ ⓓ ⓔ	42. ⓐ ⓑ ⓒ ⓓ ⓔ	

This page intentionally left blank.

Practice Answer Sheet

Section 30

Reproduction

Fill in a circled letter to indicate your answer choice.

1. ⓐ ⓑ ⓒ ⓓ ⓔ	25. ⓐ ⓑ ⓒ ⓓ ⓔ	49. ⓐ ⓑ ⓒ ⓓ ⓔ	73. ⓐ ⓑ ⓒ ⓓ ⓔ
2. ⓐ ⓑ ⓒ ⓓ ⓔ	26. ⓐ ⓑ ⓒ ⓓ ⓔ	50. ⓐ ⓑ ⓒ ⓓ ⓔ	74. ⓐ ⓑ ⓒ ⓓ ⓔ
3. ⓐ ⓑ ⓒ ⓓ ⓔ	27. ⓐ ⓑ ⓒ ⓓ ⓔ	51. ⓐ ⓑ ⓒ ⓓ ⓔ	75. ⓐ ⓑ ⓒ ⓓ ⓔ
4. ⓐ ⓑ ⓒ ⓓ ⓔ	28. ⓐ ⓑ ⓒ ⓓ ⓔ	52. ⓐ ⓑ ⓒ ⓓ ⓔ	76. ⓐ ⓑ ⓒ ⓓ ⓔ
5. ⓐ ⓑ ⓒ ⓓ ⓔ	29. ⓐ ⓑ ⓒ ⓓ ⓔ	53. ⓐ ⓑ ⓒ ⓓ ⓔ	77. ⓐ ⓑ ⓒ ⓓ ⓔ
6. ⓐ ⓑ ⓒ ⓓ ⓔ	30. ⓐ ⓑ ⓒ ⓓ ⓔ	54. ⓐ ⓑ ⓒ ⓓ ⓔ	78. ⓐ ⓑ ⓒ ⓓ ⓔ
7. ⓐ ⓑ ⓒ ⓓ ⓔ	31. ⓐ ⓑ ⓒ ⓓ ⓔ	55. ⓐ ⓑ ⓒ ⓓ ⓔ	79. ⓐ ⓑ ⓒ ⓓ ⓔ
8. ⓐ ⓑ ⓒ ⓓ ⓔ	32. ⓐ ⓑ ⓒ ⓓ ⓔ	56. ⓐ ⓑ ⓒ ⓓ ⓔ	80. ⓐ ⓑ ⓒ ⓓ ⓔ
9. ⓐ ⓑ ⓒ ⓓ ⓔ	33. ⓐ ⓑ ⓒ ⓓ ⓔ	57. ⓐ ⓑ ⓒ ⓓ ⓔ	81. ⓐ ⓑ ⓒ ⓓ ⓔ
10. ⓐ ⓑ ⓒ ⓓ ⓔ	34. ⓐ ⓑ ⓒ ⓓ ⓔ	58. ⓐ ⓑ ⓒ ⓓ ⓔ	82. ⓐ ⓑ ⓒ ⓓ ⓔ
11. ⓐ ⓑ ⓒ ⓓ ⓔ	35. ⓐ ⓑ ⓒ ⓓ ⓔ	59. ⓐ ⓑ ⓒ ⓓ ⓔ	83. ⓐ ⓑ ⓒ ⓓ ⓔ
12. ⓐ ⓑ ⓒ ⓓ ⓔ	36. ⓐ ⓑ ⓒ ⓓ ⓔ	60. ⓐ ⓑ ⓒ ⓓ ⓔ	84. ⓐ ⓑ ⓒ ⓓ ⓔ
13. ⓐ ⓑ ⓒ ⓓ ⓔ	37. ⓐ ⓑ ⓒ ⓓ ⓔ	61. ⓐ ⓑ ⓒ ⓓ ⓔ	85. ⓐ ⓑ ⓒ ⓓ ⓔ
14. ⓐ ⓑ ⓒ ⓓ ⓔ	38. ⓐ ⓑ ⓒ ⓓ ⓔ	62. ⓐ ⓑ ⓒ ⓓ ⓔ	86. ⓐ ⓑ ⓒ ⓓ ⓔ
15. ⓐ ⓑ ⓒ ⓓ ⓔ	39. ⓐ ⓑ ⓒ ⓓ ⓔ	63. ⓐ ⓑ ⓒ ⓓ ⓔ	87. ⓐ ⓑ ⓒ ⓓ ⓔ
16. ⓐ ⓑ ⓒ ⓓ ⓔ	40. ⓐ ⓑ ⓒ ⓓ ⓔ	64. ⓐ ⓑ ⓒ ⓓ ⓔ	88. ⓐ ⓑ ⓒ ⓓ ⓔ
17. ⓐ ⓑ ⓒ ⓓ ⓔ	41. ⓐ ⓑ ⓒ ⓓ ⓔ	65. ⓐ ⓑ ⓒ ⓓ ⓔ	89. ⓐ ⓑ ⓒ ⓓ ⓔ
18. ⓐ ⓑ ⓒ ⓓ ⓔ	42. ⓐ ⓑ ⓒ ⓓ ⓔ	66. ⓐ ⓑ ⓒ ⓓ ⓔ	90. ⓐ ⓑ ⓒ ⓓ ⓔ
19. ⓐ ⓑ ⓒ ⓓ ⓔ	43. ⓐ ⓑ ⓒ ⓓ ⓔ	67. ⓐ ⓑ ⓒ ⓓ ⓔ	
20. ⓐ ⓑ ⓒ ⓓ ⓔ	44. ⓐ ⓑ ⓒ ⓓ ⓔ	68. ⓐ ⓑ ⓒ ⓓ ⓔ	
21. ⓐ ⓑ ⓒ ⓓ ⓔ	45. ⓐ ⓑ ⓒ ⓓ ⓔ	69. ⓐ ⓑ ⓒ ⓓ ⓔ	
22. ⓐ ⓑ ⓒ ⓓ ⓔ	46. ⓐ ⓑ ⓒ ⓓ ⓔ	70. ⓐ ⓑ ⓒ ⓓ ⓔ	
23. ⓐ ⓑ ⓒ ⓓ ⓔ	47. ⓐ ⓑ ⓒ ⓓ ⓔ	71. ⓐ ⓑ ⓒ ⓓ ⓔ	
24. ⓐ ⓑ ⓒ ⓓ ⓔ	48. ⓐ ⓑ ⓒ ⓓ ⓔ	72. ⓐ ⓑ ⓒ ⓓ ⓔ	

This page intentionally left blank.

Practice Answer Sheet

Section 31

Surgical Nursing

Fill in a circled letter to indicate your answer choice.

1. ⓐ ⓑ ⓒ ⓓ ⓔ	31. ⓐ ⓑ ⓒ ⓓ ⓔ	61. ⓐ ⓑ ⓒ ⓓ ⓔ	91. ⓐ ⓑ ⓒ ⓓ ⓔ
2. ⓐ ⓑ ⓒ ⓓ ⓔ	32. ⓐ ⓑ ⓒ ⓓ ⓔ	62. ⓐ ⓑ ⓒ ⓓ ⓔ	92. ⓐ ⓑ ⓒ ⓓ ⓔ
3. ⓐ ⓑ ⓒ ⓓ ⓔ	33. ⓐ ⓑ ⓒ ⓓ ⓔ	63. ⓐ ⓑ ⓒ ⓓ ⓔ	93. ⓐ ⓑ ⓒ ⓓ ⓔ
4. ⓐ ⓑ ⓒ ⓓ ⓔ	34. ⓐ ⓑ ⓒ ⓓ ⓔ	64. ⓐ ⓑ ⓒ ⓓ ⓔ	94. ⓐ ⓑ ⓒ ⓓ ⓔ
5. ⓐ ⓑ ⓒ ⓓ ⓔ	35. ⓐ ⓑ ⓒ ⓓ ⓔ	65. ⓐ ⓑ ⓒ ⓓ ⓔ	95. ⓐ ⓑ ⓒ ⓓ ⓔ
6. ⓐ ⓑ ⓒ ⓓ ⓔ	36. ⓐ ⓑ ⓒ ⓓ ⓔ	66. ⓐ ⓑ ⓒ ⓓ ⓔ	96. ⓐ ⓑ ⓒ ⓓ ⓔ
7. ⓐ ⓑ ⓒ ⓓ ⓔ	37. ⓐ ⓑ ⓒ ⓓ ⓔ	67. ⓐ ⓑ ⓒ ⓓ ⓔ	97. ⓐ ⓑ ⓒ ⓓ ⓔ
8. ⓐ ⓑ ⓒ ⓓ ⓔ	38. ⓐ ⓑ ⓒ ⓓ ⓔ	68. ⓐ ⓑ ⓒ ⓓ ⓔ	98. ⓐ ⓑ ⓒ ⓓ ⓔ
9. ⓐ ⓑ ⓒ ⓓ ⓔ	39. ⓐ ⓑ ⓒ ⓓ ⓔ	69. ⓐ ⓑ ⓒ ⓓ ⓔ	99. ⓐ ⓑ ⓒ ⓓ ⓔ
10. ⓐ ⓑ ⓒ ⓓ ⓔ	40. ⓐ ⓑ ⓒ ⓓ ⓔ	70. ⓐ ⓑ ⓒ ⓓ ⓔ	100. ⓐ ⓑ ⓒ ⓓ ⓔ
11. ⓐ ⓑ ⓒ ⓓ ⓔ	41. ⓐ ⓑ ⓒ ⓓ ⓔ	71. ⓐ ⓑ ⓒ ⓓ ⓔ	101. ⓐ ⓑ ⓒ ⓓ ⓔ
12. ⓐ ⓑ ⓒ ⓓ ⓔ	42. ⓐ ⓑ ⓒ ⓓ ⓔ	72. ⓐ ⓑ ⓒ ⓓ ⓔ	102. ⓐ ⓑ ⓒ ⓓ ⓔ
13. ⓐ ⓑ ⓒ ⓓ ⓔ	43. ⓐ ⓑ ⓒ ⓓ ⓔ	73. ⓐ ⓑ ⓒ ⓓ ⓔ	103. ⓐ ⓑ ⓒ ⓓ ⓔ
14. ⓐ ⓑ ⓒ ⓓ ⓔ	44. ⓐ ⓑ ⓒ ⓓ ⓔ	74. ⓐ ⓑ ⓒ ⓓ ⓔ	104. ⓐ ⓑ ⓒ ⓓ ⓔ
15. ⓐ ⓑ ⓒ ⓓ ⓔ	45. ⓐ ⓑ ⓒ ⓓ ⓔ	75. ⓐ ⓑ ⓒ ⓓ ⓔ	105. ⓐ ⓑ ⓒ ⓓ ⓔ
16. ⓐ ⓑ ⓒ ⓓ ⓔ	46. ⓐ ⓑ ⓒ ⓓ ⓔ	76. ⓐ ⓑ ⓒ ⓓ ⓔ	106. ⓐ ⓑ ⓒ ⓓ ⓔ
17. ⓐ ⓑ ⓒ ⓓ ⓔ	47. ⓐ ⓑ ⓒ ⓓ ⓔ	77. ⓐ ⓑ ⓒ ⓓ ⓔ	107. ⓐ ⓑ ⓒ ⓓ ⓔ
18. ⓐ ⓑ ⓒ ⓓ ⓔ	48. ⓐ ⓑ ⓒ ⓓ ⓔ	78. ⓐ ⓑ ⓒ ⓓ ⓔ	108. ⓐ ⓑ ⓒ ⓓ ⓔ
19. ⓐ ⓑ ⓒ ⓓ ⓔ	49. ⓐ ⓑ ⓒ ⓓ ⓔ	79. ⓐ ⓑ ⓒ ⓓ ⓔ	109. ⓐ ⓑ ⓒ ⓓ ⓔ
20. ⓐ ⓑ ⓒ ⓓ ⓔ	50. ⓐ ⓑ ⓒ ⓓ ⓔ	80. ⓐ ⓑ ⓒ ⓓ ⓔ	110. ⓐ ⓑ ⓒ ⓓ ⓔ
21. ⓐ ⓑ ⓒ ⓓ ⓔ	51. ⓐ ⓑ ⓒ ⓓ ⓔ	81. ⓐ ⓑ ⓒ ⓓ ⓔ	111. ⓐ ⓑ ⓒ ⓓ ⓔ
22. ⓐ ⓑ ⓒ ⓓ ⓔ	52. ⓐ ⓑ ⓒ ⓓ ⓔ	82. ⓐ ⓑ ⓒ ⓓ ⓔ	112. ⓐ ⓑ ⓒ ⓓ ⓔ
23. ⓐ ⓑ ⓒ ⓓ ⓔ	53. ⓐ ⓑ ⓒ ⓓ ⓔ	83. ⓐ ⓑ ⓒ ⓓ ⓔ	113. ⓐ ⓑ ⓒ ⓓ ⓔ
24. ⓐ ⓑ ⓒ ⓓ ⓔ	54. ⓐ ⓑ ⓒ ⓓ ⓔ	84. ⓐ ⓑ ⓒ ⓓ ⓔ	114. ⓐ ⓑ ⓒ ⓓ ⓔ
25. ⓐ ⓑ ⓒ ⓓ ⓔ	55. ⓐ ⓑ ⓒ ⓓ ⓔ	85. ⓐ ⓑ ⓒ ⓓ ⓔ	115. ⓐ ⓑ ⓒ ⓓ ⓔ
26. ⓐ ⓑ ⓒ ⓓ ⓔ	56. ⓐ ⓑ ⓒ ⓓ ⓔ	86. ⓐ ⓑ ⓒ ⓓ ⓔ	
27. ⓐ ⓑ ⓒ ⓓ ⓔ	57. ⓐ ⓑ ⓒ ⓓ ⓔ	87. ⓐ ⓑ ⓒ ⓓ ⓔ	
28. ⓐ ⓑ ⓒ ⓓ ⓔ	58. ⓐ ⓑ ⓒ ⓓ ⓔ	88. ⓐ ⓑ ⓒ ⓓ ⓔ	
29. ⓐ ⓑ ⓒ ⓓ ⓔ	59. ⓐ ⓑ ⓒ ⓓ ⓔ	89. ⓐ ⓑ ⓒ ⓓ ⓔ	
30. ⓐ ⓑ ⓒ ⓓ ⓔ	60. ⓐ ⓑ ⓒ ⓓ ⓔ	90. ⓐ ⓑ ⓒ ⓓ ⓔ	

This page intentionally left blank.

Practice Answer Sheet

Section 32

Terminology

Fill in a circled letter to indicate your answer choice.

1. ⓐ ⓑ ⓒ ⓓ ⓔ	27. ⓐ ⓑ ⓒ ⓓ ⓔ	53. ⓐ ⓑ ⓒ ⓓ ⓔ	79. ⓐ ⓑ ⓒ ⓓ ⓔ
2. ⓐ ⓑ ⓒ ⓓ ⓔ	28. ⓐ ⓑ ⓒ ⓓ ⓔ	54. ⓐ ⓑ ⓒ ⓓ ⓔ	80. ⓐ ⓑ ⓒ ⓓ ⓔ
3. ⓐ ⓑ ⓒ ⓓ ⓔ	29. ⓐ ⓑ ⓒ ⓓ ⓔ	55. ⓐ ⓑ ⓒ ⓓ ⓔ	81. ⓐ ⓑ ⓒ ⓓ ⓔ
4. ⓐ ⓑ ⓒ ⓓ ⓔ	30. ⓐ ⓑ ⓒ ⓓ ⓔ	56. ⓐ ⓑ ⓒ ⓓ ⓔ	82. ⓐ ⓑ ⓒ ⓓ ⓔ
5. ⓐ ⓑ ⓒ ⓓ ⓔ	31. ⓐ ⓑ ⓒ ⓓ ⓔ	57. ⓐ ⓑ ⓒ ⓓ ⓔ	83. ⓐ ⓑ ⓒ ⓓ ⓔ
6. ⓐ ⓑ ⓒ ⓓ ⓔ	32. ⓐ ⓑ ⓒ ⓓ ⓔ	58. ⓐ ⓑ ⓒ ⓓ ⓔ	84. ⓐ ⓑ ⓒ ⓓ ⓔ
7. ⓐ ⓑ ⓒ ⓓ ⓔ	33. ⓐ ⓑ ⓒ ⓓ ⓔ	59. ⓐ ⓑ ⓒ ⓓ ⓔ	85. ⓐ ⓑ ⓒ ⓓ ⓔ
8. ⓐ ⓑ ⓒ ⓓ ⓔ	34. ⓐ ⓑ ⓒ ⓓ ⓔ	60. ⓐ ⓑ ⓒ ⓓ ⓔ	86. ⓐ ⓑ ⓒ ⓓ ⓔ
9. ⓐ ⓑ ⓒ ⓓ ⓔ	35. ⓐ ⓑ ⓒ ⓓ ⓔ	61. ⓐ ⓑ ⓒ ⓓ ⓔ	87. ⓐ ⓑ ⓒ ⓓ ⓔ
10. ⓐ ⓑ ⓒ ⓓ ⓔ	36. ⓐ ⓑ ⓒ ⓓ ⓔ	62. ⓐ ⓑ ⓒ ⓓ ⓔ	88. ⓐ ⓑ ⓒ ⓓ ⓔ
11. ⓐ ⓑ ⓒ ⓓ ⓔ	37. ⓐ ⓑ ⓒ ⓓ ⓔ	63. ⓐ ⓑ ⓒ ⓓ ⓔ	89. ⓐ ⓑ ⓒ ⓓ ⓔ
12. ⓐ ⓑ ⓒ ⓓ ⓔ	38. ⓐ ⓑ ⓒ ⓓ ⓔ	64. ⓐ ⓑ ⓒ ⓓ ⓔ	90. ⓐ ⓑ ⓒ ⓓ ⓔ
13. ⓐ ⓑ ⓒ ⓓ ⓔ	39. ⓐ ⓑ ⓒ ⓓ ⓔ	65. ⓐ ⓑ ⓒ ⓓ ⓔ	91. ⓐ ⓑ ⓒ ⓓ ⓔ
14. ⓐ ⓑ ⓒ ⓓ ⓔ	40. ⓐ ⓑ ⓒ ⓓ ⓔ	66. ⓐ ⓑ ⓒ ⓓ ⓔ	92. ⓐ ⓑ ⓒ ⓓ ⓔ
15. ⓐ ⓑ ⓒ ⓓ ⓔ	41. ⓐ ⓑ ⓒ ⓓ ⓔ	67. ⓐ ⓑ ⓒ ⓓ ⓔ	93. ⓐ ⓑ ⓒ ⓓ ⓔ
16. ⓐ ⓑ ⓒ ⓓ ⓔ	42. ⓐ ⓑ ⓒ ⓓ ⓔ	68. ⓐ ⓑ ⓒ ⓓ ⓔ	94. ⓐ ⓑ ⓒ ⓓ ⓔ
17. ⓐ ⓑ ⓒ ⓓ ⓔ	43. ⓐ ⓑ ⓒ ⓓ ⓔ	69. ⓐ ⓑ ⓒ ⓓ ⓔ	95. ⓐ ⓑ ⓒ ⓓ ⓔ
18. ⓐ ⓑ ⓒ ⓓ ⓔ	44. ⓐ ⓑ ⓒ ⓓ ⓔ	70. ⓐ ⓑ ⓒ ⓓ ⓔ	96. ⓐ ⓑ ⓒ ⓓ ⓔ
19. ⓐ ⓑ ⓒ ⓓ ⓔ	45. ⓐ ⓑ ⓒ ⓓ ⓔ	71. ⓐ ⓑ ⓒ ⓓ ⓔ	97. ⓐ ⓑ ⓒ ⓓ ⓔ
20. ⓐ ⓑ ⓒ ⓓ ⓔ	46. ⓐ ⓑ ⓒ ⓓ ⓔ	72. ⓐ ⓑ ⓒ ⓓ ⓔ	98. ⓐ ⓑ ⓒ ⓓ ⓔ
21. ⓐ ⓑ ⓒ ⓓ ⓔ	47. ⓐ ⓑ ⓒ ⓓ ⓔ	73. ⓐ ⓑ ⓒ ⓓ ⓔ	99. ⓐ ⓑ ⓒ ⓓ ⓔ
22. ⓐ ⓑ ⓒ ⓓ ⓔ	48. ⓐ ⓑ ⓒ ⓓ ⓔ	74. ⓐ ⓑ ⓒ ⓓ ⓔ	100. ⓐ ⓑ ⓒ ⓓ ⓔ
23. ⓐ ⓑ ⓒ ⓓ ⓔ	49. ⓐ ⓑ ⓒ ⓓ ⓔ	75. ⓐ ⓑ ⓒ ⓓ ⓔ	
24. ⓐ ⓑ ⓒ ⓓ ⓔ	50. ⓐ ⓑ ⓒ ⓓ ⓔ	76. ⓐ ⓑ ⓒ ⓓ ⓔ	
25. ⓐ ⓑ ⓒ ⓓ ⓔ	51. ⓐ ⓑ ⓒ ⓓ ⓔ	77. ⓐ ⓑ ⓒ ⓓ ⓔ	
26. ⓐ ⓑ ⓒ ⓓ ⓔ	52. ⓐ ⓑ ⓒ ⓓ ⓔ	78. ⓐ ⓑ ⓒ ⓓ ⓔ	

This page intentionally left blank.

Section 33

Toxicology

Fill in a circled letter to indicate your answer choice.

1. ⓐ ⓑ ⓒ ⓓ ⓔ	7. ⓐ ⓑ ⓒ ⓓ ⓔ	13. ⓐ ⓑ ⓒ ⓓ ⓔ	19. ⓐ ⓑ ⓒ ⓓ ⓔ
2. ⓐ ⓑ ⓒ ⓓ ⓔ	8. ⓐ ⓑ ⓒ ⓓ ⓔ	14. ⓐ ⓑ ⓒ ⓓ ⓔ	20. ⓐ ⓑ ⓒ ⓓ ⓔ
3. ⓐ ⓑ ⓒ ⓓ ⓔ	9. ⓐ ⓑ ⓒ ⓓ ⓔ	15. ⓐ ⓑ ⓒ ⓓ ⓔ	
4. ⓐ ⓑ ⓒ ⓓ ⓔ	10. ⓐ ⓑ ⓒ ⓓ ⓔ	16. ⓐ ⓑ ⓒ ⓓ ⓔ	
5. ⓐ ⓑ ⓒ ⓓ ⓔ	11. ⓐ ⓑ ⓒ ⓓ ⓔ	17. ⓐ ⓑ ⓒ ⓓ ⓔ	
6. ⓐ ⓑ ⓒ ⓓ ⓔ	12. ⓐ ⓑ ⓒ ⓓ ⓔ	18. ⓐ ⓑ ⓒ ⓓ ⓔ	

We Welcome Your Comments

We value your opinion and encourage you to send us your comments, flattering or critical. Please let us know if you detect any errors or ambiguous statements, or if there is any way in which we can make *Review Questions & Answers For Veterinary Technicians* more useful to you.

Paul W. Pratt, VMD
Editor and Publisher

Return to:
American Veterinary Publications
5782 Thornwood Drive
Goleta, CA 93117

Detach, fold and seal with tape.
No postage needed in the United States.

FOLD HERE

NO POSTAGE NECESSARY IF MAILED IN THE UNITED STATES

BUSINESS REPLY MAIL

FIRST CLASS MAIL PERMIT NO. 770 SANTA BARBARA, CA

POSTAGE WILL BE PAID BY ADDRESSEE

American Veterinary Publications
5782 Thornwood Drive
Goleta, CA 93117-9942

FOLD HERE

You may use this as a return envelope. Detach at right and fold as indicated. If a check is enclosed, please tape the sides.

Other Books For Veterinary Technicians

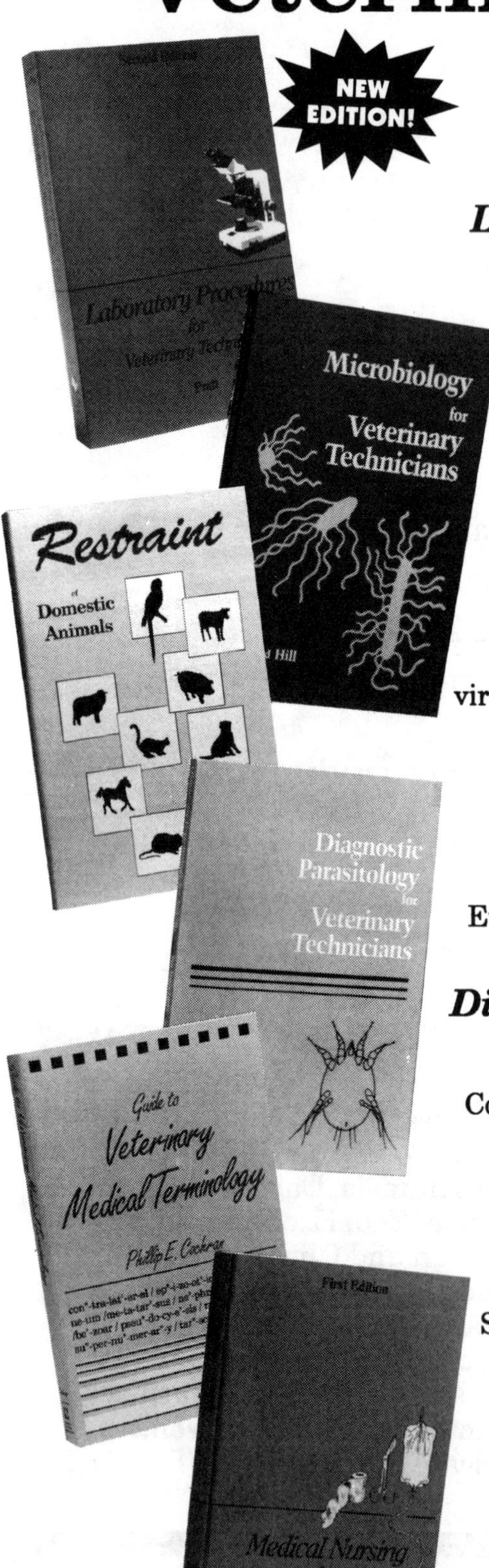

Laboratory Procedures for Veterinary Technicians

NEW 2ND EDITION, Edited by PW Pratt, 1992, 602 pages, Paperback, Illustrated, **$29**

As an introductory manual for new technicians, or as a valuable daily reference for experienced ones, this benchmark text will save hours of training and provide excellent guidance in improving patient care. Written in the same practical "cookbook" style as the first edition. Coverage for all domestic species.

Microbiology for Veterinary Technicians

by M Ikram and E Hill, 1991, 211 pages, Paperback, Illustrated, **$24.50**

Concise yet comprehensive information on bacteriology, mycology and virology. Describes procedures used in isolating and identifying pathogens in all domestic species.

Restraint of Domestic Animals

by TF Sonsthagen, 1991, 145 pages, Paperback, Illustrated, **$21.50**

Everything technicians need to know about restraint of domestic species.

Diagnostic Parasitology for Veterinary Technicians

Edited by J Colville, 1991, 266 pages, Paperback, Illustrated, **$24.50**

Contains information on how to detect and identify internal and external parasites. Complete coverage for all domestic species.

Guide to Veterinary Medical Terminology

by PE Cochran, 1991, 274 pages, Paperback, Illustrated, **$24.50**

Step-by-step primer explains surgical, medical, anatomic and directional terms. Highly recommended for technicians and receptionists.

Medical Nursing for Animal Health Technicians

Edited by PW Pratt, 1985, 464 pages, Paperback, Illustrated, **$26.50**

Easy-to-read "how-to" book on nursing procedures. Complete coverage for all domestic species. Widely used.

Order Form

Mailing Information

Name ____

Street ____

City/State/Zip ____

Telephone (__________) ______________________________

Merchandise

Qty	Title	Price	Total
______	______________________	_______	$ _______
______	______________________	_______	$ _______
______	______________________	_______	$ _______
______	______________________	_______	$ _______

Merchandise Total $ _______

California residents add 7.25% sales tax $ _______

Shipping Charge (see below) $ _______

GRAND TOTAL $ _______

Payment

☐ Check enclosed *(U.S. funds only)*

☐ Please charge my ______ VISA ______ MasterCard

Card # ______________________________ Exp ______________

Signature ______________________________

Shipping Charge *(Canadian and Foreign shipments, add $2 per item to charges below.)*

Merchandise Total	Shipping Charge
$0-30	$4
$31-65	$5
$66-100	$6
$101-150	$7
Over $150	$8

Terms

U.S. funds only, please. Prices are in U.S. dollars. Check or credit card information must accompany your order. Sorry, we cannot bill you or ship COD. Prices subject to change without notice. Satisfaction guaranteed or full purchase price refunded (less shipping).

Delivery

Books are shipped via UPS within the continental 48 states. Include street address (not PO Box) for UPS delivery. Hawaii, Alaska, Canada and Foreign shipments are via Book Post. Please allow 2-3 weeks for UPS delivery. Book Post and Foreign orders may take longer. All items may not arrive in the same shipment.

Send completed order form, with payment or credit card information, to:

American Veterinary Publications, 5782 Thornwood Dr, Goleta, CA 93117

For fastest service, call (805) 967-5988, 8 AM – 4 PM, M-F, Pacific Time

FOLD HERE

NO POSTAGE NECESSARY IF MAILED IN THE UNITED STATES

BUSINESS REPLY MAIL

FIRST CLASS MAIL PERMIT NO. 770 SANTA BARBARA, CA

POSTAGE WILL BE PAID BY ADDRESSEE

American Veterinary Publications
5782 Thornwood Drive
Goleta, CA 93117-9942

FOLD HERE

You may use this as a return envelope. Detach at right and fold as indicated. If a check is enclosed, please tape the sides.